29.95

D0606522

CQ Researcher on
Teens in America

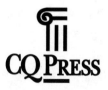

A Division of Congressional Quarterly Inc.
Washington, D.C.

CQ Press
A Division of Congressional Quarterly Inc.
1414 22nd Street, N.W.
Washington, D.C. 20037

(202) 822-1475; (800) 638-1710

www.cqpress.com

Printed and bound in the United States of America

04 03 02 01 00   5 4 3 2 1

⊚ The paper used in this publication meets the minimum requirements of the American National Standard for Information Sciences—Permanence of Paper for Printed Library Materials, ANSI Z39.48-1992.

Library of Congress Cataloging-in-Publication Data
CQ researcher on teens in America.
       p.   cm.
    Includes bibliographical references and index.
    ISBN 1-56802-628-5 (alk. paper)
       1. Teenagers—United States.   2. Parent and teenager—United States.   3. School violence—United States.   4. Journalism, School—United States.   5. School choice—United States.   6. Sex instruction for teenagers—United States.   7. Drug testing—United States.   I. Title: Teens in America.   II. CQ researcher.

HQ796.C214 2000
305.235'0973—dc21
                                                                                                        00-045526

Photo credits: 19, 23, 135, 141, 150, Reuters; 39, 46, Pacers Photography; 41, The Freedom Forum/Judy G. Rolfe; 59, Bobby Neel Adams; 63, Ericka McConnell; 66, BISON; 71, Austin CEO Foundation; 77, 81, 89, 90, Davidson College; 79, 83, George Washington University; 95, Best Friends; 115, AP; 138, KRT Photo.

Text credits: 15, The Family Research Council, 801 G Street, NW, Washington, DC 20001, www.frc.org; 26, National School Safety Center; 40, Freedom Forum; 42, 44, Journalism Kids Do Better; 64, CEO America; 78, 80, National Association of Scholars; 100, 111, National Center for Health Statistics, Centers for Disease Control and Prevention; 109, Reprinted with permission from *Insight*. Copyright 1997 News World Communications Inc. All rights reserved; 116, Quest Diagnostics; 117, Department of Health and Human Services; 129, Reprinted with permission of *HR News*, published by the Society of Human Resource Management, Alexandria, VA; 136, U.S. Department of Education; 137, 148, The Applied Research Center; 140, Chicago Public Schools.

Appendix: The publisher wishes to thank Kathryn L. Schwartz for permission to use *A+ Research and Writing for High School and College Students*, copyright 1997 by Kathryn L. Schwartz. Published by the Internet Public Library: http://www.ipl.org.

Contents

Introduction

The youth of today live in an era that is much more complex than that of their parents or grandparents. As recently as a generation ago, "school violence" meant a fistfight on the playground; today, it might mean a carefully planned ambush. The marijuana that first struck fear into the establishment in the 1930s seems tame in comparison with today's array of potentially deadly drugs. Just one generation ago, a high school diploma was a ticket to a job that paid a decent wage, and an undergraduate degree put you into a small elite; today, an undergraduate degree is a basic starting point, and curriculum is all-important.

Not only have the issues become more complex and the stakes higher, but more individuals, organizations, and institutions are affecting the lives of American teenagers. Congress, the president, the courts, the schools, and all manner of private organizations are trying to mold teen behavior by offering carrots for "good" behavior and sticks for "bad." And every aspect of young Americans' lives—education, extracurricular activities, even sex life—is now a matter of public policy.

One thing, however, has changed very little: Whether from their inattention or lack of empowerment, young Americans have little input into the decisions that so greatly affect them. Read between the lines of the *Researcher*s reprinted here, and you will note that teens—most of them not of voting age, and few that are of voting age actually casting a ballot—are the object of studies, debates, polls and manipulation but seldom inject themselves into the policy-making process. Perhaps a better understanding of the issues and policy-making process will inspire their participation.

This books aims to add context to the debates relevant to teenagers in America by reprinting eight articles from *The CQ Researcher,* a weekly magazine that focuses on issues of public concern. Each *Researcher* examines a single topic, such as parental rights or school journalism. It gives the reader a broad overview of the subject, including the historical background and a discussion of the current controversies and initiatives.

The *Researcher,* which was founded in 1923 under the name *Editorial Research Reports,* is distributed primarily to libraries and media offices. Each article is as long as 11,000 words, which could be the length of a term paper. It is based on intensive research, drawing on information from interest groups, universities, and the government. Each piece generally uses at least 15 interviews.

An Overview of the Chapters

The eight *CQ Researcher* articles in this book have been reproduced essentially as they appeared when first published. In some cases, important developments have taken place since the original publication.

Each chapter follows a similar format. It begins with an overview of the topic, then poses several key questions, or "issue questions." These may include: "Should youths who commit adult crimes be tried as adults?" and "Is a liberal arts education the best way to prepare for the workplace?" The answers to these questions are never conclusive because the issues are so controversial. Instead, they highlight the range of opinions among experts.

Next comes the "Background" section, which provides a history of the issue, including important government actions and court decisions. Then there is an examination of existing policy (under the heading "Current Situation") and an "Outlook" section, which gives a sense of what might happen in the near future.

All the chapters also contain an "At Issue" section in which two experts provide opposing answers to a relevant question. Finally, each chapter has sidebars on matters related to the main issue, a chronology of key events and a bibliography that explains the usefulness of each source.

The chapters are:

Parental Rights

Conservative lawmakers and the Religious Right say that legislation, court decisions and bureaucratic meddling have caused parents to lose authority over their children to teachers, school boards, child-welfare agencies, psychologists, physicians, birth-control counselors and any number of other surrogates. They have mounted an aggressive campaign to win new parental rights guarantees in state constitutions and federal law. Opponents argue that parental rights laws are dangerous and unnecessary. Such laws, they say, would throw schools into gridlock, lead to costly lawsuits and open children to parental abuse.

School Violence

In response to growing violence by students—including coldly calculated ambushes and mass murders—schools have cracked down. Many are quick to expel potential troublemakers and have established hot lines for threat tips, installed metal detectors and instituted dress codes. However, many people believe school violence stems from the easy availability of guns. Others see the problem as one of moral decline, which is better remedied by principled leadership in the family, the community and the nation than by gun-control measures. (Whereas this issue of the *CQ Researcher* focuses on the causes of school violence, "Zero Tolerance," the final selection in this book, examines the constitutionality, implications and efficacy of the remedy.)

Student Journalism

Ten years after the Supreme Court gave school administrators broad powers to censor student journalists, unflinching stories in student publications continue to cause consternation among administrators and even among increasingly diverse student bodies. Moreover, many observers believe journalism education to be facing a crisis of direction. Critics contend that students would be better served pursuing a degree in another discipline—say, political science or economics—and then learning the craft of journalism in graduate school or on the job. Supporters counter that journalism curriculums do emphasize the liberal arts and are often more rigorous and coherently structured than alternative courses of study. (See "Liberal Arts Education," below, for a broader debate on the merits of vocational education.)

School Choice Debate

School choice advocates believe that only radical reform can fix the nation's failing public schools and that providing parents with tuition vouchers—redeemable at the school of their choice—must be the cornerstone of the reform. Choice, they say, will inject a healthy dose of competition in education, thereby improving a public education system that is monopolistic and resistant to change. But opponents say that vouchers will siphon money away from schools that are already underfunded. Moreover, they argue, using taxpayer dollars to send children to sectarian schools violates the constitutional prohibition on government support for religion.

Liberal Arts Education

The liberal arts—the humanities, social sciences and natural sciences—were the foundation of higher learning until the early twentieth century. Their advocates believe that learning to read and think critically should be at the core of undergraduate studies. Over the past century, however, students and the educational institutions that minister to them have increasingly turned to career-oriented curricula—engineering, journalism, marketing and the like. Advocates of the liberal arts contend that universities have become too consumer-driven, offering students what they want instead of what they need. Yet they do not agree among themselves whether a liberal education should focus on Western culture or more broadly on world culture.

Encouraging Teen Abstinence

Although the overall U.S. teen birthrate is declining, out-of-wedlock births are skyrocketing in the United States and throughout the industrialized world. To reverse this trend, Congress and the states are spending $837.5 million over five years to encourage teenagers and unmarried adults to abstain from sexual intercourse, without teaching them about contraception or disease prevention. Critics say that abstinence-only education leaves youths "defenseless."

Drug Testing

Until recently, only adults working in occupations affecting public safety—airline pilots, for example—were tested for drug use. Nowadays, many state and local governments require random testing of high school students participating in after-school activities, among other groups. Proponents say drug testing deters drug use, but opponents say that cannot be proven and believe drug testing to be a serious erosion of civil liberties.

Zero Tolerance

A series of schoolyard shootings in recent years has prompted school officials and lawmakers to impose mandatory punishments for a variety of misbehaviors, many of them seemingly minor. Proponents credit tough disciplinary policies with driving school crime rates down. But critics question their effectiveness and worry about the impact the policies are having on individual rights. And civil rights advocates say the policies are affecting minority, disabled and academically challenged students disproportionately.

1 Parental Rights

THOMAS J. BILLITTERI

John Burrington of Colorado Springs has seen too much ugliness in his years as a pediatric surgeon. Children with bones fractured by angry parents. Children with welts from electric cords. Children who have been burned and scarred, and worse.

And now Burrington thinks he sees something every bit as abhorrent: a proposed amendment to the Colorado Constitution that would give parents the "inalienable" right "to direct and control the upbringing, education, values and discipline of their children." Indeed, Burrington worries that the amendment — to be decided by voters Nov. 5 — has the potential to shield child abusers.

On the surface, Colorado's "parental rights" initiative seems as uncontroversial an election-year issue as clean air and full employment. "To vote no is like voting no to mom, apple pie and the flag," Burrington acknowledges.

But Burrington thinks the proposal, by sanctioning parental discipline, would put children at greater risk for abuse and neglect. Moreover, he fears, it would encourage parents to sue teachers, principals or other government representatives over school curricula and many other decisions affecting their children that the parents didn't like.

"It's fairly difficult to prosecute child abuse cases now," Burrington says. If parents have an "inalienable" right to discipline their children, "then it will be almost impossible to prosecute child abuse short of mayhem or murder." The amendment, he says, "is absolutely criminal and will set things back 100 years."

Amendment supporters, including conservative lawmakers and the Christian Right, call such statements non-

From *The CQ Researcher,*
October 25, 1996.

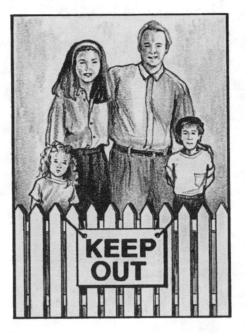

sense. The measure grants no new rights, they argue, but simply codifies existing ones that lower courts, bureaucracies, school boards and legislators have taken away. A short, clearly worded amendment would give parents a more streamlined and economical means than they have now to challenge government intrusion into family decisions — such as how a child learns about sex or whether a parent may spank a misbehaving child.

"Like many Coloradans, I'm concerned about what appears to be an assault on the American family," said Denver lawyer Mike Norton, a former U.S. attorney in the Reagan administration and a spokesman for the Coalition for Parental Responsibility, which is leading the initiative drive. "This would give parents a [legal] basis on which to argue that they are in the best position to control the upbringing of their children." [1]

Norton views as "outrageous" arguments that the measure would protect child abusers. "Everybody knows what discipline is and what child abuse is," he said. "Our parental rights

amendment is not going to supersede the Criminal Code." [2]

As the first state to bring a parental rights amendment to a vote, Colorado is at the epicenter of an emerging nationwide movement. Proponents hope that codifying parental rights will help limit how far government can "intrude" on children's lives and parents' right to raise their children as they see fit. The outcome could have profound consequences for public education, family law and child protection — and any other area where government and the rights of children and parents intersect. [3]

Approval of Colorado's initiative could give momentum to nascent efforts in more than two dozen other states, and perhaps rekindle interest in parental rights in Congress, where two such bills were introduced in 1995. (*See map, p. 2.*)

"Once we win in Colorado in November, it will prove this is a successful concept," says Greg D. Erken, executive director of "Of the People," an Arlington, Va., group that has been pushing parental rights amendments nationwide since 1993. "We expect that a number of states in 1997 and 1998 will renew their efforts to adopt their own parental rights amendments."

Those backing parental rights measures include such conservative stalwarts as the Christian Coalition (which had a parental rights plank in its 1995 Contract With the American Family), the Traditional Values Coalition, the Home School Legal Defense Association and the Heritage Foundation.

Supporters claim that the Supreme Court long ago classified parental rights as "fundamental," thus giving them the same strict level of judicial protection as free speech and religion and racial equality. That hotly contested claim rests largely on a pair of high court rulings from the 1920s (*see p. 12*).

Status of Parental Rights Amendments in the States

Proposed parental rights amendments to state constitutions have been introduced or sponsored in more than half the states, according to Of the People. In Colorado, an amendment proposal is on the Nov. 5 ballot.

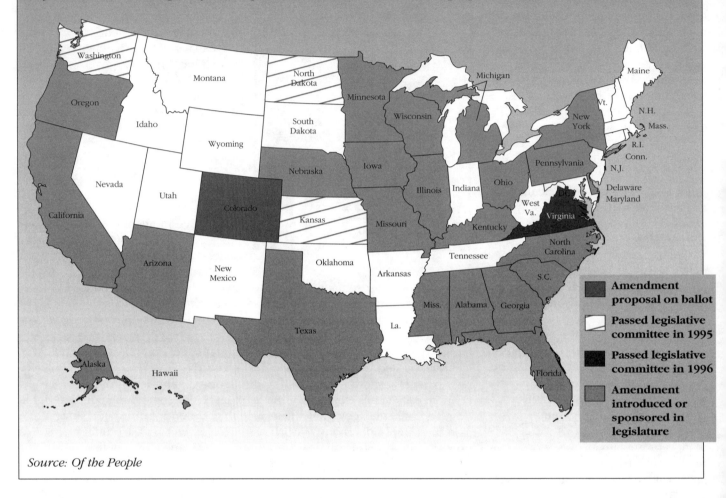

Amendment proposal on ballot

Passed legislative committee in 1995

Passed legislative committee in 1996

Amendment introduced or sponsored in legislature

Source: Of the People

Proponents of new parental rights laws say teachers, school boards, child-welfare agencies, lower courts, bureaucrats and professional "elites" such as psychologists, physicians and birth-control counselors have ignored the court's intentions and chopped away at parental authority.

"All of our institutions of authority in this country have been undermined, and in some cases been under frontal assault, for some time — schools, government, law enforcement, churches, families. . . . Parents are no different," says Rep. Steve Largent, R-Okla., who

with Sen. Charles E. Grassley, R-Iowa, introduced the "Parental Rights and Responsibilities Act" in Congress last year *(see p. 5)*. "We literally see hundreds, if not thousands, of cases across the country [in which] parents' ability to direct the upbringing of their children is undermined or usurped by a government agency."

Parental rights advocates point to a litany of perceived intrusions, especially in the schools, including birth-control counseling, condom distribution and lessons about homosexuality, as well as the abrupt separation of chil-

dren from parents accused of abuse. [4]

"We really believe legislation is needed to address the growing attack against the parent-child relationship," says Andrea Sheldon, director of government affairs at the Traditional Values Coalition. "You can see that in so many different ways: When the federal government says, 'It doesn't matter what your parents say, we're going to give you money to go off and get an abortion, and your parents don't need to weigh in,' [and when] children are given questionnaires about their family, about their sexual activities, and parents don't know about it."

Psychologist James C. Dobson, a conservative radio broadcaster and founder of Colorado Springs-based Focus on the Family, sees the struggle for parental rights as a "contest between two world views. There are those of us who . . . believe that we should bring our children up to worship God and understand his principles . . . including the sanctity of life and premarital chastity [and] those on the other end of the continuum who hold to no eternal truths. . . .

"This contest . . . is [being] played out . . . throughout government, in the educational system and everywhere else decisions are being made for the culture. It is especially relevant to children because we all know children are the prize to the winner. You know, those who are able to tell children what is right and wrong, those who are able to write the curricula for kids, will necessarily determine the future of the culture because in just 20 years those youngsters will be adults and will be taking over. And so there is an intense struggle for the hearts and minds of kids. That's what's behind this invasion of parental rights." [5]

Dozens of professional organizations and liberal advocacy groups are fighting the parental-rights push. They include groups as diverse as The National PTA, the National Education Association (NEA), the American Civil Liberties Union, Planned Parenthood Federation of America, the American Academy of Pediatrics and the National Council of Churches of Christ. They argue that codifying parental rights into an "ambiguous" new law would have catastrophic consequences: gridlock in the public education system; greater incidence of child abuse and teen pregnancy; soaring government legal bills; and a virtual dismantling of child-protection safeguards.

"By giving parents a new cause of action to assert their views in court, this legislation would open to challenge virtually any governmental action or policy involving the health, safety and welfare of children," warned the Academy of Pediatrics. [6]

"None would [disagree] that active parental involvement in the care, upbringing and education of our children is the cornerstone of a strong, healthy society," Sammy J. Quintana,

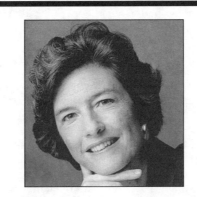

"The question is: Who is in charge of public education? It is the job of educators and schools to determine the curriculum that is going to best [produce] a learned citizen."

— *Anne Bryant, executive director, National School Boards Association*

president of the National School Boards Association, told a Senate Judiciary subcommittee hearing last December on the proposed Parental Rights and Responsibilities Act. "[But] this bill is about making it more difficult for public schools to teach our children. It is about lining the pockets of lawyers and draining the scarce educational resources in our schools. It is about putting the health and safety of our children in jeopardy. It is about

playing politics with our children." [7]

Some opponents also charge that parental rights activists are engaged in a "stealth" effort to gain greater control of the public schools, erode the wall of separation between church and state and win approval for tax-paid vouchers to fund private or parochial schooling.

The strict legal test in the bills proposed in Congress requires government to show a "compelling interest" in any action it takes impinging on "parental rights." That troubles Rebecca Isaacs, director of public policy for People for the American Way, a seasoned liberal advocacy group that is heading up an opposition coalition.

"The law would let any parent sue over something that they believe in an extremely vague, broad way interferes with their right to bring up their child," Isaacs says. "You can't have any [law] with a lower threshold or broader right with a harder burden for government to meet. It's unprecedented."

Public support for codifying parental rights is, in some ways, difficult to predict. A *Rocky Mountain News* poll of registered Colorado voters in early September found a 76 percent approval rate for the state's constitutional amendment (72 percent of Democrats approved and 83 percent of Republicans). [8]

While foes of Colorado's parental rights amendment acknowledged the difficulty of making their case on such a complex and emotional issue, they predicted that much of the support would evaporate once voters learned the implications of the simply worded measure.

"My experience in focus groups is that as soon as you start talking about what this [Colorado measure] could mean, the support drops off very rap-

From Peyote to Religious Freedom ...

It was an obscure religious practice involving the hallucinogenic drug peyote, but it touched off a national controversy that now involves parental rights.

In 1990, the U.S. Supreme Court affirmed Oregon's denial of unemployment benefits to two Native Americans dismissed from their jobs at a private drug rehabilitation center. The reason for their dismissal: ingesting peyote as part of tribal religious rituals.

The Native Americans claimed the First Amendment's guarantee of religious freedom made the state's action unconstitutional. But Oregon argued that they had been fired for "work-related misconduct" — and thus didn't deserve jobless benefits — because using peyote was a criminal offense under state law. [1]

Fearing the Smith decision could curtail religious freedoms far beyond peyote use, an unusually broad coalition of religious groups — from the liberal National Council of Churches of Christ to the National Association of Evangelicals — helped push a bill through Congress to preclude such rulings in the future. President Clinton signed the Religious Freedom Restoration Act (RFRA) in 1993. [2]

Now, some parental rights advocates are saying that the parental rights act proposed last year by Sen. Charles E. Grassley, R-Iowa, and Rep. Steve Largent, R-Okla., is the secular complement to RFRA, with both protecting fundamental rights guaranteed by the Constitution. [3]

A leading proponent of that view is Michael P. Farris, president of the Home School Legal Defense Association. Farris co-chaired the drafting committee on RFRA and was a chief architect of the Grassley-Largent legislation.

"Religious liberty was undermined by a single stroke of a Supreme Court guillotine" in the peyote case, Farris said in congressional testimony last year. "Parental liberty is dying from the cuts of a thousand switchblades." [4]

To Farris, the disconnect between parents' secular and religious rights became abundantly clear in a pair of home-schooling cases he brought before the Michigan Supreme Court in the early 1990s. [5]

In the cases, consolidated for oral arguments, two families contended that a Michigan law requiring all teachers to be certified was an unconstitutional infringement on their rights. One family, the DeJonges, wanted to home school for religious reasons. The other, the Bennetts, had non-religious reasons.

In the DeJonge case, the court "used the fundamental rights test and concluded that the [Michigan] statute was unconstitutional because it violated the principles of religious freedom when combined with parental rights," Farris told the congressional hearing.

In the Bennett case, Farris said he argued that the parents' rights "to direct the upbringing of their children was also a fundamental right." But the Bennetts lost.

The court, rendering both decisions on the same day in 1993, said in the Bennetts' case that "the fundamental rights analysis did not apply to a parental rights claim standing alone without a religious component," Farris testified.

And that brings Farris back to his RFRA argument. "The difficulty that parents face in court when they're trying to

idly. The devil is really in the details," says Michael Hudson, vice president of People for the American Way, a leading member of the Protect Our Children Coalition, which is opposing the Colorado initiative.

Outside Colorado, similar amendments have found sponsors in 27 state legislatures, to a large extent due to the efforts of the group Of the People, which has support from the American Legislative Exchange Council, a group of conservative state lawmakers.

Central to the debate over parental rights are several high-profile cases that proponents say reflect the growing usurpation of parental authority by government: Parents who say they were told it was "none of your business" after they objected to their teen daughters being taken by a school counselor to a clinic where birth-control materials were dispensed; students who say they were unable to "opt out" of sex-education courses; parents outraged by a school-sponsored physical exam that included genital inspections of sixth-grade girls.

Foes claim parental rights backers are exaggerating or altering details of cases, and in some instances using "bogus horror stories" to wage a disinformation campaign, according to Americans United for Separation of Church and State. [9]

Movement backers "specialize in lurid, tabloid-type anecdotes to try to show there is some broad, sweeping problem, rather than [a problem] that should be — and could be — taken care of in the local community," says Isaacs.

"In my experience, the Chicken Little, sky is falling phenomenon is occurring," says Gloria Feldt, president of Planned Parenthood. "I would not want to say no parent has ever been treated unfairly; the justice system is sometimes imperfect. But those of us who have been teachers and worked with youth and families in different situations tend to know that there is seldom a clear black and white" picture of what happens when children are involved.

But parental rights advocates counter that it is the liberals who are engaging in hyperbole, predicting dire consequences from parental rights measures in attempts to derail the movement. Not only are courts and

... to the Fight Over Parental Rights

litigate their cases is exactly the same" as that faced by claimants after the peyote case, he says. "Courts are using the wrong standards for evaluating their rights. Nobody denies parents have rights — the question is, what level: fundamental or non-fundamental?"

In the Smith decision, Farris says, "The Supreme Court decided religious freedom was not a fundamental right. In parental rights cases (without a religious dimension), a lot of appellate and lower courts in the federal and state system have decided parents' rights are not fundamental. RFRA gives all religious-based claims in public schools fundamental-rights status. So what's left to be established are secular-based claims."

And that is why those who argue that the parental rights movement is a stealth attempt to inject religion into the schools "can be proven almost silly in their arguments," Farris maintains.

"It's the secular parents who are the only ones who stand to win anything (from parental rights laws) in terms of their interaction with the public schools," he says. Religious parents, he adds, already have RFRA.

Opponents of the parental rights movement reject Farris' argument that a parental rights bill is the needed complement to RFRA. "It's a snow job," says Rebecca Isaacs, director of public policy at People for the American Way.

Isaacs and other critics say RFRA is unlike the Parental Rights and Responsibilities Act because RFRA provides a narrow remedy whereas the parental rights bill takes a broad-brush approach.

Under RFRA, they say, a person could be individually exempted from a law that substantially infringes on his religious freedom. Under the parental rights bill, an aggrieved party could suspend some government functions for all citizens.

Not only that, critics say, a parental rights measure would allow individual parents to manipulate local policy to reflect their personal religious beliefs. And unlike RFRA, where the individual has to prove the government took away his religious freedom, a parental rights measure would put an onerous burden of proof on government, critics say.

"Under parental rights legislation, all you have to show is that you're a parent and that you think some activity a local institution is doing interferes with your newly named fundamental rights," Isaacs says. "Then the government has to show a compelling interest for that activity and that it was accomplished by the least restrictive means."

For schools, child-abuse workers and health and safety agencies, she says, that burden of proof "is going to wreak havoc."

---

[1] Kermit L. Hall, ed., *The Oxford Companion to the Supreme Court* (1992), p. 725. The case is *Employment Division v. Smith*.

[2] See *1993 CQ Almanac*, p. 315.

[3] The bills died when the 104th Congress ended and must be reintroduced next year.

[4] Farris testified before the Senate Judiciary Subcommittee on Administrative Oversight and the Courts, Oct. 26, 1995.

[5] For background, see "Home Schooling," *The CQ Researcher*, Sept. 9, 1994, pp. 769-792.

---

bureaucracies usurping parental authority, parental rights advocates counter, but liberals are engaging in hysteria of their own.

"It's Chicken Little, the sky is falling," says Sheldon of the Traditional Values Coalition, echoing Feldt from across the ideological chasm. "It doesn't matter what the issue is."

But if parental rights pass, Sheldon adds, courts and bureaucracies will think twice about usurping parental authority, and school personnel and other government workers "will have to be more careful" about how they deal with students' rights. "They're not careful now — they don't have to be."

As the debate continues over parental rights, these are some of the questions being asked:

Is it necessary to codify parental rights into law?

A parental rights law or amendment is needed, advocates insist, because lower courts, school boards and legislators have chipped away at the rights established long ago by the Supreme Court.

While parental rights may still exist on paper, they say, the "little guy" can't afford to pursue them against powerful groups like the NEA and well-organized bureaucracies such as school boards and child protective services. Even members of the "humane professions" — educators, lawyers, doctors, social workers and school counselors — have usurped the role of parents, critics contend.

The answer, according to parental rights backers, is a variety of legal tacks that critics say would be destructive and unnecessary.

The Grassley-Largent parental rights bills that died in the 104th Congress could well resurface next year. They guaranteed parental rights in education, health decisions, discipline (including "reasonable corporal discipline") and religious instruction. The measures excluded abuse, neglect and custody disputes from their scope, and prevented parents from withholding medical treatment in cases involving serious harm.

The Colorado initiative, bearing the characteristic brevity of most constitutional amendments, contains no stated exclusions, and supporters say its reference to "discipline" is tied to existing state definitions. The Grassley version of the federal bill required a parent to try to settle a dispute out of court, but Colorado's measure has no such stipulation.

Many other proposed state constitutional amendments are even more broadly written. The key portion of the model language proposed by Of the People simply says: "The right of parents to direct the upbringing and education of their children shall not be infringed."

The federal bills sought to erect the highest legal hurdle for the "government" — be it a kindergarten teacher, child-welfare bureau or federal agency. To justify an action that impinged on parental rights, the government would have to demonstrate that the action was essential to "accomplish a compelling governmental interest" and that it used "the least restrictive means of accomplishing" that interest. Parents who believed their rights were trampled could sue in state or federal court.

In requiring the government to show "clear and convincing" evidence that an action was necessary, Grassley's proposed federal standard is even stricter than the "preponderance" of evidence standard called for in racial-discrimination cases. But critics of the bill say the cases cited by parental rights proponents do not warrant imposing draconian legal burdens on school boards and juvenile-welfare boards.

Proponents frequently point to the controversial 1995 case *Brown v. Hot, Sexy and Safer Productions Inc.,* in which parents in Massachusetts charged they were not given an opportunity to review or remove their children from a graphic high school "AIDS-awareness" assembly. According to the parents' suit, the program's

speaker allegedly used profane language to describe body parts and excretory functions and advocated oral sex, masturbation, gay sexual activity and condom use.

The appeals court found no violation of family rights protections, adding fuel — and another oft-used anecdote — to the parental rights debate.

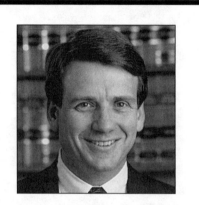

"There's a clear move in this country to outlaw spanking. We want to say that parents always have a right to reasonable spanking."

— *Michael P. Farris, president, Home School Legal Defense Association*

bate. "It is this type of unbending governmental abuse of authority in transgressing the fundamental right of the family that requires the 'compelling interest' standard to be applied in these situations," declared the American Center for Law and Justice, a Christian legal advocacy group in Virginia Beach, Va. [10]

Of the People founder Jeffrey Bell agrees. He says that the model state amendment proposed by Of the People is intentionally broad to spark a debate about parental rights and responsibilities. He says the group

wants to leave the details of the amendment to be worked out at the community level — and, if need be, in the courts. "It doesn't argue each and every controversial educational practice," Bell told the Christian Coalition in September. "It gets it back to a sovereignty issue: populism vs. elitism. Who is in charge? Who should be in charge?"

Critics of the proposed parental rights legislation argue, however, that imposing a compelling-interest standard on government would lead to an explosion of destructive social consequences and the nullification of dozens of state laws that carefully balance parental rights and the needs of children.

"Communities would be paralyzed under the threat of lawsuits about virtually all the services and programs they provide," said People for the American Way. "Child protective services would be discouraged from investigating reports of abuse. . . . Basic health care in schools, such as hearing and vision testing and sports physicals, could be prohibited. Local decisions between parents and educators about curriculum content, textbook selection and student assessments could be overturned." [11]

"This bill does not 'codify' existing law," the NEA says. It "creates a *new* fundamental right and will have dire consequences for this country's public schools. [12]

Besides, the NEA and other opponents argue, parents already have a wide array of rights and options to fight what they consider unreasonable government interference. Pediatric surgeon Burrington notes, for example, that parents in Colorado can home-school their children. [13] "The problem is parental responsibility," he says. "You can't legislate responsibility."

Would a federal Parental Rights and Responsibilities Act or similar state laws produce educational gridlock?

Critics call parental rights legislation a train wreck waiting to happen. "The legislation is so broad that it could be read to give [parents] a veto over everything that's done in the school," said Gwen Gregory, deputy general counsel for the National School Boards Association. "Schools would come to a screeching halt." [14]

The 2.4-million-member NEA, the nation's largest teachers' union, claims the federal Parental Rights and Responsibilities Act would, among other things, force schools to provide a "designer" curriculum for each student, allow parents to sue a teacher for saying anything in class the parents don't like, give parents the right to opt their children out of required courses and allow parents to win suits challenging such policies as "no pass/no play" rules and teacher grading standards.

"This legislation is disruptive, intrusive, expensive and unnecessary, and will wreak havoc in the public schools," the NEA declared in a recent statement.

Many educators also claim that parental rights laws would destroy the traditional democratic underpinnings of the public school system, making litigation the preferred engine of change instead of traditional approaches such as school board elections, referendums and parent-teacher negotiations.

Shirley Igo, the National PTA's vice president for legislation, also worries that parental rights initiatives could chill parental involvement in the schools because volunteers would fear being dragged into court. "It would destroy the level of trust the PTA has been working to build over the past 100 years," Igo says.

With parental rights laws in place, control of curricula decisions, ancillary services such as drug and birth-control counseling, sex education and even choice of library books would be in the hands of a religious or ultra-conservative minority rather than professional educators, opponents say.

"The question is, who is in charge of public education?" says Anne Bryant, executive director of the school boards association. "It is the job of educators and schools to determine the curriculum that is going to best [produce] a learned citizen."

Critics say the proposed measures would also discourage school districts and public health agencies from making pregnancy and drug counseling available to teens, resulting in higher rates of illegitimacy, drug abuse and disease.

"A major concern," says Feldt of Planned Parenthood, "is that parental rights measures would gut confidentiality laws that now protect teens seeking sensitive services such as prenatal care, birth control and treatment for sexually transmitted disease. "Obviously in the ideal world, teens would be communicating with parents about these issues," Feldt says. "We'd support programs to further that, but laws that are punitive in nature don't further that parent-child relationship. Not every family comes from the 'Ozzie and Harriet' mold."

Some also see a hidden agenda in the movement: supporting tax-paid vouchers for private religious schools. [15] "It's going to be an easy move from this to vouchers, because the schools won't be able to comply with all the requests for designer curriculum," Isaacs says.

But backers of parental rights dismiss warnings of dire consequences or nefarious motives, saying groups like the NEA are trying to protect their power base and advance an ultra-liberal agenda.

"There's nothing in this legislation," Grassley says of his bill, "that's going to change traditional control of education."

Adds Largent, "There is no coalition of moms and dads that has [a lobbying] office on K Street in Washington. The principal opponent to this bill is the education bureaucracy. It's understandable why. This is threatening their power because we're saying, 'Let's empower parents to become partners in education decisions.'"

Of the People founder Bell says the NEA and other parental rights foes "believe parents aren't competent to raise their child, but they don't talk about that." Instead, he says, they claim parental rights laws will lead to increased child abuse, designer curricula, even a ban of Shakespeare's Romeo and Juliet, which contains references to teen love and suicide, and Macbeth, with its themes of witchcraft and murder.

Such fears are off base, Bell told the Christian Coalition forum. Besides, he said, "I thought the school system had been doing a pretty good job already of taking Shakespeare out of [education]."

Would children be at greater risk for abuse and neglect from proposed parental rights laws?

Marilyn Van Derbur, Miss America in 1958, has said she was sexually abused by her father. Now she sees a similar threat to a new generation of youngsters — from the proposed federal parental-rights bill.

"Do not make it more difficult than it already is for child-protection services" to investigate abuse, she urged a House Judiciary subcommittee hearing last year. [16]

It's a plea being repeated by a battalion of child-welfare organizations, from the National Child Abuse Coalition to the National Safe Kids Campaign, chaired by former Surgeon General C. Everett Koop. They argue the measure would dismantle health and safety protections that courts, legislatures and other public bodies have carefully constructed over the decades. (See "At Issue," p. 15.)

"Proponents [of parental rights legislation] cite instances of children being summarily removed from the care of protective parents," says the Chicago-based American Professional Society on the Abuse of Children. "Cer-

Sex Education Fires Controversy ...

In the battle over parental rights, no issue is more incendiary than sex education.

Conservative advocates of stronger parental rights believe public schools have gone too far in efforts to teach youngsters about the hazards of teen pregnancy, sexually transmitted disease and the availability and use of contraceptives. "Government officials have no right to form moral beliefs in children that contradict the beliefs of parents," declares the Heritage Foundation. Under parental rights laws, the group says, school officials would either refrain from teaching about issues like contraception and abortion, or parents would have the "clear right to opt out from the official imposition of 'values' hostile to their beliefs." [1]

But foes of new parental rights guarantees, such as proposed federal legislation, say too many parents are ignoring the harsh realities of life in the late 20th century. Competent sex education and confidential sex-related health services are among the most effective ways of stemming teen pregnancy rates and the spread of AIDS and other sexually transmitted diseases among young people, they argue.

"When I look at what this legislation is about," says Gloria Feldt, president of Planned Parenthood Federation of America, "it really seems to me an attempt to play on the fear parents have of being out of control of their kids. That's not an altogether unfounded fear, but not one that can really be solved by legislation of this nature."

Clearly, sexual mores and differing notions about sex education are driving forces of the parental rights movement. It was former New York City school chief Joseph A.

Fernandez's ill-fated program to distribute condoms in the schools that helped launch the parental rights movement — and led to his firing in 1993. And cases such as *Brown v. Hot, Sexy and Safer Productions Inc.* — in which parents protested the sexual explicitness of an AIDS awareness assembly presented to Massachusetts high school students — gave the movement important momentum.

"It is not bad for a loving mother — whether secular or religious — to tell her 13-year-old daughter that she will not take her to a doctor for birth control pills," wrote Rep. Steve Largent, R-Okla. "It is bad to let an immature child or an uninformed government official veto a good parent's best judgment." [2]

Under parental rights bills proposed in Congress last year by Largent and Sen. Charles E. Grassley, R-Iowa, parents could oppose "government officials handing out condoms and prescribing contraceptives for their children," just as "religious parents" can object now under the Religious Freedom Restoration Act (RFRA), Largent wrote. [3] (*See story, p. 4.*)

"Under the Parental Rights and Responsibilities Act, laws which interfere with the rights of secular parents would be evaluated under the compelling interest standard," Largent wrote. "A law permitting all 13-year-old girls to consent to birth control pills would likely fail this test. It would unnecessarily interfere with the rights of responsible parents to make health-care decisions for their children." [4]

Grassley, Largent and other supporters of parental rights say that the Supreme Court has clearly classified parental rights as "fundamental," thus giving them the same strict

tainly, mistakes of overintervention occur." But "American children are killed and maimed every day by parents who have not been adequately restrained by the state." [17]

Opponents of parental rights laws are especially worried that health and abuse agencies would hesitate to report or treat cases for fear of being sued. Even if the government eventually could prove a compelling interest in a case and that its actions were the least restrictive, time-consuming legal proceedings could intensify the risk to the child, opponents argue.

"Communities would be virtually paralyzed in the child protection services they provide, including vital counseling services to troubled or despondent youth," the American

Humane Association said. [18]

The Safe Kids campaign, in a June 4 letter to Sen. Orrin G. Hatch, R-Utah, chairman of the Judiciary Committee, said the federal bill would let parents sue "over virtually any public rule or law that affects children" — including bike helmet, smoke detector, child-safety seat and seat-belt laws.

The Academy of Pediatrics also noted the bill's corporal punishment provision. "It forces courts to decide whether child abuse applies and opens a wedge to challenge and relitigate issues of child maltreatment in a separate cause of action apart from the original case," the group said in a March statement.

In the Colorado amendment, there is no explicit exemption for abuse. Advocates say "discipline" is defined

by existing state law. The amendment's broad language bothers Hudson of People for the American Way. "It will be a lawyer's field day to argue what those terms like discipline, values and education mean," he says.

"No parent has a right to abuse a child," the Heritage Foundation responds. "The truth is that this [federal] bill would reinforce the right of states to protect children from abuse." [19]

"This [bill] does not alter, amend or change any current child-protective service's ability to remove a child from a home" or report abuse or neglect, Largent says. Criticism from child-welfare advocates "is really a red-herring argument against parental rights."

Of the People's Erken echoes the point in reference to the Colorado

... Over Teaching 'Hostile' Values

level of judicial protection as free speech and racial equality. But, they say, school boards, teachers and professional "elites," to name a few, have ignored the court's intentions and assaulted parental authority.

Yet critics of the parental rights movement say curbs on education or availability of professional help could have devastating consequences. "Adolescents seeking family planning services, screening and treatment for sexually transmitted diseases, and prenatal care might have no other alternatives to school and public clinics," the American Public Health Association said. The proposed federal Parental Rights and Responsibilities Act "could result in poor health outcomes for adolescents including unintended pregnancy, sterility, HIV infection and unhealthy pregnancies." [5]

The Alan Guttmacher Institute, a reproductive-health policy organization in New York City, noted recently that many states have laws authorizing minors to consent to health care related to sexual activity. The group said, for example, that 23 states and the District of Columbia have laws authorizing minors to give consent for contraceptive services. Twenty-seven states and the District allow pregnant minors to obtain prenatal care and delivery services without parental consent or notification, and 49 states plus the District allow minors to consent to the diagnosis and treatment of sexually transmitted disease. [6]

Referring to Largent's parental rights legislation, the institute said, "Although the proposal seems eminently reasonable at first glance, in practice it would override longstanding efforts by both the states and Congress to reconcile the right of

parents to guide and protect their minor children and minors' need and desire for confidentiality in certain situations." [7]

But the Family Research Council says the legislation is needed more than ever today because of changing policies in schools regarding sex education. "Public schools are ... increasingly adopting policies whereby an entire class is subjected to mandatory psychological testing or explicit sex education [that] contradicts the values taught at home. Psychological testing of children is often performed under the guise of standardized tests which include intrusive questions about the child's emotional state and sexual experiences, the child's relationship with his or her parents, and values and habits within the home." [8]

---

[1] Heritage Foundation, "How Congress Can Protect the Rights of Parents to Raise Their Children," *Issue Bulletin No. 227,* July 23, 1996, p. 26.

[2] Rep. Steve Largent, "Questions and Answers About the Parental Rights and Responsibilities Act, p. 23.

[3] *Ibid.*

[4] *Ibid.*

[5] "Parental Rights and Responsibilities Act Fact Sheet," American Public Health Association.

[6] "Lawmakers Grapple with Parents' Role in Teen Access to Reproductive Health Care," *Issues in Brief,* November 1995, published by Alan Guttmacher Institute.

[7] *Ibid.*

[8] Cathleen A. Cleaver and Greg Erken, "Who Decides How Children Are Raised?" *Family Policy,* August 1996, published by Family Research Council. Cleaver is the council's director of legal studies; Erken is executive director of Of the People.

---

measure. "The rude misunderstanding is that we are legislating an absolute right for parents," he says. "If that were the case, sure, then there would be gridlock in the schools, and government would be prevented from acting to protect the children's welfare. However, parental rights are not absolute."

Erken and Bell say legal precedents clearly establish that a parent can't abuse a child and then claim "parental rights."

Michael P. Farris, president of the Home School Legal Defense Association, says that while "real abuse is exempted wholesale" from the federal bill he helped to shape, what opponents don't like is that "parents have a federally recognized right to spank their children. [That's] not real abuse."

"There's a clear move in this coun-

try to outlaw spanking," Farris says. "We want to say that parents always have a clear recognition that they have a right to reasonable spanking. We don't want our prisons any fuller than they are. We don't want our kids doing drug abuse. We want kids to obey the law. My belief is that children who are disciplined are better citizens."

Of course, many cases of alleged child abuse or neglect fall into gray areas that could become arenas of increased controversy under a parental rights measure. Consider, for example, parents who withhold or alter medical treatment and child-welfare workers who disagree.

That scenario occurred late last summer in Dallas after doctors told the parents of 10-year-old Rachel Stout that she could die unless her ulcerated

colon was removed. The parents refused, child protective authorities stepped in and Rachel's father took her to Canada for treatment by a practitioner of holistic medicine. After a blood infection halted the alternative treatment, Rachel's parents consented in October to the surgery. [20]

Other conflicts arise over government efforts to stem child abuse and neglect. The Heritage Foundation cites a set of 1995 guidelines in Durham, N.C., for judging the presence of child abuse. "Though most of these 'Minimum Standards of Care' make sense," the foundation says, "a number of them indicate a dangerous overreach by bureaucrats." For example, a parent could be investigated for child abuse for confining a child to his room or for violating government standards "governing the supervision, nutrition, clothing, cleanliness and even the bedtime of children," the foundation says. [21]

Durham County Social Services Director Daniel Hudgins dismisses the foundation's characterization, noting the standards of care are guidelines and not regulations, and were developed by community representatives to help doctors, teachers and others better evaluate reports of potential abuse.

The idea was to help the community "screen out reports that didn't meet any level of maltreatment or abuse," Hudgins says. "Taken alone, none of those guidelines would result in any kind of action by the department against a parent. They were [developed] to improve the quality of what we do and reduce [government] intervention. As opposed to government coming up with standards, this was an attempt to involve the community."

Would parental rights laws lead to an explosion in costly litigation?

Supporters see parental rights laws reducing litigation by encouraging parents to become more involved in school and other community decisions, thereby stemming conflicts before they explode into expensive legal battles.

"It's going to end up in a lot less lawsuits," Grassley claims. "It's going to promote dialogue between educators and parents."

Furthermore, Grassley says, the 90-day "administrative remedy" procedure that he added to his bill was designed expressly to settle disputes between parents and bureaucrats before they get to court.

Besides, Farris points out, parents have long been able to sue in state or federal court if they feel their rights have been violated. And since 1993, they have been able to sue under the Religious Freedom Restoration Act. On Oct. 15, the Supreme Court agreed to rule on the constitutionality of the far-reaching law,

which makes government infringement on religious practices more difficult. [22] (*See story, p. 4.*)

"Where's the avalanche of cases?" Farris asks.

Advocates also say that because those rights are not absolute — consider cases of abuse, for example — parents wouldn't be assured of winning every case under a parental rights law.

Noting that the high court has delineated rights for school boards as well as parents, the Heritage Foundation says, "If parents raised ridiculous claims under [a federal bill], their cases would be thrown out of court. . . . Frivolous litigation would be costly for parents and of no benefit to them." [23]

Opponents of the parental rights movement find little comfort in such assurances. They contend parental rights laws would benefit lawyers because parents would be able to sue at the drop of a hat, and the government would have to clear exceedingly high legal hurdles to win. Moreover, says the Academy of Pediatrics, suits involving parental rights laws "would decimate the resources of a community [earmarked to] safeguard children and support families, and put more children at risk of abuse and neglect."

"The bill allows parents to file an action in state or federal court, even if that parent is also arguing before another tribunal," Quintana of the school boards association testified last December. "A school district would be forced to fight on both fronts, doubling the costs." Not only that, Quintana said, the federal bill would award attorney's fees to the victor — discouraging mediation or mutual agreement. [24]

Isaacs of People for the American Way calls the 90-day administrative remedy in Grassley's bill "a joke," saying it is a pressure tactic rather than a means of conflict resolution. "Say [I'm a parent who claims] teaching evolution interferes with my right to raise my child as I see fit," she says. "So the administrative remedy kicks in. It means the

school must stop teaching evolution to everybody during the period — or does it mean only my kid would be taken out of that class? It's completely unclear — it has to be litigated," she says. Or, she says, a parent could simply wait 90 days and then sue.

The NEA estimates the cost in the billions just to hire more teachers to meet the demands of the federal bill. "An enormous, unfunded federal mandate," the teachers' union called the Grassley-Largent proposal. "Depending on how widely parents exercise this new fundamental right . . . the costs to school districts of providing such 'designer' curricula will be exorbitant. If, for example, [a parental rights act] forces school districts to hire just *one* extra teacher for each school, the annual cost will be . . . $3,346,330,650." [25]

Parental rights advocates scoff at the NEA's resistance to the movement, saying the big union is running scared from demands for accountability while trying desperately to protect its power base in the public school system.

Besides, Grassley says, the NEA's unfunded-mandates argument doesn't hold water. "They've got to be joking," he says. "They opposed the unfunded mandates bill we got passed in 1995. They're talking out of both sides of their mouth." ∎

BACKGROUND

A 'Fundamental' Right

The Founding Fathers didn't mention parental rights in the Constitution and Bill of Rights, but their silence on the matter is not surprising.

In early America, children had few if any rights. There was little question of parents' rights to freely direct their offspring.

Conservatives argue, nonetheless, that the Ninth and 14th amendments to the

Chronology

1700s-1800s

Formation of the new nation's constitution sets the stage for battles over parental rights.

Dec. 15, 1791
The first 10 amendments to the Constitution take effect. They include the First Amendment, which guarantees religious freedom, and the 9th, which says listing of certain rights in the Constitution "shall not be construed to deny or disparage others retained by the people."

July 9, 1868
Ratification of the 14th Amendment, which says no state may deprive a person of "life, liberty, or property, without due process of law."

———— • ————

1900-1980

Parental rights become an issue in the courts and schools.

June 4, 1923
Supreme Court says a state law limiting the teaching of foreign languages in public schools violates the Constitution's "liberty" guarantee, which includes right "to marry, to establish a home and bring up children." (*Meyer v. Nebraska*).

June 1, 1925
Supreme Court says Oregon law requiring children to attend public school unreasonably interferes with parents' liberty to direct the education and upbringing of their children (*Pierce v. Society of Sisters*).

1960s
A ban on school prayer signals courts' increasing involvement in issues of values, religion and family life.

June 25, 1962
Supreme Court bars use of prayer written by New York state Board of Regents in public school classrooms (*Engel v. Vitale*).

May 15, 1967
Supreme Court expands juvenile rights (*In re Gault*).

1976
Supreme Court rejects Missouri law requiring parental consent for a minor to have an abortion (*Planned Parenthood of Central Missouri v. Danforth*).

1979
Supreme Court supports rights of parents to commit their children to mental institutions (*Parham v. J.R.*).

———— • ————

1980s
Courts and policy-making bodies enhance the rights of children, opening the door for a parental rights movement among conservatives.

Dec. 4, 1980
Washington state Supreme Court allows troubled teen to remain in alternative residential placement, saying interests of the state and child are sufficient to justify "relatively minor degree of intrusion" on parents' constitutional rights (*In re the Welfare of Sheila Marie Sumey*).

Nov. 20, 1989
U.N. Convention on the Rights of the Child unanimously approved by U.N. General Assembly.

1990s
Parental rights activists push for changes in Congress and the states.

1990
Supreme Court denies Native Americans unemployment compensation after they are fired for using the drug peyote in tribal religious rituals. The ruling leads to the Religious Freedom Restoration Act in 1993 (*Employment Division v. Smith*).

1992-1993
New York City diversity curriculum touches off grass-roots protest that helps inspire parental rights movement.

Dec. 30, 1993
New York appeals court finds New York City's condom distribution program unconstitutional without a parental opt-out provision (*Alfonso v. Fernandez*).

1993
Arlington, Va.-based Of the People begins promoting parental rights amendments to state constitutions.

May 17, 1995
Christian Coalition introduces its "Contract With the American Family," which calls for a parental rights act and rejection of the U.N. Convention on the Rights of the Child.

June 1995
Sen. Charles E. Grassley, R-Iowa, and Rep. Steve Largent, R- Okla., introduce parental rights bills.

Nov. 5, 1996
Ballot initiative for parental rights constitutional amendment set for vote in Colorado.

The Case of the Troubled Teenager

The Sheila Marie Sumey case offers a textbook example of how interpretations can vary in an emotional issue such as parental rights. Supporters of efforts to codify parental rights say the state of Washington trampled on the rights of Sheila Marie's parents. Opponents say the parents never lost their rights in the first place.

The basic facts are not in dispute: In 1978, Sheila Marie was a troubled 15-year-old. She flouted rules set by her parents, ran away from home and did not benefit from counseling. In June 1978, to prevent Sheila Marie from running away again, her mother called police and had her placed in a juvenile-care facility. The teenager later requested placement in an alternative residential facility; her request was granted, against the parents' wishes. The parents appealed, contending their parental rights had been violated.

In the indignant view of Rep. Steve Largent, R-Okla., who introduced parental rights legislation last year, "the Supreme Court of Washington ruled that it was not a violation of constitutional parents' rights to remove a child from the home because she objected to her parents' reasonable rules. The parents had grounded their eighth-grade daughter because she wanted to smoke marijuana and sleep with her boyfriend. The Supreme Court found that it was reasonably within the lower court's jurisdiction to remove the girl from her family home. No strict standards were applied. The parents' rights were completely terminated for simply grounding their daughter to stop her from using illegal drugs and engaging in illicit activity!" [1]

Michael P. Farris, president of the Home School Legal Defense Association, calls the ruling "perhaps the most infamous decision in the history of American parental rights." When the parents had trouble getting their daughter to obey their rules, they asked the state for help, he said in congressional testimony last year. "Rather than telling this girl she was required to follow her parents' instructions," Farris said, "the state of Washington took this girl from her parents." [2]

Foes of parental rights laws say that a close reading of the Washington Supreme Court opinion indicates Sheila Marie's parents' rights were never terminated. "That's totally false," says Rebecca Isaacs of People for the American Way. "The parents' rights were not terminated. It couldn't be more explicit."

Critics also note that the court granted the teenager's request to live in the second juvenile facility, where the parents had visiting rights, as a last resort, in view of the severely strained relations between the teenager and her parents. The foes also point out that it was not until Sheila Marie was permitted to be moved to the second facility that the parents sued, claiming violation of their constitutional rights.

While the state's Supreme Court did not find the parents unfit, it held in December 1980 that the "interests of [the] state and child supporting the alternative residential placement procedure were sufficient to justify [a] relatively minor degree of intrusion upon [the] parents' constitutional rights to [the] care, custody and companionship of the child."

As things turned out, parental rights activists say, Sheila Marie years later came to agree with her parents.

After the courts and welfare agency backed the girl, her "teenage and early adult years were extraordinary troubled," the Heritage Foundation wrote in a passage critical of the court's decision. "Now an adult and mother herself, she sees the wisdom of her parents' approach and says that she wishes the local and state authorities had backed them instead of her." [3]

---

[1] Rep. Steve Largent, "Why Do We Need the Parental Rights and Responsibilities Act?" position paper. The case is *In re the Welfare of Sheila Marie Sumey.*

[2] Testimony before Senate Judiciary Subcommittee on Administrative Oversight and the Courts, Dec. 5, 1995.

[3] Patrick F. Fagan and Wade F. Horn, "How Congress Can Protect the Rights of Parents to Raise Their Children," *Heritage Foundation Issue Bulletin No. 277,* July 23, 1996.

Constitution leave no doubt that parental rights are on a par with freedom of speech, press and religion.

The Ninth Amendment, as interpreted by parental rights backers, means that a right doesn't have to be explicitly mentioned in the Constitution to merit judicial protection.

"This constitutional presumption in favor of the traditional rights of citizens was recognized and in place at the time of the adoption of the Bill of Rights," Farris wrote. "Parental rights have long been recognized as 'implicit in the concept of ordered liberty.' " [26]

Indeed, many conservatives reach back to English legal theorist Sir William Blackstone, who wrote in 1769 that parental power includes the "restraint and correction" of children. His ideas helped shape those of the Founders and live on today.

Key Cases From the 1920s

Besides the Ninth Amendment, movement backers rest their argument on the 14th Amendment's Due Process clause and its protection of "life, liberty, or property." The clause figures prominently in a number of cases cited by conservative activists, most notably a pair of decisions from the 1920s that are the legal pillars of today's parental rights movement.

In *Meyer v. Nebraska,* the Supreme Court in 1923 struck down a state law banning the teaching of foreign languages to elementary school pupils. Writing for the majority, Associate Justice James Clark McReynolds cited the Due Process guarantee of liberty, which includes, he wrote, the right of the individual "to marry, to establish a home and bring up children."

According to Rep. Largent, the court invalidated the foreign language ban because it "did not 'promote' education but rather 'arbitrarily and unreasonably' interfered with 'the natural duty of the parent to give his children education suitable to their station in life.' The court chastened the legislature for attempting 'materially to interfere . . . with the power of parents to control the education of their own.' " [27]

Two years later, in *Pierce v. Society of Sisters,* the court struck down an Oregon statute that required parents to send children ages 8-16 to public schools. Again citing the Due Process clause, McReynolds wrote that Oregon's initiative undermined the right of parents and guardians "to direct the education and upbringing of their children" — language adopted verbatim by today's parental rights advocates.

"The child is not the mere creature of the state; those who nurture him and direct his destiny have the right and high duty to recognize and prepare him for additional obligations," the court also said.

Though critics say the court never described parental rights as "fundamental" in the *Meyer* or *Pierce* decisions, advocates say the two cases — taken with other high court rulings in ensuing decades — clearly establish the constitutional supremacy of parents' rights.

Opponents view the *Meyer* and *Pierce* legacies quite differently than parental rights activists, arguing that the Supreme Court has never deemed parental rights "fundamental." And they say that courts traditionally have sought to balance parental rights with those of children and to allow the state to step in to protect children when a situation warrants it.

"The lower courts have not misconstrued the law, because the U.S. Supreme Court has *never* recognized parental rights as fundamental," The National PTA argues. "The lower courts have simply followed suit by refusing to apply a 'compelling state interest' test to parental rights claims." [28]

Isaacs of People for the American Way says conservatives are reading way too much into *Meyer* and *Pierce.* The court took "very specific [and] limited fact situations and . . . ruled against certain kinds of legislation as an infringement on parents rights," she says.

But, she emphasizes, the court's decisions were "not some wholesale, across-the-board" characterization of parental rights as fundamental, as many conservatives argue. "That view is a fantasy," she says.

U.N. Treaty

Conservatives are troubled by an other legal issue: the United Nations Convention on the Rights of the Child, which President Clinton signed in 1995 and now awaits Senate action. The convention's 54 articles, which lay out a comprehensive charter of civil, social and economic rights for children, left conservatives worried about how the treaty would affect U.S. laws on abortion, capital punishment and other sensitive issues.

The treaty, already ratified by more than 175 nations, "would virtually undermine parents' rights as we know them in the United States," the Christian Coalition said in its Contract With the American Family. "Parents no longer would have the basic right to control what their children watch on television, whom they associate with and what church they attend."

The Heritage Foundation calls the treaty "incompatible with traditional Western conceptions of the liberty of parents and with the U.S. Supreme Court's settled view of parental rights as 'beyond debate.' Worse, the state is the only other entity whose rights are made clearly superior to the domestic life of the family as an institution." [29]

John C. Green, director of the Ray C. Bliss Institute of Applied Politics at the University of Akron and an expert on the Christian Right, says

conservatives are hostile to the treaty partly because it contains "liberal values and liberal code words," such as "village." The word upset the Christian Right when first lady Hillary Rodham Clinton used it to describe community influence on family formation in her best-selling book *It Takes A Village.*

In addition, Green says Christian conservatives are "very suspicious of things international," such as talk of a "new world order," because their eschato-logical views — their ideas about the end of the world and the process of salvation — emphasize the threat of an Antichrist and a final battle between the forces of good and the evil rulers of the world. With the U.N. treaty, "You're reducing parental authority along with national sovereignty," Green says. "It's a double whammy."

The Rev. Jay Lintner, a policy official in Washington for the United Church of Christ, a liberal Protestant denomination, says those who back parental rights measures are trying to "absolutize the rights of parents" and give "no weight to the rights of the community or the rights of children."

Lintner calls the movement "a thinly disguised attack on the public school system," and adds: "While the radical Christian Right who is pushing this bill says parents' rights are not absolute, in fact, the way this is written would make it extremely difficult for many child welfare agencies to protect children." ■

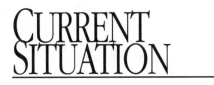

An Ironic Approach?

The parental rights movement may seem, at first glance, like it emerged from nowhere to take the ideological stage in America. But observers say it is of a piece with many other conservative and religious causes of the recent and distant past.

"Seeking to protect rights in law or in constitutions is a very American thing, and something that conservatives have always identified with," says Green at the University of Akron. "So in that sense, people are pushing these parental rights laws out of a conservative tradition that is many centuries old."

Still, Green and others see an incongruity in conservative advocates of limited government seeking a legal remedy that involves federal authority in local issues. "There's a powerful irony" in going to higher levels of government to deal with local affairs, says Green.

That's not the only unusual aspect of the parental rights movement, Green says. While seeking full "rights" for all Americans has traditionally been the province of liberals — rights for gays and people with disabilities, for example — conservatives have, in recent years, taken the same approach.

"The Christian Right has adopted the [approach] of liberalism," Green says, noting, for example, the quest for tax-funded vouchers for private school tuition. "That to me is just powerfully ironic."

Some politicians see an irony, too. Rep. Barney Frank, D-Mass., called the federal bill "the most direct assertion of federal superiority over the states I have ever seen." [30]

And David Blankenhorn, president of the Institute for American Values and an adviser to Of the People, has conceded being troubled by "the notion that we're to solve our problem by creating more rights," though he has endorsed the parental rights push. [31]

But proponents say they are not seeking a top-down solution to local issues. Grassley says he has sought a "floor, not a ceiling" for parental rights, with plenty of room left for states and localities to set higher boundaries. [32]

"The PRRA does not manufacture a single new federal program or create a need for new bureaucrats at any level of government," Largent wrote. [33] "Rather, it simply establishes the legal standard to be employed in judging cases where the right of parents comes in conflict with the decisions or policies of government officials."

"This is not a big-government issue," Farris argues. "It's about limiting the power of all governments."

Battles in the States

Limiting the power of government is indeed the key objective in Colorado and many other states where conservatives are fighting for stronger parental rights guarantees. In Colorado, advocates tried unsuccessfully to attach parental rights wording to the Colorado children's code.

Backers of the constitutional amendment drive subsequently gathered more than 83,000 signatures to put the measure on the ballot. As of late September, proponents had raised nearly $150,000 (including about $137,000 from Of the People). The opposing Protect Our Children Coalition had collected almost $65,000. [34]

Democratic Colorado Gov. Roy Romer has blasted the amendment, saying it is "absolutely unnecessary" because parents already can control the upbringing of their children. "It is a constitutional amendment proposed by a group on the far right of our culture," he told reporters. "I think its intent is to have the government have its hands off children almost totally, and I worry about this heavy-handed, generalized use in the constitution." [35]

In other states, meanwhile, the battle to pass amendments is just beginning. "We expect the momentum to continue" regardless of what happens in Colorado, says Of the People's Erken.

Already, a number of state Republican platforms reflect parental rights language, and in August such wording was inserted into the Republican national platform.

"Fourteen of the 22 [state] platforms reviewed by People for the American Way included so-called 'parental rights' language," the group said in August. [36]

There is other evidence of the movement's growth. In Kansas this year, the legislature passed legislation making it the "public policy" of the state "that parents shall retain the fundamental right to exercise primary control over the care and upbringing of their children" and "that children shall have the right to protection from abuse and neglect."

And Of the People said in late May that constitutional amendment proposals had found legislative sponsors in 28 states, including California, Florida, New York and Texas. Yet few of those measures have seen floor action, and even conservative supporters of parental rights have balked in some states at the notion of changing constitutional language.

Both Erken and Bell cite Michigan as fertile ground for the parental rights movement, and there's little wonder why. Parental rights language has already been added to Michigan's school code; the state has a conservative Republican governor, John Engler; and Elisabeth "Betsy" DeVos, Of the People's national co-chairman, chairs the Michigan Republican Party, serves as a Republican national committeewoman and is married to Dick DeVos, chief executive officer of the Amway Corp., a generous backer of conservative causes.

Yet the sponsor of Michigan's proposed parental rights amendment, state Sen. Joanne Emmons, R-Big Rapids, has shifted strategies. She says "concerns by friends on my side" caused her to "back off" and first pursue a legislative rather than a constitutional approach. Among other things, she says, there was the worry that the amendment "might be used in ways we

At Issue:

Would the Parental Rights and Responsibilities Act undercut established legal protections for children?

AMERICAN CIVIL LIBERTIES UNION
FROM A LETTER TO THEN SENATE MAJORITY LEADER BOB DOLE, JAN. 25, 1996.

*a*s an organization that has consistently defended family integrity against unwarranted government intrusion, we are painfully aware of the need for vigilance in this sensitive area. However, although we agree with one of the major premises of this legislation — that the vital role that parents play in the raising of their children is of critical importance and must be respected — we have seen no evidence warranting this broadly written federal statute that undermines longstanding protections for children.

This legislation [would forbid] federal, state and local governments and their officials from "interfer[ing] with or usurp[ing] the right of a parent to direct the upbringing of the child of the parent." Parents would be able to assert this right in lawsuits in either federal or state courts. . . . A government or official may only prevail in such a suit by proving that the government actions were "essential to accomplish a compelling governmental interest," which is an extraordinarily high standard of proof.

This legislation will make it especially difficult for the government to assist children in situations in which their health is endangered because of their parents' actions or inaction. It prohibits a government official or agency from becoming involved in health-care decisions, no matter how injurious the parent's actions may be to the child, unless the very strict "compelling government interest" test is met. . . .

This bill could make it impossible for education professionals to design and implement public school curricula. [It] permits any parent of a public school student to file a lawsuit challenging almost any aspect of the school's curriculum or extracurricular activities. . . .

This bill will reduce protections for children who are physically disciplined by their parents. . . . The language explicitly condoning a parent's right to physically discipline a child is, to our knowledge, without precedent in federal law. . . .

This bill could put children who are victims or potential victims of child abuse and neglect at great risk. Currently child abuse and neglect cases are handled almost exclusively by our state courts. This bill, however, creates a two-tiered system where parents may ask a federal judge to second-guess the decision of a child welfare agency official in a lawsuit alleging that the agency's action "interferes" with the parents' rights.

This dual track will create unnecessary lawsuits, and will create expensive litigation costs for child welfare agencies forced to defend their actions in federal court. The existence of this new cause of action will also have a chilling effect on child protective service workers and government officials.

CATHLEEN A. CLEAVER, DIRECTOR OF LEGAL STUDIES, FAMILY RESEARCH COUNCIL, GREG D. ERKEN, EXECUTIVE DIRECTOR, OF THE PEOPLE
FROM "PARENTAL RIGHTS: WHO DECIDES HOW CHILDREN ARE RAISED?" FAMILY POLICY, AUGUST 1996.

*c*ritics of both the federal parental rights bill and the state constitutional amendments typically claim that parental rights laws would make it tougher for the state to protect children from abuse and would give one parent the right to dictate school curriculum for everyone else's child, leading to education gridlock.

These and most other criticisms are grounded in the mistaken notion that these proposals would provide an absolute right for parents, which would override any state interest in the welfare and education of children. But . . . the well-established limits to parental rights under this doctrine would continue to apply.

For example, in *Prince v. Massachusetts* (1944), the high court made it clear that "neither the right of religion nor the rights of parents are beyond limitation." *Prince* identified numerous areas in which the state may set limits on parental rights, such as compulsory school attendance, mandatory vaccination policies and child labor laws. And in *Runyon v. McCrary* (1976), the Supreme Court held that parents "have no constitutional right to provide their children with education unfettered by reasonable government regulation." All constitutional rights have their limits, and parental rights are no exception.

The clash over parental rights proposals begs the fundamental question: Who decides what's in the best interests of children? Parents? Or the government? Are ordinary parents generally competent to raise their children or should parents defer to elite authorities backed by state power? . . .

If successful, the parental rights movement will provide parents with greater legal standing to ensure that government respects their rights through its policies, and when necessary, in the courts. But beyond this immediate, practical benefit, a national debate on parental rights also has great potential to foster more parental responsibility.

The key to encouraging greater parental responsibility is to explicitly recognize the link between rights and duties upon which this nation was founded, and to renew our optimism in the ability of the people to manage their own affairs, as citizens and as parents. Indeed, [as G.K. Chesterton observed in *Orthodoxy*], "the most terribly important things must be left to ordinary men themselves," including the right of parents to protect their children from harmful influences and to direct their children's upbringing. Recognizing the irreplaceable role of parents is essential to keeping the power of the state in check, revitalizing citizenship and ensuring that children receive the love, protection and guidance only a parent can provide.

FOR MORE INFORMATION

American Center for Law and Justice, P.O. Box 64429, Virginia Beach, Va. 23467; (757) 226-2489; www.aclj.org. Founded in 1990, ACLJ is dedicated to the promotion of pro-liberty, pro-life and pro-family causes. It engages in litigation, provides legal services and supports attorneys who are involved in defending religious and civil liberties.

Focus on the Family, 8605 Explorer Dr., Colorado Springs, Colo. 80920; (719) 531-5181; www.family.org. Founded in 1977, the nonprofit Christian organization works to preserve traditional values and the institution of the family.

National Child Abuse Coalition, 733 15th St. N.W. Suite 938, Washington, D.C. 20005; (202) 347-3666. The coalition contends that amendments and legislation aimed at codifying parental rights would put children at risk of abuse from abusive parents.

National Education Association, 1201 16th St. N.W. Washington, D.C. 20036-3290; (202) 833-4000; www.nea.org. The NEA is the largest teachers' union and views laws designed to bolster parents' rights as potentially detrimental to school quality.

National School Boards Association, 1680 Duke St., Alexandria, Va. 22314; (703) 683-7590; www.nsba.org. This federation of school board associations is interested in such issues as local governance and quality of education programs.

People for the American Way, 2000 M St., N.W., Suite 400, Washington, D.C. 20036; (202) 467-4999; www.pfaw.org. This nonpartisan organization promotes protection of First Amendment rights. It is leading a coalition of groups opposed to parental rights laws.

Traditional Values Coalition, 139 C St. S.E., Washington, D.C. 20003; (202) 547-8570; www.traditionalvalues.org. The coalition is a legislative interest group that supports conservative Judeo-Christian values.

could not anticipate by a judge, and then you have no legislative redress."

A constitutional amendment would be harder to fix if problems arose, Emmons acknowledges. "Once it goes into the constitution, it will have to have another vote of the people to change it."

In Illinois, state Sen. Patrick O'Malley, R-Palos Park, cosponsored a parental rights amendment with Rep. Al Salvi, now a Republican candidate for the U.S. Senate. "The intrusion of government into our personal lives is stifling our individual freedom and discouraging personal responsibility," O'Malley declared in April. "With this amendment, we reassert the importance of parental authority and responsibility as a means of balancing parental rights with other interests compet-

ing for the control of family life." [37]

O'Malley's proposed measure passed the Executive Committee of the Republican-controlled Senate, but it did not make it onto the Illinois ballot this fall. "The groups most interested in its passage felt on balance they needed to do more public education," O'Malley says. "We intend to go back at it in [January] and get it on the ballot at the next available date."

In Virginia, whose conservative leanings make it another bellwether in the parental rights movement, Republican Gov. George F. Allen supported an amendment that passed the Senate Privileges and Elections Committee 8-2 last February and moved to the Senate floor. But Democratic Lt. Gov. Donald S. Beyer Jr. voted against the bill, kicking the proposal back to committee.

Such setbacks don't seem to discourage the movement's chief backers. "The parental revolt a year from now is going to be much bigger than it is today," a confident Bell predicted at the Christian Coalition's September conference. ■

OUTLOOK

'Building Momentum'

Former pro football receiver Largent uses a sports metaphor to analyze the future of the parental rights movement. "This is a marathon," he says. "It's not a 100-yard dash."

That marathon won't be an easy one for parental rights backers to win in Congress, beginning with the November elections. Largent is up for re-election this year, and the loss of the Republican majority in either chamber could cripple the conservative parental rights cause.

Indeed, support for the measures falls largely along partisan lines. Of the 140 sponsors of Largent's bill, for example, all but about a dozen were Republicans. Largent concedes that if Republicans lose the House, his bill "will go nowhere." Nonetheless, Largent plans to reintroduce the measure in the 105th Congress, even if Republicans lose control of Congress in November.

Grassley seems less definite. "I would like to reintroduce" the bill in the next Congress, he says, "and at the same time I would like to garner more bipartisan support for the initiative in the Senate. Right now, our job is to continue building grass-roots support and educating the public about the goal of the legislation, in the face of disinformation from special interests in Washington, D.C."

Grassley's bill faced tough opposition from Democrats. The Senate

Subcommittee on Administrative Oversight and the Courts, chaired by Grassley, voted in April to send the bill to the full Judiciary Committee after it had been through significant revision, including addition of the 90-day administrative process clause.

But heavy resistance came from Sen. Howell Heflin, D-Ala., a former school board president and ranking Democrat on the subcommittee. The bill, he said, "is premised on a false idea: that the rights of parents are being vastly undermined across the country." The measure would "open the floodgates of litigation," Heflin added, and "could impose chaos in matters relating to curriculum content, textbook selection, dress codes and home schooling, just to name a few." [38]

As for Largent's bill, which died in a House Judiciary subcommittee, legislative aide Paul Webster says subcommittee Chairman Charles T. Canady, R-Fla., had concerns about use of the legislation by a liberal judge. "I think his primary concern [was] that some federal court judge could begin decreeing all manner of family law that's not consistent" with the bill, Webster says. "[He] has a real concern that a very liberal federal judge could just say [children's] reproductive rights are outside the fundamental rights of parents [to oversee] and . . . in one judicial act" gut a significant portion of the bill's intent.

Of the People Chairman Bell said at the Christian Coalition meeting that Canady had bottled up the bill because he thought parental rights should be a state rather than federal issue. (Canady's press aide did not respond to phone calls.)

Even if parental rights legislation were to reach the marathon finish line, backers expect that it would be tripped at the end by a presidential veto, assuming Bill Clinton remains in the White House.

Still, Grassley is sanguine about the long-term prospects. "We're in the first step of promoting an important national debate," he says. "Our job is to continue building momentum."

Adds Sheldon of the Traditional Values Coalition: "Just because you introduce a bill doesn't mean you expect it to become law that year," she says. "A public-policy debate — that's what we want." ■

Notes

[1] Quoted in *The Rocky Mountain News,* Sept. 22, 1996.

[2] Quoted in *The Denver Post,* Sept. 22, 1996.

[3] See "Parents Rights Amendment Foils Colorado Senate Race," *The Washington Post,* Oct. 20, 1996, p. A1. For background, see "Children's Legal Rights," *The CQ Researcher,* April 23, 1993, pp. 337-360.

[4] For background, see "Parents and Schools," *The CQ Researcher,* Jan. 20, 1995, pp. 49-72.

[5] Dobson's remarks were made during a discussion of parental rights on his syndicated show, "Focus on the Family Radio Hour," June 17-18, 1996.

[6] Letter to U.S. senators from Dr. Maurice E. Keenan, president of the American Academy of Pediatrics, March 19, 1996.

[7] Testimony before Senate Judiciary Subcommittee on Administrative Oversight and the Courts, Dec. 5, 1995.

[8] The poll of 482 voters was taken in conjunction with the Scripps-Howard News Service.

[9] See "The Parent Trap: Relying on Bogus Horror Stories And Mega-Bucks Backing, The 'Parental Rights' Movement Is Luring Americans Into An Attack On Public Schools And Church-State Separation," *Church & State,* June 1996, published by Americans United for Separation of Church and State.

[10] "Commentary on Protections Which Should Be Afforded Parental Rights and Responsibilities," position paper, The American Center for Law and Justice, undated, p. 10.

[11] From "Oppose H.R. 1946/S. 984: The 'Parental Rights And Responsibilities Act,'" People for the American Way, September 1996.

[12] "Statement of the National Education Association Regarding The Parental Rights and Responsibilities Act," February 1996, p. 2.

[13] For background, see "Home Schooling," *The CQ Researcher,* Sept. 9, 1994, pp. 769-792.

[14] Quoted in "Parental-Rights Advocates Push for Constitutional Amendment," *Insight on the News,* Sept. 9, 1996, p. 40.

[15] For background, see "School Choice," *The CQ Researcher,* May 10, 1991, pp. 253-276, and "Attack on Public Schools," *The CQ Researcher,* July 26, 1996, pp. 662-663.

[16] Quoted in *The Washington Times,* Oct. 27, 1995.

[17] Letter to U.S. senators, March 19, 1996.

[18] Letter to U.S. senators from Adele Douglass, director, Washington office, American Humane Association, March 19, 1996.

[19] Heritage Foundation, "How Congress Can Protect the Rights of Parents to Raise Their Children," *Issue Bulletin No. 227,* July 23, 1996, p. 23.

[20] For background, see *The New York Times,* Oct. 14, 1996.

[21] Heritage Foundation, *op. cit.,* pp. 13-14.

[22] See "High Court to Rule on Religion Law," *The Washington Post,* Oct. 16, 1996, p. A1.

[23] Heritage Foundation, *op. cit.,* p. 25.

[24] Testimony before Senate Judiciary Subcommittee on Administrative Oversight and the Courts, Dec. 5. 1995.

[25] National Education Association, *op. cit.*

[26] Michael P. Farris, "The Parental Rights and Responsibilities Act: Establishing a Standard of Liberty," National Center for Home Education Special Report, undated, p. 2.

[27] Steve Largent, "Questions and Answers About the Parental Rights and Responsibilities Act," undated, p. 1.

[28] "Oppose the Parental Rights and Responsibilities Act," position paper of The National PTA.

[29] Heritage Foundation, *op. cit.,* p. 19.

[30] Quoted in *The Washington Times,* Oct. 27, 1995.

[31] Quoted in "Parental-Rights Advocates Push for Constitutional Amendment," *op. cit.*

[32] Opening statement of Sen. Charles E. Grassley on the Parental Rights and Responsibilities Act of 1996, Senate Judiciary Subcommittee on Administrative Oversight and the Courts, April 17, 1996.

[33] Largent, *op. cit.,* p. 14.

[34] *The Denver Post,* Sept. 22, 1996.

[35] Quoted in *The Daily Camera,* Sept. 21, 1996.

[36] People for the American Way, "The Republicans and the Religious Right: A Study of 1996 State Republican Party Platforms," Aug. 2, 1996, p. 6.

[37] Press release, April 18, 1996.

[38] Quoted in *School Board News,* published by the National School Boards Association, April 30, 1996.

Bibliography
Selected Sources Used

Books

Bates, Stephen, *Battleground: One Mother's Crusade, the Religious Right, and the Struggle for Control of Our Classrooms,* Poseidon Press, 1993.

Bates, formerly a senior fellow at the Annenberg Washington Program of Northwestern University, chronicles the case of Vicki Frost, a Tennessee mother who sued school officials after she found such themes as evolution, feminism and telepathy in her children's schoolbooks. The high-profile case, dubbed "Scopes II" by journalists, pitted two powerful advocacy groups against each other: Concerned Women for America and People for the American Way.

Christian Coalition, *Contract With the American Family,* 1995.

This book lays out the political priorities of one of the nation's most powerful conservative religious organizations, including enactment of a parental-rights measure and defeat of the U.N. Convention on the Rights of the Child.

Hawes, Joseph M., *The Children's Rights Movement: A History of Advocacy and Protection,* Twayne Publishers, 1991.

Hawes, a professor of history at Memphis State University, provides a well-organized overview of children's rights from the establishment of child aid societies in the 1800s and the creation of broader government programs in the early 20th century to the maturing of the children's rights movement beginning in the 1960s. The book includes a useful chronology and a nine-page bibliographic essay.

Nelkin, Dorothy, *The Creation Controversy: Science or Scripture in the Schools,* Beacon Press, 1982.

Nelkin, a Cornell University professor, provides a broad overview of the evolution vs. creationism controversy in American schools.

Samuels, Sarah E., and Mark D. Smith, eds., *Condoms in the Schools,* Kaiser Family Foundation, 1993.

The authors provide a useful overview of a key point of contention in the parental rights debate: making condoms available to public school students. The book includes a survey of condom programs, the views of school officials and discussions of funding and policy options and legal issues.

Articles

Applebome, Peter, "Array of Opponents Battle Over 'Parental Rights' Bills," *The New York Times,* May 1, 1996.

This front-page overview of the parental rights movement surveys the issues and quotes the chief spokesmen on either side of the debate.

Glanzer, Perry L., "Parental Rights and Public Education," *Focus on the Family,* July 1996.

Glanzer is an education policy analyst at Focus on the Family, a conservative Christian organization in Colorado Springs, Colo. This 29-page booklet surveys "current rights and threats" to parental rights in education and securing parental rights through legislative reform, among other issues.

Green, John C., James L. Guth, Lyman A. Kellstedt and Corwin E. Smidt, "Evangelical Realignment: The Political Power of the Christian Right," *Christian Century,* July 5-12, 1995.

Green, director of the Ray C. Bliss Institute of Applied Politics at the University of Akron, and his colleagues provide a wide-ranging and incisive look at the Christian Right's influence in the 1994 Republican triumph in Congress and at evangelical politics at the dawn of a new millennium.

Grunes, Rodney A., "Creationism, the Courts and the First Amendment," *Journal of Church and State,* fall 1989.

Grunes, associate professor of political science at Centenary College, examines the political and legal contexts of the creationism controversy and analyzes Louisiana's 1981 "Balanced Treatment" Act mandating that creationism be given equal time whenever evolution was taught in the public schools.

O'Connor, Karen, and Gregg Ivers, "Education At Risk?: Creationism, Evolution and the Courts," *Political Science and Politics,* winter 1988.

O'Connor and Ivers, both of Emory University, give a useful history of the creationism controversy and address the impact of a series of "creationism-evolution" cases on the place of religion in the public schools.

Stepp, Laura Sessions, "Who's in Charge?: A Parents' Rights Movement Is Stirring Controversy," *The Washington Post,* July 15, 1996.

Reporter Stepp provides an overview of the emerging parental rights movement and quotes many of the principal players.

Reports and Studies

People for the American Way, *The Republicans and the Religious Right: A Study of 1996 State Republican Party Platforms,* Aug. 2, 1996.

The liberal advocacy group analyzes Republican platforms and various issues, including parental rights, concluding that the "Christian Coalition is well on its way to its stated goal of taking over the Republican Party."

2 School Violence

KATHY KOCH

When 11-year-old Logan Hamm of Seattle went to a weekend sleepover party recently, he stuffed his water pistol into his backpack along with his pajamas.

But in the school cafeteria the next Monday, when he reached into his bag for his lunch, out tumbled the gun, which he had painted black to look more realistic. Classmates alerted school authorities, who promptly expelled the middle-schooler. [1]

Seattle schools spokesman Trevor Neilson said the district's zero-tolerance weapons policy applies to toy guns as well as real ones. "In the wake of what happened in Jonesboro, Springfield and West Paducah," he said, "we take these things very, very seriously." [2]

Five times within eight months last year, troubled boys — some as young as 11 — brought guns to school and fired on their classmates. Eleven students and two teachers were killed, and 47 were wounded in the high-profile, small-town mass murders in Pearl, Miss., West Paducah, Ky., Jonesboro, Ark., Edinboro, Pa., and Springfield, Ore.*

When experts gather at the White House on Oct. 15 to discuss school safety, they will be haunted by the riveting television images of schoolyards cordoned off by yellow police tape, paramedics rushing gurneys to waiting ambulances and police leading adolescent boys away in handcuffs and leg irons.

President Clinton called for the meeting after the massacres left a stunned nation asking how such incidents could have occurred.

---

*Four other multiple murders occurred at schools last year, but they involved murder/suicides by jealous boyfriends, including two by adults and a dispute between rival "party crews" at a school in California. In a separate incident at a high school in Stamps, Ark., 14-year-old Joseph Colt Todd randomly shot and wounded two students, claiming he was tired of being bullied.

From *The CQ Researcher,*
October 9, 1998.

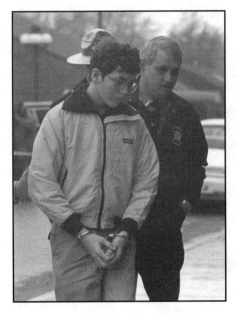

"The recent series of killings in our schools has seared the heart of America about as much as anything I can remember in a long, long time," Clinton said on July 7.

At the daylong meeting, conferees will devise ways to prevent recurrences and contingency plans for the grim possibility that it might happen again. They will also grapple with the many questions prompted by the shootings. How did the boys get access to firearms? Did they give off signals indicating that they had reached the breaking point? Who is ultimately responsible for these tragedies?

In the wake of the shootings, school officials have been tightening up on security, stringently enforcing their weapons policies and trying to ensure that such horrific incidents don't happen again. Although 1997-98 was not the bloodiest year in school history — more violent school deaths occurred in 1992-93 — it will be remembered as the year that youngsters in America's heartland turned to mass murder to solve adolescent problems.

The most reliable statistics on school deaths come from the National School Safety Center (NSSC), which surveys press accounts of incidents each year. [3] The center counted 42 "school-associated violent deaths" in the last academic year — a 68 percent jump from the previous year's total of only 25. But that was still fewer than the 55 deaths in 1992-93, the same year that juvenile crime peaked nationwide. *(See graph, p. 26.)* In the past, most violent school deaths occurred in urban secondary schools, involved firearms and both the victims and offenders tended to be male, according to the NSSC. The motives most commonly cited were interpersonal disputes. The victims last year were predominantly female.

But as many experts point out, despite the intense media attention surrounding the recent shootings, schools are the safest places for children — safer even than their own homes. "Kids are safer in schools than they are anywhere else in America," says William Modzeleski, director of the Education Department's Safe and Drug-Free Schools Program.

Shootings at schools account for less than 1 percent of the more than 5,000 firearms-related deaths of children under 19 in the U.S. each year. Juveniles are murdered outside of schools — and overwhelmingly by adults in or around the home — 40 times more often than they are killed in school, according to a study by the Justice Policy Institute (JPI), a Washington think tank. Indeed, American children are twice as likely to be struck by lightning as they are to be shot in school, the report said. [4]

Nevertheless, nearly a million students — some as young as 10 — packed guns into their backpacks along with their homework last year, according to an annual survey released June 18 by the anti-drug advocacy group PRIDE. The good news, says PRIDE, is that the number of students bringing guns to school has dropped 36 percent over the last five years.

Under federally mandated zero-tolerance policies instituted in 1994, some 6,100 students were expelled for bringing a gun to school in 1996-97, says a Department of Education report released last May 8. "Our nation's public schools are

Crime in Public Schools, 1996-97

Only 10 percent of the nation's public schools reported at least one serious, violent crime in the 1996-97 school year, based on a survey of 1,200 school principals. Almost half reported at least one less serious or non-violent incident.

Violence in Schools

At least one serious, violent crime ** 10%

At least one serious, non-violent crime *** 47%

No crime * 43%

* Did not report any crimes listed in the questionnaire to the police. Other crimes could have occurred or crimes that occurred were not reported.

** Includes murder, rape/sexual battery, suicide, attack or fight with weapon, robbery.

*** Includes attack or fight without weapon, theft/larceny, vandalism.

Source: U.S. Department of Education, National Center for Education Statistics, "Violence and Discipline Problems in U.S. Public Schools: 1996-97," February 1998

cracking down on students who bring guns to school," said U.S. Secretary of Education Richard W. Riley. [5]

But while students might be less likely to be murdered at school compared with the outside world, they can also be robbed, assaulted or raped at school. It is difficult to ascertain whether non-homicidal school violence has increased or decreased over the years, because no one has kept comprehensive statistics in a consistent manner. Existing studies portray different snapshots of the problem.

According to the *1996 Sourcebook of Criminal Justice Statistics*, the number of high school seniors who reported being injured or threatened by someone with a weapon was actually lower in 1996 than 20 years ago. For example, 3.4 percent of seniors in 1976 said they had been injured by someone with a weapon, compared with 2.8 percent in 1996. Such assaults apparently peaked in 1991 at 3.9 percent and have been declining since.

Yet, another study released last April by the Education and Justice departments found that the number of students physically attacked or robbed at school increased 23.5 percent between 1989 and 1995, from 3.4 percent to 4.2 percent. The increase occurred even as overall school crime rates remained steady, at about 14 percent, during the six-year period. [6]

Gang presence in schools nearly doubled during the same period, according to the report released last April 12 by the Bureau of Justice Statistics and the National Center for Education Statistics. While almost none of the 10,000 students interviewed admitted taking a gun to school, 12.7 percent said they knew of another student carrying a gun to school.

President Clinton called the trend unacceptable. "Gangs and the guns, drugs and violence that go with them must be stopped from ever reaching the schoolhouse door," Clinton said

in a statement released with the report. He urged Congress to approve initiatives against gangs and youth violence that he proposed last year.

Although the NSSC's review of news reports found that 25 violent deaths occurred in schools during the 1996-97 school year, more than 1,200 public school principals surveyed in a nationally representative sampling by the Education Department found that no murders occurred in their schools during that year, and only four had any suicides on campus. [7]

Ninety percent of public schools had no "serious, violent crime" that year, but those that did reported 4,170 rapes, 7,150 robberies and 10,950 physical attacks or fights with weapons, according to the Education Department report. Only 4 percent of those incidents occurred in elementary schools. By far, most school crime was of a less violent nature, including 190,000 physical attacks or fights without a weapon, 116,000 thefts or larcenies and 98,000 cases of vandalism.

The report also found that most schools have a zero-tolerance policy toward weapons on campus, and 78 percent have a violence-prevention or reduction program in place. Further, violent crimes occur most often in schools with classroom discipline problems and in large schools in central cities.

Indeed, last year's high-profile shootings received overblown press coverage because of the "man-bites-dog" nature of the story: They occurred in rural schools and were perpetrated by white adolescent boys "as opposed to urban kids of color," contends JPI Diretor Vincent Schiraldi. As a result, public officials "from the school house to the state house to the White House" have overreacted to the shootings, he says. [8]

"We are witnessing a tragic misdirection of attention and resources . . . even though the real threat may lie elsewhere," the report said. To remedy the so-called "crisis of classroom violence," politicians have put extra police in schools, eliminated minimum ages at which children can be tried as adults and proposed expanding the death penalty to juveniles and eliminating after-school programs, the JPI report said. "If we want to reduce the overall number of childhood gun deaths we should be expanding after-school programs and restricting gun sales," Schiraldi said.

Since the shootings, many schools have adopted a no-nonsense, zero-tolerance policy on threats, similar to the attitude taken at airports if passengers make even joking references to highjacking. Teachers now report any mention of violence, even references in short stories, journal entries, notes passed between students and drawings of violent acts.

The new measures acknowledge the fact that in nearly all of last year's rampages, the shooters had made numerous threats or dropped hints that they were contemplating violent action. The perpetrators also had a history of violence or anti-social behavior.

"The major challenge for schools is how to react without overreacting," says Ronald D. Stephens, executive director of the California-based NSSC. He says most schools are developing comprehensive "safe school" plans, beefing up their security operations, and training their staff to recognize early warning signs of potential troublemakers. To help them do that the Education Department issued a checklist for school officials trying to sort out which threats are youthful pranks and which are coming from students likely to erupt into violence. (See story, p. 22.)

"Schools want to find these kids and defuse the anger before the time bomb goes off," says Barbara Wheeler, president of the National School Boards Association.

Other schools have set up hot lines for tips about threats by students so that friends worried about "ratting" on their buddies can report threats anonymously. Others have installed metal detectors, instituted uniform dress codes and hired additional school psychologists.

Yet what has profoundly shaken most parents, policy-makers, scholars, ethicists and clergy, was the detached, premeditated, cold-blooded nature of the recent incidents.

"These attacks were planned," said Gary Goldman, author of *Books and Bullets: Violence in the Public Schools*. "This wasn't a spur-of-the-moment thing. These boys had a chance to think things over. Calmly, coolly, they decided to take care of matters with pistols and rifles." [9]

"You could spend the next five years trying to figure out if big schools or single parents or a violent movie drove these kids to this," he continues. "But the only real common thread is that they saw the way to get rid of their problem was to get rid of other people. I'm not sure there is a simple way to explain a tragedy like that." [10]

As citizens and lawmakers try to make sense of recent school shootings, these are some of the questions they are asking:

Would tighter gun control reduce school violence?

In the Jonesboro shooting, when Andrew Golden and Mitchell Johnson couldn't break into Andrew's father's steel gun vault with a blow torch, they found three guns he had left unsecured, including a .357 Magnum. Then they broke into Andrew's grandfather's house and stole four more handguns and three rifles, which were kept in unlocked storage cases.

Gun control advocates say the case clearly demonstrates the need for nationwide safe-storage laws requiring gun owners to keep their weapons locked and unloaded.

"The boys were unable to blow-torch their way into the father's gun safe," notes Nancy Hwa, a spokeswoman for the Center to Prevent Handgun Violence. But they were able to get their hands on 10 other guns that had not been locked up, she points out.

Her group advocates child access prevention (CAP) laws, requiring gun-owners to store their firearms so they are inaccessible to kids. Sixteen states already have such laws, which also hold gun owners criminally liable if they fail to store their guns properly and those guns are then used by a juvenile committing a crime. The Clinton administration has urged Congress and the states to pass CAP laws. [11] The five states where the recent school mass murders occurred — Mississippi, Arkansas, Oregon, Kentucky and Pennsylvania — do not have CAP laws.

Supporters say such laws also prevent accidental shootings by children, a claim backed up by a recently published study. It found that accidental deaths of children dropped an average of 23 percent in states with CAP laws. [12]

In June, after the fifth mass shooting, Education Secretary Riley challenged the 2.8 million-member National Rifle Association (NRA) to help keep guns out of the hands of unsupervised children.

"Unsupervised gun use and children do not mix," Riley told 450 school officials attending a Safe and Drug-Free Schools conference June 9 in Washington, D.C. The NRA needs to "help keep our children from becoming the victims of gun violence in our schools, in our homes and in our streets. I challenge the NRA to direct its attention to getting guns out of the hands of unsupervised children," he continued.

Partly in response to the school shootings, Sen. Richard J. Durbin, D-Ill., tried to attach federal CAP language to the Justice appropriations bill. "It's time for the adults who own the guns to act responsibly, to store them safely and to take responsibility for the guns in their possession," Durbin said as he

How to Spot a Potential Killer

Most of the boys who went on school shooting rampages last year fit profiles of what kind of youngster is likely to erupt into violence. Most had been picked on and bullied. Luke Woodham, the Pearl, Miss., shooter, said, "I'm not insane. I am angry. I killed because people like me are mistreated every day." [1] Many came from troubled homes, and most had given clear warnings and threats to friends.

The National School Safety Center in Westlake Village, Calif., has developed a checklist of characteristics common among youths who have committed murders at schools. School staff should alert the parents and guidance counselors, or law enforcement agencies in some cases, if a child exhibits these characteristics:

- Has a tantrums and angry outbursts.
- Resorts to name calling, cursing or abusive language.
- Makes violent threats when angry.
- Has previously brought a weapon to school.
- Has serious disciplinary problems at school and in the community.
- Has drug, alcohol or other substance abuse or dependency.
- Is on the fringe of his/her peer group with few or no close friends.
- Is preoccupied with weapons, explosives or other incendiary devices.
- Has previously been truant, suspended or expelled.
- Is cruel to animals.
- Has little or no supervision and support from parents or a caring adult.
- Has witnessed or been a victim of abuse or neglect in the home.
- Has been bullied and/or bullies or intimidates peers or younger children.
- Tends to blame others for difficulties and problems he causes himself.
- Prefers TV shows, movies or music expressing violent themes and acts.
- Prefers reading materials dealing with violent themes, rituals and abuse.
- Reflects anger, frustration and the dark side of life in school essays or writing projects.
- Is involved with a gang or an anti-social group on the fringe of peer acceptance.
- Is often depressed and/or has significant mood swings.
- Has threatened or attempted suicide.

The American Academy of Child and Adolescent Psychiatry's (AACAP) Web-site fact sheet lists many of the same characteristics in describing violent behaviors that bear watching. [2] Its list also includes fire-setting and intentional destruction of property and vandalism. Factors cited by the AACAP as increasing the risk of violent behavior include brain damage from a head injury, firearms being present in the home and stressful family socioeconomic factors, such as poverty, marital breakup, single parenting or unemployment.

The U.S. Department of Education's "Guide to Safe Schools" also lists many of the same warning signs. In addition, it lists: excessive feelings of rejection, feelings of being picked on and persecuted, poor academic achievement and intolerance and prejudicial attitudes.

The guide warns school officials to avoid "labeling" or stereotyping children as troublemakers, and to use the list judiciously. "Know what is developmentally typical behavior, so that behaviors are not misinterpreted," it says.

The Education Department also recommends that school authorities intervene immediately if a child has a weapon or has presented a detailed plan to harm or kill others.

Many experts advise against simply expelling a troubled youth from school because such children already feel that no one cares about them. Keeping the child engaged in school activities is more likely to avert disaster, some psychologists say. For instance, Northwestern University has a program that offers suspended local high school students the option of going to a therapist instead of being expelled.

If a child exhibits troubling behaviors, says the AACAP, the parents should seek a comprehensive psychological evaluation. "Most important, efforts should be made to dramatically decrease the exposure of children and adolescents to violence in the home, community and through the media," says the AACAP's Web site. "Clearly, violence leads to violence."

---

[1] Scott Bowles, "Armed, alienated and adolescent," *USA Today*, March 31, 1998.

[2] American Academy of Child and Adolescent Psychiatry Web site, "Understanding Violent Behavior in Children and Adolescents."

---

introduced the amendment. [13] The Senate resoundingly rejected the provision (69-31), along with three other gun-control measures on July 22 — two days before Russell E. Weston Jr. entered the Capitol building and shot two Capitol Hill policemen.

Curt Lavarello, executive director of the National Association of School Resource Officers, says tightening up gun laws and requiring parents to keep guns locked up would help prevent the proliferation of guns among teens that he has witnessed during 12 years as a po-

lice officer working in schools.

"A lot of the issues that kids get into fights over are the same as they were 25 years ago," he says. "What's changed drastically is the availability and accessibility of weapons and firearms, and the desire to turn to weapons to end a dispute."

Rep. Carolyn McCarthy, D-N.Y., whose husband was killed by a gunman on a Long Island commuter train, recently introduced sweeping legislation requiring that guns be stored safely, that child safety locks be sold with all new guns and that manufacturers produce guns with improved childproof safety features.

"We lose 14 children a day to gun violence in this country," McCarthy says. "That's a classroom full of kids every two days. We need comprehensive federal legislation that will keep guns out of the hands of children who are unsupervised." Congress was not expected to consider her legislation this session, which is scheduled to end Oct. 9. (See At Issue, p. 33.)

In 1995 about 5,300 American children under 19 were killed with firearms. Of those, about 4,700 were suicides and homicides (most committed by adults) and 440 were accidental shootings. [14] The Children's Defense Fund says that children under 15 in the United States die from gunfire 12 times more often than in 25 other industrialized countries — combined.

Further, between 1985 and 1994, the number of juveniles murdering with a gun quadrupled, while the number killing with all other types of weapons remained constant. [15]

Although it is illegal for anyone under 18 to possess a handgun, guns are easily accessible for juveniles in America, says Dennis Henigan, director of legal affairs for Handgun Control Inc. The primary route by which juveniles buy illegal guns is through high-volume gun sales, he says.

"In most states it's perfectly legal for a licensed dealer to sell 15 to 20 handguns to a single purchaser," he says. "Then the purchaser sells those guns in the black market." He noted the "spectacular success" of Virginia's new one-gun-a-month law, which has already resulted in a 61 percent decline in guns traced back to Virginia from crimes committed in New York City. Besides Virginia, Maryland and South Carolina are the only other states that limit gun sales to 12 a year.

But John Velleco, a spokesman for the Gun Owners of America, says, "It's not access to guns that is the driving force behind juvenile violence." Because the Ten Commandments have been "ordered off the walls of our schools . . . our children are growing up in an ethical never-never land, and don't know the differ-

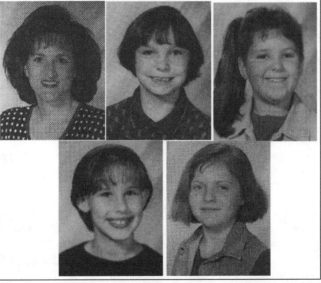

The four students and a teacher slain March 24 at a school in Jonesboro, Ark., are (top, from left) Shannon Wright, 32; Brittany Varner, 11; Paige Ann Herring, 12; (bottom, from left) Natalie Brooks, 12, and Stephanie Johnson, 12.

Reuters

ence between right and wrong," he says.

If more gun laws would solve the problem, then juvenile gun-related crimes should have plummeted after the 1968 passage of the Gun Control Act, which made it illegal for juveniles to possess guns, he says. "If the gun control theory had any merit, we should have had more shootings by juveniles before 1968 and then it should have declined. But that didn't happen."

Alan Gottlieb, chairman of the 650,000-member Citizens Committee for the Right to Keep and Bear Arms, argues that "the knee-jerk reaction to impose more gun controls in the wake of these incidents fails to address the underlying problem. Gun control is a Band-Aid approach to a potentially serious hemorrhage." [16] Instead of gun control, the Congress should boost intervention and psychological counseling for anyone caught carrying a gun to school, he said.

Chief NRA lobbyist Tanya Metaksa says that additional laws are not needed because under the Gun-Free Schools Act of 1994 it is already illegal for anyone to bring a firearm to school. Pointing out that the Jonesboro shooters tried to blow-torch their way into a gun safe, she says, "No amount of laws are going to stop a juvenile or adult from illegally procuring a gun or knife or anything else."

Laws making gun owners responsible for crimes committed by a juvenile who breaks into their homes and steals their gun are akin to prosecuting a legitimate automobile owner whose car is stolen and used by criminals in a crime, she says.

The NRA opposes "one-size-fits-all" federal gun storage laws. "We think responsible gun storage comes from each gun owner looking at their environment and making an educated, informed decision," Metaksa says. That decision would be different for an elderly woman living in a high-crime area and a household where there are young children, she says.

Regarding mandatory purchase and use of trigger locks, Metaksa says, "The recent shootings in schools have troubled and saddened us all, but it is unsound and ultimately unsafe to prescribe a single federal gun storage standard." She also stated, "When fatal firearms accidents are at an all-time low and violent crime is on the decline, it is senseless to propose in-

Society's Glorification of Violence . . .

Even after the verdicts were handed down last summer in the Jonesboro, Ark., school shootings, many of the survivors were still asking, "Why?" For many observers, the trial of 11-year-old Andrew Golden and 13-year-old Mitchell Johnson did not answer the question perhaps most often asked since the five deadly shooting sprees at American schools last year: Why would teenagers murder classmates in such a pre-meditated, seemingly remorseless, random fashion?

"These are cold-blooded, evil children," said Lloyd Brooks, the uncle of slain Jonesboro schoolgirl Natalie Brooks. [1]

But experts say it's not quite that simple. There are plenty of theories and plenty of adult blame to go around, according to most child-behavior experts.

Many say adults who create today's envelope-pushing violent culture and then allow guns to easily fall into underage hands are to blame. "The violence in the media and the easy availability of guns are what's driving the slaughter of innocents," said Barry Krisberg, president of the National Council on Crime and Delinquency in San Francisco. [2]

"There are now four privately owned guns in the U.S. for every child," notes Kevin Dwyer, president-elect of the National Association of School Psychologists. "At the same time, kids are being trained by video games to be more impulsive, less prone to think things through."

"These [school shootings] are symptoms of a changing culture that desensitizes our children to violence," President Clinton said after the incidents last spring. [3]

"Schools are being asked to pick up the pieces" from an excessively violent society, Education Secretary Richard W. Riley said. "I visit 60-70 schools a year. The message I hear again and again is that schools are being asked to 'detox' young people from the glorification of violence and to sensitize children about the value of life itself."

Many educators, psychologists and parents complain that movies and TV give kids the message that violence is an acceptable solution to complex problems, and that violence is normal behavior. They complain that children today are being taught "acceptable behavior" from the likes of shock-rocker Marilyn Manson, talk-show host Jerry Springer and the young, male techies who create the increasingly realistic, ultra-violent video games.

"We've redefined deviancy," says Ronald D. Stephens, executive director of the National School Safety Center.

"Raise your kids better or I'll raise them for you," warned Manson, the self-described anti-Christ, who simulates sado-masochistic sex acts on stage and whose songs deal with occultism, suicide, torture and murder. [4]

But parents aren't the only ones who need to more closely monitor what kids are watching and hearing. After public outcry this past summer, the controversial school-based commercial television network Channel One apologized for playing Manson's music on its news shows, which often run during homeroom in 12,000 schools nationwide.

Some Manson fans are Goths, members of a suburban youth cult who wear black garb and like his death-rock music. In 1997 two Goths charged with committing a "thrill" murder in Washington state cited a passion for Manson's music.

Another group listed on school-sponsored Channel One's Web site is Bone Thugs-N-Harmony, whose rap lyrics explicitly refer to rapes, murder, sex and reproductive organs. Critics of Channel One say kids who learn about a musical group through TV at school probably think their music is appropriate. Jonesboro assailant Johnson was reportedly obsessed with the group's songs about gun massacres.

Some now fear that violent music lyrics may be more harmful than TV or movies. "It's not like watching a movie, which they might view once or twice," says Barbara Wyatt, president of the Parents Music Resource Center. "They listen to music over and over. It's like listening to a foreign language over and over until it becomes part of your subconscious."

Youths listen to about 10,500 hours of music during their teen years, she says. Parents complain that even if they monitor all the CDs their kids buy, they cannot control what kids hear on the radio.

Cable and broadcast TV representatives say parents are responsible for what their kids watch. "You can't put everything on the backs of broadcasters," says John Earnhardt, director of media relations for the National Association of Broadcasters. "Parents definitely have a role."

Parents should use the new TV ratings system to monitor what kids watch, he says. But the National Institute on Media and the Family says most parents find the new standards too weak. In a recent survey, the institute found that only 12 percent of parents agreed that TV-14 programs (unsuitable for those under 14) were appropriate for teenagers over 14.

"The people doing the rating seem to be out of touch with America's parents," institute President David Walsh said. [5]

Parents complain it is a full-time job filtering out all the violence inundating kids in today's music, videos, movies, advertisements and television. Many overworked parents rue the lack of quality after-school programs, causing thousands of "latchkey" kids to be left without supervision from 3-7 p.m., often with only the TV for company.

Earnhardt contends that broadcast television is not as violent as cable television. "Compared with cable, there isn't a lot of violence on broadcast television," he says.

Tell that to Topeka, Kan., teacher and mother of two Deborah Parker. She is furious that her local broadcast station has recently scheduled the fist-fighting, hair-pulling, chair-swinging "Jerry Springer Show" at 4 p.m., the time when working parents cannot supervise their adolescent kids' TV watching. She has collected 500 signatures in three weeks asking the station to schedule the show at least an hour later, when more parents are home. So far

... Gets Blame for Children's School Shootings

the broadcaster has refused, saying that to compete with cable TV's kid-friendly after-school lineup he must run the show, which is the highest-rated syndicated talk show in the country.

The aggressively tasteless program — which has dealt with such subjects as bestiality and cross-dressing and often erupts into on-stage violence between guests — is irresistible to many adolescents, who make up much of the audience. In May, a New York teacher was beaten, scratched and spat upon by 11- and 12-year-old girls when she tried to prevent them from watching the show on a classroom TV.

"Such shows contribute to the mean-spiritedness we see in so many different contexts today," says Charles P. Ewing, forensic psychologist at the State University of New York and author of *Kids Who Kill*. "There's much less civility in our society, much less empathy for people. It teaches kids that it's OK not to have respect for other human beings."

Just a few years ago "The Simpsons" was considered outrageous, he points out. "But it seems mainstream now," he says. "That's how quickly our social values are changing."

The Rev. Michael Pfleger of Chicago's St. Sabina Catholic Church worries that "when vulgar language and fistfights are portrayed as the natural response to settle disagreements, children begin to think such bizarre behavior is appropriate. This is particularly dangerous when the producers admit that young people are the primary group they seek to attract." [6]

Rev. Pfleger has picketed Springer's Chicago headquarters for months and threatened to lead a national boycott of his advertisers. Springer claims that for every advertiser who might pull its ad, "There are 20 more dying to get on — and probably willing to pay more." [7]

Politicians, psychologists and child experts are becoming increasingly worried about the long-term impact of excessively violent video games. In recent Senate hearings experts suggested that "murderous video games — more than television and movies — may do the most harm in desensitizing children to the consequences of violence," said Sen. Joseph I. Lieberman, D-Conn., who has sought a rating system for video games. [8]

"I'm not one to blame all juvenile violence on the media," psychologist Ewing says. "But I think video games are maybe the worst offenders. You win by counting the number of people you kill, and that's considered enjoyable entertainment."

Others say the fast-paced, kill-or-be-killed mentality of violent video games, which rewards those quickest on the trigger, teaches kids to be impulsive. "When a kid is watching violence on TV, he is an observer," Walsh says. "With video games he is a participant." He likens such games to the video techniques used by the military to desensitize soldiers.

A core group of video companies "keeps pushing the envelope" using cutting-edge graphics and digital technology to make the violence increasingly realistic, Walsh says. "The games are moving closer and closer to virtual reality. Unfortunately, the most violent games — like Duke Nukem, Primal Rage and Postal — are the most popular with 8- to 13-year-old boys."

Lieberman announced July 22 that he and Sen. Herb Kohl, D-Wis., had persuaded coin-operated video game-makers and amusement arcade owners to voluntarily reduce the amount of violence in new games. The companies have also devised a voluntary, industrywide rating system allowing individual owners to limit access by younger patrons to the most violent games.

"Without some kind of access policy," Lieberman said, "these ratings may amount to little more than mayhem magnets for kids." He asked cartridge and computer game makers to also "take a hard look at some of the worst stuff they are marketing to kids and to stop making violent games that violate our values and put our children at risk."

But most kids who play video games do not go around shooting classmates. "Just because they are not taking out guns and killing people doesn't mean they're not affected by these games," Ewing says. "It normalizes violence. It gives kids the idea that violence is a normal part of everyday life."

Ewing noted that even older youths exhibit an increasing level of meanness and cruelty, citing recent deaths at fraternity and military hazings. "Hazing used to be things like paddling or humiliating pledges," he says. "Now people are actually dying."

Laws lowering the age at which adolescents can be tried as adults are "a way of appearing to do something about a social problem that adults have created," he says. "It's easier to pass a bill like that or build a new prison than to finance programs that we know work," like after-school or youth development programs.

"We've got to sit down as a community and acknowledge that our society has a problem,'" says Barbara Wheeler, president of the National School Boards Association. "We need to figure out where we lost touch with civility. Maybe we need to take the train back to that fork in the road, and take the other path."

---

[1] Nadya Labi, "The Hunter And The Choirboy," *Time*, April 6, 1998.

[2] Richard Lacayo, "Toward the Root of the Evil," *Time*, April 6, 1998.

[3] "Clinton Says School Shooting Incidents Reflect 'Changing Culture,'" *The Washington Post*, May 24, 1998.

[4] Quoted in "This Man Wants to Raise Your Children," *Entertainment Monitor*, May/June 1996, p. 19.

[5] Press release, April 23, 1998, issued with the release of the survey.

[6] Steve Brennan, "Chicago priest out to collar 'Springer,'" BPI Entertainment News Wire, Aug. 26, 1998.

[7] Leslie Ryan, "Springer not worried about ads," *Electronic Media*, Sept. 21, 1998.

[8] Press conference, July 22, 1998.

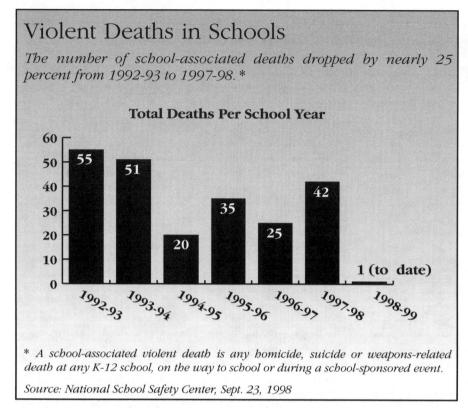

Violent Deaths in Schools

The number of school-associated deaths dropped by nearly 25 percent from 1992-93 to 1997-98. *

Total Deaths Per School Year

1992-93: 55
1993-94: 51
1994-95: 20
1995-96: 35
1996-97: 25
1997-98: 42
1998-99: 1 (to date)

* *A school-associated violent death is any homicide, suicide or weapons-related death at any K-12 school, on the way to school or during a school-sponsored event.*

Source: National School Safety Center, Sept. 23, 1998

effective laws that will only restrict the freedoms of law-abiding citizens and the fundamental right of self-defense."

One way to prevent kids from murdering at school, she says, is to "take threats more seriously. The kids involved last year gave lots of warning signs that nobody took seriously."

Should youths who commit adult crimes be tried as adults?

Shortly after the Jonesboro shootings, an elderly man sipping coffee at a Waffle House in a nearby town said, "I don't care how old they are; if they kill somebody, they ought to die. I don't care if they're 5 years old. The Bible says an eye for an eye and a tooth for a tooth. They need to change the law." [17]

He was referring to an Arkansas law under which the Jonesboro shooters, who were 11 and 13 when they were arrested, could not be tried as adults. Even though they have since been convicted, they can only be held until age 18 in a juvenile facility. The state has

vowed to build a special facility to hold them until they reach 21, when they must be released.

Yet in Pearl, Miss., Luke Woodham, 17, was tried as an adult for killing his mother the same day that he opened fire on classmates. He won't be eligible for parole until he is 65.

The two cases show how state laws differ in the way they treat violent juveniles. In recent years many states have lowered the age at which violent youths can be tried as adults, and Arkansas legislators say they'll do the same.

For much of this century, the juvenile justice system subscribed to the notion that children committing crimes should be treated rather than punished. That attitude began changing in the late 1980s as crack cocaine entered the American scene, and the nature of juvenile crime changed from truancy, vandalism and joy-riding in stolen cars to assault, rape and murder.

Juveniles under 18 accounted for 13 percent of all violent crimes "cleared" by arrest in 1996, according to the FBI,

and juvenile violent crime increased much faster than adult violent crime. Further, juvenile lawbreakers are getting younger and younger. Since 1965, the number of 12-year-olds arrested for violent crimes has doubled, and the number of 13- and 14-year-olds has tripled, according to the FBI. [18]

"Those statistics are a major reason why we need to revamp our antiquated juvenile justice system," wrote Linda J. Collier, a Pennsylvania juvenile court lawyer, who teaches on juvenile justice at Cabrini College in Radnor, Pa. "Too many states still treat violent offenders under 16 as juveniles who belong in the juvenile system."

Since 1994, the laws in 43 states have been changed to make it easier to prosecute juveniles as adults.

Proponents of the "adult-crime, adult-time" philosophy blame much of today's juvenile crime rate on an overly permissive juvenile justice system at which too many teenagers thumb their noses. The NRA says, "The young criminal's closest accomplice is a juvenile justice system that fails to mete out adult time for adult crime." [19]

School resource officer Lavarello says that when he warns kids about possible jail terms if they commit a crime, they don't believe him. "They tell me, 'That's not true, because I have a friend who did that, and he's not in jail,'" says Lavarello.

Under the current system, 40 percent of juveniles age 15 and older do not serve any time when they commit crimes, Rep. Mark Souder, R-Ind., said on Sept. 15, encouraging the House to pass a bill that would allow juveniles as young as 14 to be tried as adults for violent or drug crimes.

"There should be a price to pay if someone shoots somebody, if they rape somebody or if they use a gun in an armed robbery," he said. "We have spent too much time worrying about these juveniles without thinking about the people, who are terrorized by these young people."

Lavarello agrees. "Kids as young as 12 know the dangers of shooting a gun," he says. "They need to know that there will be consequences."

Opponents of trying youths as adults say teens do not really understand the long-range implications of their actions. Sending them to an adult prison, where they are more likely to be beaten or raped, only transforms them into even harder criminals, creating more and worse crime in the long run, they argue.

"Juveniles who come from dysfunctional families need more than being locked up," said Texas Democratic Rep. Sheila Jackson-Lee, arguing against the bill. The legislation eventually passed the House, 280-126, and is awaiting conference action.

"It's just another step towards dismantling the juvenile justice system," says Charles P. Ewing, a forensic psychologist at the State University of New York at Buffalo and author of *Kids Who Kill.* "Children don't have the cognitive capacity of adults," he continues. "That's why we limit their rights to marry, drive, drink and buy cigarettes. But yet we're saying, 'Oh, but, by the way, if you commit a crime, you're suddenly an adult.'

"It's a way of appearing to do something about a problem that adults created," he adds, namely a society that inundates youths with violence in music, movies, video games and television, and allows them easy access to guns. "It's a social problem that we've all created."

It is more politically popular to try kids as adults and build more prisons than to fund programs known to work, like after-school recreational programs, youth development programs and crime prevention and intervention programs, he says.

Criminologist Jeffrey Fagan, of the Center for Violence Research and Prevention at Columbia University's School of Public Health, agrees. "These laws are about symbolism, not about substance," he says, noting that juveniles retained in adult jails have higher recidivism rates than those kept in juvenile court.

Ironically, he points out, Congress

and the states are lowering the minimum ages just as juvenile crime is declining, after peaking in 1994. "The laws are targeting a problem that is far less of a problem than it was five years ago," Fagan says. "So the public is being sold a bill of goods."

Some states are successfully fighting juvenile crime by taking an innovative approach that combines heavy-duty early intervention for at-risk youths, while making sure juveniles are held accountable for even minor first-offenses. Then if juveniles become violent offenders despite the early interventions, they are tried as adults.

"If the attempt to rehabilitate juvenile delinquents is unsuccessful," said Harry L. Shorstein, state attorney for Florida's 4th Judicial Circuit in Jacksonville, "then it is my firm belief that we should treat habitual and violent juvenile criminals like adults." [20]

Shorstein's innovative program, however, does not just toss juveniles into adult jails, where they are more likely to be beaten and raped. Juveniles are tried as adults but are then segregated into juvenile jail facilities, where they must attend school and meet with an adult mentor. The program has resulted in a 78 percent drop in juvenile homicide, a 53 percent reduction in rapes committed by juveniles and a 58 percent drop in juvenile auto theft. [21]

"Prevention efforts cannot succeed if those not abiding by the law do not believe there is a consequence to criminal behavior," Shorstein told a Senate subcommittee hearing on Sept. 10. ■

BACKGROUND

Unruly Students

School violence is not new. Schoolchildren in 17th-century France were

often armed, and dueled, brawled, mutinied and beat teachers, according to Alexander Volokh, author of "Making Schools Safe," a study of school violence conducted for the Reason Public Policy Institute (RPPI).

"Schoolmasters were afraid for their lives, and other people wouldn't walk past schools because they were afraid of being attacked," said Volokh. [22]

Student mutinies, strikes and violence were also common in English public schools between 1775 and 1836, forcing schoolmasters to seek help from the military, he said. In 1797 when one group of British boys was ordered to pay for damages they had done to a tradesman, they blew up their headmaster's office door, set fire to his office and withdrew to an island in a nearby lake. "British constables finally took the island by force," said Volokh.

Early American schools had their share of unruly students. In Colonial times, students mutinied at more than 300 schools each year, often chasing off or locking out the teacher. In 1837, nearly 400 schools in Massachusetts were vandalized.

Yet in modern times, standards for classroom discipline and the definition of what is acceptable student behavior have changed dramatically in America. Corporal punishment doled out by ruler- and rod-wielding pioneer teachers is much less common today, having been replaced by judicial due process, concern for students' rights and efforts to build self-esteem.*

The classroom began changing in the early 1900s with the advent of the "progressive" education movement, which eschewed authoritarian methods of discipline and encouraged teachers to recognize students as individuals. Progressive education, although criticized as too permissive,

---

*Corporal punishment is still allowed in 23 states, but it has been outlawed in more than half of the individual school districts in those states.

was first embraced by experimental private schools and eventually gained wide acceptance during the first 50 years of this century. [23]

Students' Rights

In the 1960s, the anti-war, anti-establishment rebellion of college students spilled over into the high schools, leading students to question authority and the status quo. Then in 1967, the Supreme Court held in *Gault v. Arizona* that juveniles in court must be given the same rights and protections as adults. [24] The decision made schools and law enforcement officials more reluctant to send kids away to training schools, especially for offenses like truancy or misbehavior, which would not be crimes if committed by an adult.

In 1975, two precedent-setting developments made it extremely difficult for teachers to kick violent or disruptive students out of class. The first was a landmark ruling in *Goss v. Lopez*, in which the Supreme Court said students could not be suspended without due process of law.

"Many central-city schools have tended to abandon expulsion as the ultimate enforcer of discipline," wrote Jackson Toby, director of Rutgers University's Institute for Criminological Research. [25]

Secondly, Congress passed the Education for All Handicapped Children Act, which mandated that all children be educated in the "least restrictive environment" possible. That law required that handicapped students be "mainstreamed" into regular classrooms, along with emotionally disturbed students with severe behavioral and disciplinary problems.

"Youngsters who in the past would not have gone to regular school because of their negative behavior are now attending mainstream schools," writes Connecticut school counselor Carl Bosch, in his book *Schools Under Seige, Guns, Gangs and Hidden Dangers.* [26]

At the same time, school officials became skittish about sending kids to alternative schools, designed for students with severe discipline problems and those expelled for carrying weapons. The schools were criticized as "dumping grounds" for minorities.

"Schools in most big cities have given up and keep kids in school who are sufficiently troublesome that it's very difficult to maintain an educational program," wrote Toby.

Over time, lack of discipline in the classroom translates into violence in the hallways, according to several studies. "In most schools it's not the sensational acts of violence, but the smaller acts of aggression, threats, scuffles, constant back talk that take a terrible toll on the atmosphere of learning, on the morale of teachers on the attitudes of students," said Clinton, in a July 20 speech before the American Federation of Teachers.

Guns and Gangs

In 1990 Congress created "gun-free school zones," making it a felony to bring guns within 1,000 feet of any school. Then in 1994, Congress passed the Gun-Free Schools Act, requiring mandatory one-year expulsion for any student caught with a firearm at school.

Nonetheless, of the nearly 1 million kids who carried a gun to school last year, almost half of them attended school armed on six or more occasions, according to PRIDE. More than half those who carried guns to school said they had threatened to harm a teacher, and two-thirds said they had threatened to harm another student. Of the students who carried a gun to school, 59 percent were white, 18 percent were black and 12 percent were Hispanic. [27]

"These chilling numbers suggest that for every classroom of 30 students, in every school in America, on average one student has attended school with a gun in grades six through 12," said Thomas J. Gleaton, one of the authors of the nationwide survey of 154,350 students. [28]

Experts say that most students who carry guns to school do so for protection.

The presence of gangs in schools contributes to the violence. In 1989 only 15.3 percent of students nationwide reported gangs in their schools, compared with 28.4 percent in 1995. Thirty-one percent of the public school students questioned had gangs in their schools, compared with 7 percent in private schools. [29]

Gangs were most prevalent in urban schools, where 40.7 percent of students in 1995 reported gangs in their schools, compared with 24.8 percent in 1989. In suburban schools the percent of students reporting gangs almost doubled, from 14 percent to 26.3 percent, during the same period. The largest growth in gangs occurred in rural schools, where the percent of students reporting gangs jumped from 7.8 percent to 19.9 percent.

Criminologists warn that statistics on gangs should be viewed skeptically. "What we used to call peer groups are now called gangs," said Jack Levin, director of the Program for the Study of Violence at Northeastern University in Boston. [30]

Declining Violence

JPI's Schiraldi says that even though the schoolhouse shootings last year occurred in rural schools, country towns and their schools are still relatively safe places. Three rural towns where school shootings occurred last year — West Paducah, Pearl and

Chronology

1800s *Concept of juvenile justice emerges, with "training" schools and separate courts established to keep youths out of adult jails.*

1847
The first publicly funded schools for delinquents are founded in Massachusetts.

1899
Illinois establishes the first statewide court for children.

———— • ————

1900s *Progressive education movement challenges emphasis on strict discipline in public schools.*

1918
National Education Association issues an influential report promoting the command of fundamental processes and the worthwhile use of leisure as educational goals and repudiating academic mastery as a goal for secondary education. The report has a pervasive influence on American public schools through the 1950s.

1919
Progressive Education Association is established.

———— • ————

1940s-1950s *Educators still embrace progressive education, but a rise in juvenile delinquency after World War II spurs public support school discipline.*

1955
Progressive Education Association disbands.

1957
The Soviet Union's launch of Sputnik I ignites a public uproar over concern that the United States lost the space race because of lagging educational standards.

———— • ————

1960s-1970s *Vietnam War protests trickle down to high schools. Courts begin extending human-rights and due-process protections to students. Schools hire security forces as vandalism, burglary and assault increase.*

1967
In *Gault v. Arizona*, the Supreme Court rules that children in juvenile court must be accorded the same procedural protections as adults on trial.

1975
In *Goss v. Lopez*, the Supreme Court rules that students cannot be suspended without due process. The Education for All Handicapped Children Act mandates that all children be educated in the "least restrictive environment" possible.

1978
National Institute of Education publishes "Violent Schools — Safe Schools," showing that school violence is national in scope.

———— • ————

1980s *Juvenile crime becomes more violent as crack cocaine hits the streets*

and homicide among young, black males reaches epidemic proportions.

1988
On Sept. 26, a 19-year-old gunman opens fire on a Greenwood, S.C., schoolyard, killing two and wounding nine.

1989
On Jan. 17, a man with an AK-47 assault rifle fires on a Stockton, Calif., school playground. Six die and 30 are wounded.

———— • ————

1990s *Violent juvenile crime rises to a peak in 1995 and then decreases.*

1990
Congress creates "gun-free school zones," making it a felony to bring guns within 1,000 feet of any school.

1992-93
Fifty-five violent deaths occur on school property and at school functions.

1994
Congress passes the Gun-Free Schools Act, requiring one-year expulsion for any student caught with a firearm at school.

1997-98
Students commit mass murder five times within eight months by firing on classmates in school settings, all in rural towns. Thirteen are killed and 47 wounded.

1998
On July 22 the Senate kills an amendment making it a felony if gun owners do not keep their guns locked away from children.

Jonesboro — had no juvenile homicide arrests in the year before these highly publicized cases, "strongly suggesting that they are idiosyncratic events rather than evidence of a trend," said a JPI press release. In Jonesboro, for example, the number of juveniles arrested for violent offenses dropped 39 percent between 1993 and 1996.

Noting that some states have reacted to the shootings by lowering the age at which juveniles who commit violent crimes can be tried as adults, Schiraldi said, "We continue to let the tail of a few isolated cases wag the dog of the juvenile justice system. Despite these tragic cases, the fact remains that citizens in rural communities are still very safe from violent juvenile crime."

However, FBI statistics show that violent juvenile crime has increased in the nation's rural communities, even as juvenile crime nationwide is declining. For instance, rural juveniles were arrested for murder and manslaughter 14.9 percent more often in 1996 than in 1990, while juvenile homicide/manslaughter arrests declined 14.8 percent in the cities and a dramatic 26 percent in the suburbs during that same time period.

But only 100 murders were committed by juveniles in rural areas in 1996, compared with 1,868 in the cities, notes JPI researcher Jason Ziedenberg. "There is definitely a juvenile crime problem in this country," he says, "but it is not concentrated in rural areas. It is still most predominant in the cities."

Schools all over the country must cope with the same negative influences that society as a whole grapples with, writes Bosch. "Schools cannot shut their doors and expect a safe 'castle' where outside influences don't enter," he continues. "Violence in schools . . . is brought into classrooms because it exists in society, in the home and in entertainment." [31]

Ironically, even as these bizarre school shootings were shocking the nation the overall juvenile murder rate was dropping. Federal Bureau of Investigation

(FBI) 1996 statistics show that youth violence peaked in 1994 and has declined since then. Between 1994 and 1996, the number of juveniles arrested for murder declined 30 percent, and juvenile arrests for all violent crimes dropped 12 percent.

Schiraldi attributes the drop to diminished access to handguns — such as one-gun-a-month laws enacted in three states — and improving economic conditions for teenagers. For example, between 1995 and 1997, as juvenile homicide rates were falling the unemployment rate for adolescents dropped 10 percent, he points out.

Contrary to the impression that murderers are getting younger and younger, FBI statistics show that in 1965 — 33 years ago — 25 children under the age of 13 were arrested for homicide compared with only 16 in 1996. Further, 93 percent of America's counties had either one or no juvenile homicides in 1995, up from 92 percent in 1994. [32]

Noting those encouraging statistics, JPI's Schiraldi said that while incidents like the Jonesboro shootings are "so tragic as to defy description," parents should remember that "cases like this are still very much the aberration, and not the norm." ∎

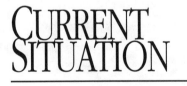

CURRENT SITUATION

Clinton's Initiatives

Citing the Education/Justice Department report on school violence last April, Clinton called the increase in violence and gangs in schools unacceptable and urged Congress to approve anti-violence initiatives he proposed in his January budget. Those initiatives focus on "what we know works: tough, targeted deterrence and

better anti-gang prevention," he said in a written statement

Among other things, Clinton has promoted greater use of school uniforms and curfews, cracking down on truancy and zero-tolerance for guns in schools. In addition, the Department of Education has issued its "early warning" handbook for identifying violence-prone students.

In a meeting with school security officers in June, Education Secretary Riley asked what single change would help end school violence. The officers unanimously said that reducing overcrowding would help the most.

In its budget proposal for fiscal 1999, the administration asked Congress to provide $12.4 billion over seven years to help school districts hire and train 100,000 new teachers, in order to reduce class size in grades one through three to an average of 18 students. Neither the House nor the Senate agreed to the request, but it was expected to be offered as an amendment before the bill is finalized.

The administration's 1999 budget also asked Congress to:

• Provide $50 million for 1,300 drug and violence prevention coordinators for 6,500 middle schools with drug and violence problems. Both the House and the Senate rejected the request.

• Dramatically increase federal funding for after-school programs, from the current $80 million level to $200 million a year. Last year the administration received 2,000 requests for after-school funds, but could only fund 300. The pending House version of the Education appropriations bill would provide only $60 million, while the Senate would provide $75 million.

• Provide $5 billion in tax credits over five years to help school districts pay for modernizing crumbling school buildings. This tax legislation is still pending, but the Senate has included $100 million in school construction funds in its Education bill.

• Boost computer-literacy among students by providing $550 million for software and teacher training initia-

Safe Schools Hotline to the Rescue

The father of a teenage girl in Ohio was worried when his daughter told him recently that she and her friends were being followed and harassed at school by a 10th-grade boy. Since August the boy had been threatening to kill her and burn down her house.

Fed up, the father finally called the Safe Schools Hotline, a privately run 800 number for reporting threats and crimes in schools. The next day the information was anonymously forwarded to his daughter's school, where authorities intervened.

The hot line is the brainchild of Pat Sullivan, president of Security Voice Inc. of Columbus, Ohio. He's offered the same service to corporate clients for years, helping them uncover embezzlement, sexual harassment or inventory theft, among other things. Four years ago he decided it might help rid schools of drugs. But since last year's school shootings more and more districts are signing up to forestall school violence as well.

"It's just taken off like crazy," Sullivan says. "We're getting a significant increase in the number of reports about guns in backpacks."

"The best defense is the kids themselves," says Paul Kitchen, assistant superintendent of Sikeston Public Schools in Missouri. "In every shooting incident last year, kids knew what was going to happen before it happened. If they had had a really good way of contacting somebody anonymously, things might have turned out differently."

His school district recently joined 800 other school systems in nine states that have signed up for the hot line service. "It's a fantastic concept. I've never seen a better program for the money," Kitchen says. "You can't get enough police officers and metal detectors to solve this problem."

The beauty of the service, which costs $1.80 per student per year, is that callers talk to a machine located in Columbus, he says. The information is then transcribed verbatim and faxed to local school authorities. If the threat is imminent, transcribers call local school officials at home — even in the middle of the night.

Students feel "very, very comfortable talking to a computer" because they feel no one will recognize their voice and they won't be identified as a snitch, Kitchen says.

Administrators also prefer Sullivan's system over traditional hot lines because it enables them to ask the tipster questions. Each caller is given a four-digit case number and is asked to call back within three days in case officials need more details.

"We can communicate back and forth to infinity to get more information if we need it," Kitchen says. The call-back feature also allows the tipster to learn the outcome of the investigation, so they know their tip was taken seriously, Sullivan says.

"It's better than metal detectors and all that junk," Kitchen says. "I don't believe any of that stuff works." Someone intent on bringing a weapon to school can sidestep metal detectors, the screening takes too long and they are too expensive, he points out.

But the hotline is "very, very inexpensive," says Kitchen, whose annual bill for the 24-hour, 365-day-per-year service comes to $3,500. "I'll write a check for $3,500 to avoid one stabbing. It's sensible, functional and practical. We could hire 50 additional security people and not get the same results."

Besides, it's good public relations, he adds. "We've had lots of unsolicited letters from parents and churches praising us for joining the program."

Richard Ross, superintendent of the Reynoldsburg, Ohio, city schools, which piloted the program, says it also teaches kids to be good citizens. "It allows students to be responsible for the safety of themselves, their friends and their school," Ross says. "It's a way to break down that don't-squeal-on-your-buddy barrier. I think that's real important."

It also empowers students and parents who may have felt victimized by bullying and threats. Half of the calls are from parents, and even some grandparents, Sullivan says.

Besides nipping violence in the bud, the service has helped schools get rid of drug-dealing. "This is snitch-proof," Kitchen says. "Pushers don't know which wallflower girl over in the corner is going to go home and call the hot line. Or a dealer's best friend could tell on him if he thinks his buddy is heading down the wrong path."

---

tives. The Senate agreed to full funding for the initiatives in its Education appropriations bill, but the House bill would fund it at lower levels.

• Provide $100 million to help support charter schools, which are public schools given "charters" allowing them flexibility in decision-making in exchange for accountability of results. The charter school movement has grown from a single school in 1992 to 1,130 today. The Senate bill contains $80 million for charter schools.

• Provide $260 million for the America Reads literacy program, which would train 30,000 reading specialists to mobilize a million volunteer reading tutors over the next five years. The program was not funded by either the Senate or the House.

"Our prisons are full of high school dropouts who cannot read. That is one reason why funding the America Reads Challenge is so important," Secretary Riley said. "Yet Congress continues to dilly-dally and dawdle." [33]

Aid for Worst Districts

The president also asked that $125 million of the annual $531 million in Safe and Drug-Free Schools block grants be specifically targeted at the 100 school districts with the worst drug and crime problems. Currently the program — which is the nation's premier program for reducing school violence — distributes block grant money to school districts based on a per capita formula rather than an as-needed basis, spreading the money across all the nation's 15,000 school districts. As a result, six out of 10 school districts receive $10,000 a year or less. One district received only $53, according to the *Los Angeles Times.* [34]

"The funds are so spread out that some school districts really don't get enough money to make a difference, and that's a problem," Riley told the Times. [35] The administration felt that the program would be more effective if at least some of the money were specifically earmarked for school districts with the most serious violence and drug problems.

The program has been criticized recently because there is little oversight over how the money is spent. In addition, the Times investigation found that the money has been spent on things such as motivational speakers, tickets to Disneyland, fishing trips, resort weekends for educators and a $6,500 remote-controlled toy car. A total of $5.7 billion has been spent on the program since its inception in 1987.

"We are wasting money on programs that have been demonstrated not to work," said Delbert S. Elliott, director of the University of Colorado Center for the Study and Prevention of Violence. [36] Nevertheless, the House refused to earmark a portion of the funds for high-crime districts, preferring to continue spreading the money over all school districts on a per-student basis. But it urged the administration to develop "specific measurable standards" to show exactly how a proposed program would reduce either drug abuse or violence before receiving funding. Secretary Riley announced such guidelines in July.

The Senate bill would set aside $150 million for a new program to combat school violence through communitywide prevention programs, such as providing alternative schools for students expelled for disciplinary problems or for bringing a gun to school, mental health counseling and other services.

Clinton also asked Congress for $95 million for juvenile crime prevention programs among "at risk" populations. The money would be earmarked for communitywide programs made up of educators, police, mental health professionals and community organizations working together to prevent juvenile crime. It could be used for mentoring, after-school programs, tutoring, teaching conflict-resolution skills and reducing truancy.

The Senate version of the Justice Department appropriations bill included funds for the prevention program, but the House version did not. Instead the House created a block grant program that would coincide with programs outlined in the House's just-passed Juvenile Justice Prevention Act.

In response to last year's shootings the Senate bill also earmarked $210 million from other programs for a new Safe Schools Initiative. The funds could be used to increase community policing in and around schools, beef up crime prevention programs, weapons detection, surveillance equipment and information systems for identifying potentially violent youths. The bill is awaiting conference action.

Testing Strategies

After a comprehensive study of school violence-prevention strategies, the Reason Public Policy Institute (RPPI) found that there is no "one-size-fits-all silver bullet" approach to school violence prevention. [37]

"What works in Queens, [N.Y.] is often going to be a waste of resources in Okla-

homa," said Richard Seder, RPPI director of education. "Policy-makers should recognize the diversity of our schools, and rather than saddle school boards with restrictions and mandates, promote community-oriented innovation." [38]

Authors Alexander Volokh and Lisa Snell found that "The ideal violence prevention policy will likely be different for each school." Thus each school should experiment with different approaches to find out what works best in their circumstances, the authors said. [39]

Beefing up security with metal detectors, security guards or surveillance cameras has worked at some schools, the authors noted. But such strategies are expensive and can be ineffective if only random checks are made with a metal detector "wand," or if surveillance cameras are not constantly monitored.

Other schools have reduced violence by requiring school uniforms. Uniforms decrease the likelihood of fights over clothing jealousy, students carrying concealed weapons, and the wearing of gang colors. It also fosters school pride and improves the learning atmosphere.

Long Beach, Calif., for instance, saw crime decrease 36 percent the year after a dress code was adopted; fights dropped 51 percent, sex offenses 74 percent, and weapons offenses 50 percent. Many other schools have reported similar results. [40]

"However, most dress codes have been at the elementary level, which isn't exactly where the violence is," the report said.

Violence is lowest in schools with effective discipline systems that mete out punishment swiftly and consistently, the researchers found. For instance, Catholic schools have been able to avoid much of the violence that exists in public schools, even among those parochial schools that cater to the difficult-to-educate, the report said. That's because public schools are "hamstrung by procedural burdens, such as hearing and notice requirements" before disciplinary action can be taken, mandated after the civil rights revolution of the 1960s.

At Issue:

Would tighter gun control reduce school violence?

REP. CAROLYN MCCARTHY, D-N.Y.

WRITTEN FOR THE CQ RESEARCHER, SEPTEMBER 1998.

*t*he school shootings we experienced last year are examples of a disturbing trend — more and more of America's children are getting their hands on guns and shooting other children. In fact, every single day, we lose 12 of our children to gun violence, either from homicides, suicides or accidental shootings. Think about that: As a country, every two days we lose a classroom of our kids to gun violence. That's a national tragedy. And it doesn't have to happen. The common strand in all gun-related deaths involving children is the child's access to a firearm. We need comprehensive federal legislation that will keep guns out of the hands of children who are unsupervised.

Last June, I, along with a coalition of Republicans and Democrats, introduced the Children's Gun Violence Protection Act, legislation designed to prevent children from gaining access to guns by increasing our commitment to responsibility, education and safety.

Responsibility: The guns children use to shoot other children all start out in the hands of adults. The Children's Gun Violence Prevention Act of 1998 shuts down the sources of guns for kids by placing increased responsibility on parents and gun dealers. Parents whose children gain access to improperly stored guns in the home will risk facing criminal penalties. Gun dealers will also have to take greater responsibility for keeping weapons out of the hands of children or risk losing their federal firearms licenses.

Education: The best way to keep our schools safe is to utilize the hands-on experience of teachers, parents and law enforcement. The legislation provides funding for grants to assist successful anti-gun violence programs designed by schools that work with local law enforcement, parent-teacher organizations and community-based organizations.

Safety: When it comes to children, the safest gun is one that a kid cannot use. This bill will require gun manufacturers to produce guns with improved safety features, such as increased trigger-resistance standards, child safety locks, manual safeties and magazine-disconnect safeties.

The bill also expands the Youth Crime Gun Interdiction Initiative. This local/state/federal gun-tracing program has already helped identify and eliminate illegal sources of guns used in juvenile crime in 27 communities. Finally, the bill establishes a youth firearms injury surveillance program at the Centers for Disease Control and Prevention. The program will provide law enforcement with strategic information on the type of weapons used to shoot children and the relationship of the victim and perpetrator.

The time has come for Congress to take responsibility for stopping gun violence involving our children.

TANYA K. METAKSA

Executive director, NRA Institute for Legislative Action; chair, NRA Political Victory Fund

WRITTEN FOR THE CQ RESEARCHER, SEPTEMBER 1998.

*i*n May 1998, three men strolled up to Candace McLallen's front door and kicked it down. *The Corpus Christi Caller-Times* reported that Mrs. McLallen immediately "grabbed her husband's .38-caliber revolver in one hand and her 1-year-old daughter in the other [then] opened fire." Called "kick burglars" for the way they enter occupied homes, the three scattered, police said, because Mrs. McLallen defended herself and her infant: "They were so scared, they left their car behind."

Criminals invade occupied American homes 500,000 times annually. That's why choices about safety and security for the American family are best made by parents, not politicians eager to prescribe a one-size-fits-all gun storage mandate. The nation's declining fatal gun accident rate — now at an all-time low — and our declining violent crime rate prove American parents make wise choices.

There's a growing consensus in America on common-sense approaches to combating youth violence. A simple call to treat threats in schools as seriously as threats at airports would make a difference. The Clinton administration's "Guide to Safe Schools" suggests no new gun restrictions. According to the Department of Education report "Violence and Discipline Problems in U.S. Public Schools," school violence is more than 23 times more likely to be unrelated to guns.

This summer on a strong bipartisan vote, the U.S. Senate rejected new gun restrictions by a 2-1 margin, opting instead for common-sense approaches like federal grants to police for gun-safety education. Tens of thousands of NRA-certified instructors are ready to help law enforcement implement that sound policy.

When people say there ought to be a gun law, chances are there already is one. "[N]early everything juveniles do with their guns is already against the law," observed sociologists Joseph Sheley and James Wright in research on youth violence commissioned by the National Institute of Justice in the early days of the Clinton administration. "The problem, it seems, is not that the appropriate laws do not exist."

The problem, say the researchers, is moral bankruptcy. The August 1998 Battleground Research poll finds "moral and religious issues" now tied with "drugs and crime" as America's top concern. Truth be told, crime and moral bankruptcy are the same disorder. Both respond to the same treatment: a bold infusion of strong, principled leadership in the family, the community and the nation.

Communities Can Avoid Chaos . . .

Without warning, newscasters break into radio and TV shows to report that a student has gone on a shooting rampage at your daughter's middle school. You try to phone the school, but the lines are jammed.

In a panic, you race to the school, but all the roads are blocked by other parents with the same idea. Even the four-lane highway nearest the school has become a parking lot, as panicked parents abandon their cars and sprint the rest of the way.

At the school, chaos reigns. Emergency crews tend the wounded; teachers scream for everyone to calm down, while frantic parents search for their children. Television reporters swarm all over the campus interviewing dazed youngsters, as police try to rope off the crime scene. Eventually, you find your child and take her home.

Some of the schools where shootings occurred last year actually experienced such scenes, says school safety expert William Reisman, but with advance planning communities can avoid such chaos. "Unfortunately, a lot of mistakes

occurred after the shootings last year," he says. "Fortunately, we learned from their mistakes."

Reisman convened a one-day conference last June in Memphis, Tenn., to review what happened with school and emergency personnel from the towns involved. He has written a handbook for schools and emergency personnel to use in tailoring crisis-management plans. [1]

"You can't have a one-size-fits-all plan because each school is different," he says.

Drawing on the experiences of those involved in the shootings last year, he outlines what to do and not do in similar school crises. The book lays out a one-day, two-step process through which a town can put a crisis-management plan in place within 24 hours. Reisman speaks at statewide meetings of school superintendents and principals around the country, many of whom are adopting his recommendations, including:

• Parents should not call the school or go to the hospital in an emergency. Because phone lines will be jammed

---

On the other hand, private schools can require certain behavioral norms and establish certain disciplinary procedures through contract as a condition of attendance. For that reason, the authors recommend charter schools and educational choice for parents. [41]

Other schools are teaching violence-prevention through conflict resolution or peer-group mediation. The Washington-based nonprofit research institute Drug Strategies "graded" dozens of such school violence-prevention programs, and only 10 out of 84 got A's. The researchers questioned violence-prevention strategies that use scare tactics, segregate aggressive students into a separate group or focus exclusively on boosting self-esteem.

Programs that work best are those that reinforce the idea that aggression and violence are not normal behavior, teach conflict-resolution skills through role-playing and involve parents, peers, media and community organizations.

"Preventing violence requires changing norms," said the report. "This is not impossible. In the past few decades, there have been dramatic changes in social

norms concerning smoking, drinking and driving, and wearing seat belts." [42]

Adding School Counselors

Many school districts are also increasing the number of school counselors, psychologists and social workers, says NSSC's Stephens. In a 1997 study on student health the National Institute of Medicine recommended that there should be one school counselor — considered the first line of defense in identifying troubled youths — for every 250 students, one social worker per 800 students and a psychologist for each 1,000 students.

However, nationwide, the actual ratios are generally well below those recommended levels, and vary widely from district to district, says Kevin Dwyer, president-elect of the National Association of School Psychologists.

For instance, Connecticut schools have one psychologist for every 750 students, while Missouri only has one per 22,000, Dwyer says. Nationwide, the average is one for each 2,200 students, well below the recommended 1/1,000 ratio. Likewise, he says, the national average for counselors is one for every 500-750

youths, instead of the recommended 1-to-250 ratio.

Since some of the shooters last year had come back onto school grounds after being expelled for weapons offenses, some schools have begun requiring detention and psychological evaluations for anyone caught with a gun at school. Others are trying to ensure that kids caught with guns at school are not simply expelled, but are referred to alternative schools.

"I urge schools to do everything possible to make sure that expelled students are sent to alternative schools," said Secretary Riley. "A student who gets expelled for bringing a gun to school should not be allowed to just hang out on the street." ∎

OUTLOOK

More Violence?

"There will be more killings," predicts Reisman, the Iowa-based

... With Crisis-Management Plan

and police will cordon off the entire school area, parents should instead go to a pre-designated location, such as a church or movie theater, where emergency personnel will keep them informed.

• All school first-aid kits should be equipped with hospital wristbands and indelible ink pens to tag wounded or dead students at the scene. A teacher with a school yearbook should be dispatched to each hospital to help identify those who were not identified at the scene.

• Principals and vice principals should have separate offices, located at opposite ends of the school building in the event hostages are taken.

• Two sets of keys and schematic drawings of the school should be stored in two separate offices, along with orange vests to be worn by those in charge of the keys and drawings.

"When the SWAT team arrives, the first person they want to see is usually the janitor, because he is the one with all the keys and knows the layout of the school," Reisman says. School and police personnel need to decide

in advance who is responsible for the plans and keys, and those two people should wear the orange vests so police can quickly identify them.

• If necessary, students should be evacuated in small groups to separate areas outside, preferably behind solid objects, so as not to make an easy target for snipers.

• The press should be given a set of rules drawn up in advance. For instance, the school grounds are an official crime scene and therefore are off-limits. Press conferences will be held twice a day at 10 a.m. and 3 p.m. in a designated place away from the school. No minors are to be interviewed without the parents' permission.

"The press should stop putting the pictures of the perpetrators on the front page," Reisman says. "They should show the suffering of the victims instead."

---

[1] Reisman's book, *The Memphis Conference: Suggestions for Preventing and Dealing with Student-Initiated Violence,* can be ordered by calling (515) 961-4814.

---

independent criminal consultant who specializes in youth violence. Reisman, who was called in as a consultant on several of the recent shootings, said future incidents may be different. Based on the "escalation, the changes and the adaptations" that occurred from one incident to the next last year, he thinks student killers may shift to bombings on school grounds, or may try to take hostages.

Reisman has already heard about at least three telephoned threats from students this school year. "One caller said he was going to make Paducah and Jonesboro look like kindergarten," Reisman says.

Reisman has written a handbook for law enforcement officials and school and hospital administrators outlining how to devise a communitywide crisis management plan, based on the findings of a conference he organized last June, attended by about 60 emergency and school personnel involved in last year's shootings.

Reisman is not the only one who thinks school violence may increase. Within the next decade, America is expected to experience a 15 percent

increase in its teen population as the last of the baby boom generation's kids reach puberty. That could mean an unprecedented surge in youth crime as those youths reach key at-risk ages of 14-17.

Without major increases in after-school activities and child care, say others, the situation is likely to worsen as new welfare reform legislation goes into effect. The law forces single mothers to find jobs after they have been on welfare for five years. Some say that will leave more kids home alone during the dangerous 3 p.m. to 7 p.m. hours when most teenage crime occurs.

"When the school bell rings, leaving millions of young people without responsible adult supervision or constructive activities, juvenile crime suddenly triples and prime time for juvenile crime begins," said a report to Attorney General Janet Reno by James Alan Fox, dean of the College of Criminal Justice, Northeastern University. [43]

Quality after-school programs reduce crime, says Fox, not only by providing a safe haven for youngsters, but by helping them develop

values and skills as a result of the positive role models and constructive activities such programs provide.

"Until the nation makes investments in after-school and other programs for children and youth, we are likely to continue to pay a heavy price in crime and violence," said the report.

Dwyer agrees that more money needs to be put into after-school programs, as well as more school counselors, remedial support and conflict resolution programs. With almost full employment in America, "Our society uses all the adults to run the economy, but we're not taking care of the kids," says Dwyer.

Others say it is time to make gratuitous violence politically incorrect, just as smoking, drinking and driving, and not wearing seat belts have become.

"We seem to have a love affair with violence and it will take a sea change in our culture to move away from this thinking," Secretary Riley said shortly after the Springfield shooting. "As long as this society continues to glorify violence, continues to make it easy for young people to get guns — and as long as we continue to hide our heads in the sand or fail to reach out when a young person is truly troubled — we will have to confront tragedies like Springfield and Jonesboro." ∎

Notes

[1] "11-year-old expelled when squirt gun falls out of bag," The Associated Press, Sept. 22, 1998.

[2] Quoted on NBC's "Today" show, Sept. 23, 1998.

[3] The Department of Education has been preparing the "First Annual Report on School Safety," to be released at the White House conference.

[4] Elizabeth Donohue, Vincent Schiraldi and Jason Ziedenberg, "School House Hype: School shootings and the real risks kids face in America," Justice Policy Institute, July 29, 1998.

[5] Quoted in a press release accompanying the "Report on State Implementation of the Gun-Free Schools Act — School Year 1996-1997," U.S. Department of Education, 1998.

[6] "Students' Reports of School Crime: 1989 and 1995," National Center for Education Statistics and the Bureau of Justice Statistics, March 1998.

[7] The report, "Violence and Discipline Problems in U.S. Public Schools: 1996-97," was conducted by the National Center for Education Statistics, a division of the Department of Education.

[8] Quoted in a July 29 JPI press release.

[9] Scott Bowles, "Armed, alienated and adolescent," USA Today, March 31, 1998.

[10] Ibid.

[11] States with CAP laws are California, Connecticut, Delaware, Florida, Hawaii, Iowa, Nevada, New Jersey, North Carolina, Maryland, Massachusetts, Minnesota, Rhode Island, Texas, Virginia and Wisconsin

[12] Peter Cummings, et. al., "State Gun-Safe Storage Laws and Child Mortality Due to Firearms," Journal of the American Medical Association, Oct. 1, 1997.

[13] Charlotte Faltermayer, "What is Justice for a Sixth-Grade Killer?" Time, April 6, 1998.

[14] National Center for Health Statistics.

[15] James A. Fox, 1996: Trends in Juvenile Violence: A Report to the United States Attorney General on Current and Future Rates of Juvenile Offending, U.S. Department of Justice.

[16] Quoted in a June 17 press release.

[17] Faltermayer, op. cit.

[18] Linda J. Collier, "Adult Crime, Adult Time," The Washington Post, March 29, 1998.

[19] From an NRA fact sheet on proposed CAP laws.

[20] Testimony before the Senate Judiciary Subcommittee on Youth Violence, Sept. 10, 1997.

[21] "An Evaluation of Juvenile Justice Innovations in Duval County, Fla.," was conducted by Florida State University economist David W. Rasmussen and released Aug. 21, 1996.

[22] Speech to Santa Barbara educators March 4, 1998.

[23] For background, see Sarah Glazer, "Violence in Schools," The CQ Researcher, Sept. 11, 1992, pp. 796-819.

[24] In Gault v. Arizona, the Supreme Court ruled that a youth in juvenile court is entitled to due process and representation by a lawyer. The case involved a 15-year-old who was sentenced to nearly six years in reform school for allegedly making an obscene phone call to a female neighbor, an offense for which an adult would have been sentenced to 30 days in jail.

[25] Jackson Toby, "Crime in the Schools," in James Q. Wilson, ed., Crime and Public Policy (1983), p. 79.

[26] Carl Bosch, Schools Under Seige, Guns, Gangs and Hidden Dangers (1997).

[27] According to the 1997-98 USA-PRIDE Summary Report, released June 18, 1998.

[28] Quoted in a press statement released with the report.

[29] "Report on State Implementation of the Gun-Free Schools Act — School Year 1996-1997," op. cit.

[30] Shannon Tangonan, "Surveys find increases in gangs, youth violence," USA Today, April 13, 1998.

[31] Bosch, op. cit., p. 6.

[32] "Crime in the United States," Federal Bureau of Investigation, 1996.

[33] In a June 9 speech to school safety officials gathered in Washington.

[34] Ralph Frammolino, "Failing Grade for Safe Schools Plan, Los Angeles Times, Sept. 8, 1998.

[35] Quoted in Frammolino, ibid.

[36] Frammolino, ibid.

[37] Alexander Volokh and Lisa Snell, "School Violence Prevention: Strategies to Keep Schools Safe," Oct. 20, 1997.

[38] Quoted in a press statement released with the report.

[39] Volokh, ibid.

[40] Volokh, ibid.

[41] For background, see Charles S. Clark, "Attack on Public Schools," The CQ Researcher, July 26, 1996, pp. 656-679 and Kenneth Jost, "Private Management of Public Schools," The CQ Researcher, March 25, 1994, pp. 282-305.

[42] "Safe Schools, Safe Students, A Guide to Violence Prevention Strategies," Drug Strategies, 1998.

[43] James Alan Fox and Sanford A. Newman, "After-School Crime or After-School Programs."

FOR MORE INFORMATION

National Institute on Media and the Family, 606 24th Ave. South, Suite 606, Minneapolis, Minn. 55454; (612) 672-5437; www.mediaandthefamily.org. The institute is a nonprofit, national resource center for research, information and education about the impact of the media on children and families. The institute's Web site rates music, television programs, movies and video games for sexual and violent content.

National School Boards Association, 1680 Duke St., Alexandria, Va. 22314; (703) 838-6722; www.nsba.org. This federation of state school board associations monitors legislation and regulations affecting the funding and quality of public education.

Office of Juvenile Justice and Delinquency Prevention, Justice Department, 810 Seventh St., N.W., Washington, D.C. 20531; (202) 307-5911; www.ojjdp.ncjrs.org. The office administers most federal programs related to prevention and treatment of juvenile delinquency and research and evaluation of the juvenile justice system.

Justice Policy Institute, 1234 Massachusetts Ave., N.W., Suite C1009, Washington, D.C. 20020; (202) 737-7270; www.cjcj.org. This policy research group, a project of the nonprofit Center on Juvenile and Criminal Justice, seeks to reduce society's reliance on incarceration as a solution to social problems.

National School Safety Center, 141 Dusenberg Drive, Suite 11, Westlake Village, Calif. 91362; (805) 373-9977; www.nssc1.org. Affiliated with Pepperdine University, the NSSC is a nonprofit training organization created by presidential directive in 1984 to promote safe schools and to help ensure quality education for all America's children.

Bibliography

Selected Sources Used

Books

Bosch, Carl, *Schools Under Seige, Guns, Gangs and Hidden Dangers*, Enslow Publishers, 1997.

Bosch, who has worked in public schools for 23 years, points out that violence is no longer just an urban school problem and looks at the reasons violence has increased in recent years. Schools are not immune from what is happening in the broader context of society, where a violent culture has desensitized youths, he says.

Articles

Bowles, Scott, "Armed, alienated and adolescent," *USA Today*, March 31, 1998.

Bowles examines the similarities among the boys who rampaged in schools last spring. One major similarity was the fact that they all hinted or warned others that they were considering violent action. Schools must teach students to take seriously any such threats, and adults must intervene immediately.

Collier, Linda J., "Adult Crime, Adult Time," *The Washington Post*, March 29, 1998.

The Pennsylvania juvenile court lawyer and professor says that outdated juvenile justice laws have not kept up with the increasingly violent nature of juvenile crime. Instead of truancy and petty thievery, juveniles are now raping and murdering. Too many states prohibit trying juveniles under 16 as adults, she argues.

Faltermayer, Charlotte, "What is Justice for a Sixth-Grade Killer?" *Time*, April 6, 1998.

In the immediate aftermath of the Jonesboro shooting, the author surveys how many states now allow juveniles to be tried as adults and how many states have enacted Child Access Prevention laws, which require adults to store their guns so they are inaccessible to children.

Frammolino, Ralph, "Failing Grade for Safe Schools Plan," *Los Angeles Times*, Sept. 8, 1998.

Frammolino shines the spotlight on the federal Safe and Drug-Free Schools block-grant program, the government's premier vehicle for fighting school crime. He gives the program a failing grade because of the way it is administered — the money is allotted on a per-capita rather than an as-needed basis, and has not been governed by strict performance guidelines. As a result, the program has been used, among other things, to pay for fishing trips, resort weekends for school personnel, a $6,500 remote-controlled toy police car and a clown act promoting bicycle safety.

Reports

Donohue, Elizabeth, Vincent Schiraldi and Jason Ziedenberg, "School House Hype: School shootings and the real risks kids face in America," Justice Policy Institute, July 29, 1998.

The authors argue that schools are the safest places for youngsters, safer even than their own homes. Rather than overreacting to the over-blown press reports about the recent schoolyard shootings, they argue, the government should fund after-school programs and pass laws to keep guns out of underage hands.

Report on State Implementation of the Gun-Free Schools Act — School Year 1996-1997, U.S. Department of Education, 1998.

This annual Department of Education report issued under the Gun-Free Schools Act reveals that some 6,100 students were expelled for bringing a gun to school in 1996-97.

Safe Schools, Safe Students, A Guide to Violence Prevention Strategies, Drug Strategies, 1998.

The Washington-based nonprofit research institute graded dozens of such school violence-prevention programs, and only 10 out of 84 received A's. Programs that work best are those that reinforce the idea that aggression and violence are not normal behavior, teach conflict-resolution skills through role-playing and involve parents, peers, media and community organizations.

Students' Reports of School Crime: 1989 and 1995, National Center for Education Statistics and the Bureau of Justice Statistics, March 1998.

This study, based on interviews with 10,000 students, by the Education and Justice departments finds that the number of students physically attacked or robbed at school increased 23.5 percent between 1989 and 1995. The increase occurred even as overall school crime rates remained steady, at about 14 percent, during the six-year period. Gang presence in schools nearly doubled during the same period.

Violence and Discipline Problems in U.S. Public Schools: 1996-97, National Center for Education Statistics, Department of Education.

This study surveyed more than 1,200 public school principals in a nationally representative sampling and found that 90 percent of public schools had no "serious, violent crime," but those that did reported 4,170 rapes, 7,150 robberies and 10,950 physical attacks or fights with weapons. By far, most school crime was less violent in nature, including 190,000 physical attacks or fights without a weapon, 116,000 thefts or larcenies and 98,000 cases of vandalism. Violence occurs most often in schools with classroom discipline problems and in large schools in central cities.

3 Student Journalism

SUSAN PHILIPS

At 14, Dan Vagasky didn't have much experience as a journalist. But as the editor of his middle school paper in Otsego, Mich., he had no doubt that the arrest of a student shoplifter during a school trip last year should be reported, as long as the student's name wasn't used. So did the *Bulldog Express'* faculty adviser.

When school administrators heard about the story, however, they killed it. And soon afterward, they shut down the paper.

"I view any piece of information that comes out of our schools as our opportunity to put our best foot forward," said Otsego School Superintendent James Leyndyke. "We would not pay to show what we do poorly." [1]

But in the view of the Newseum, a museum devoted to journalism, in Roslyn, Va., Vagasky's effort, as he put it, to "just tell the truth," warranted a Courage in Student Journalism Award, accompanied by a $5,000 college scholarship. "It made me feel [the experience] was a little worthwhile," he says.

The *Bulldog Express* is not the only paper to be affected by a 1988 Supreme Court decision giving school officials wide latitude to censor public school student publications:

• In Texas, a high school principal last year refused to let the student paper report students' plans to hold an "alternative prom," sparked by the school's warning that it would give Breathalyzer tests to those attending the official prom. [2]

• In Alaska, administrators at Chugiak High School removed newspapers from students' mailboxes last year when teachers objected to a column criticizing cheerleading as an

From *The CQ Researcher,*
June 5, 1998.

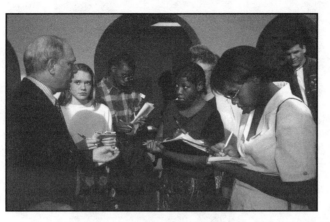

official sport. [3]

• In Chicago, a student was suspended in 1993 for writing an editorial criticizing a rule against students wearing shorts. [4]

"Educators do not offend the First Amendment by exercising editorial control over the style and content of student speech in school-sponsored expressive activities so long as their actions are reasonably related to legitimate pedagogical concerns," Justice Byron White wrote for the majority in *Hazelwood School District v. Kuhlmeier.*

Now college journalists are also facing new limitations on their First Amendment rights. Earlier this year, a Kentucky District judge cited the *Hazelwood* decision in upholding the right of Kentucky State University officials to confiscate student yearbooks deemed to be of too poor quality. The decision by Judge Joseph M. Hood marks the first time *Hazelwood* has been applied to a college publication.

"If this decision stands, I think we are opening a huge can of worms," says Mark Goodman, executive director of the Student Press Law Center in Arlington, Va. "The lesson the world has learned is that if you give those in power the authority to censor, they will use it."

Most efforts to silence the college media, however, come from students, not administrators. While college populations

have become more racially and ethnically diverse, the campus media, like their real-world counterparts, have not reflected those changes. "On so many campuses, student newspaper staffs have continued to be almost entirely Caucasian," Goodman says. "That alone perpetuates the impression that sometimes they don't understand the perspective of minority students." [5]

Protests against objectionable editorial content have become almost commonplace on college campuses in recent years, particularly the theft and destruction of offending newspapers. Last year, papers were stolen from at least seven issues of the University of California at Berkeley paper. And school papers have fueled critics' bonfires at the University of Texas in Austin, the University of North Carolina, the University of Kentucky and Cornell University.

One of the thefts at Berkeley, for example, was prompted by a column supporting legislation to end affirmative action in university admissions. And a parody of "ebonics," or black syntax, sparked one of the many attacks on the conservative *Cornell Review.*

Censorship is not the only problem student journalism faces in the post-*Hazelwood* era. There are deep divisions at the high school and college level over how journalism should be taught. And the near total disappearance of meaningful journalism instruction in many inner-city high schools suggests that for administrators under pressure to cut spending and increase test scores, student newspapers are often considered expendable.

"In some places, high school journalism isn't just dying, it's dead. In inner-city and poor, rural areas, it doesn't exist, and where it does exist it is a joke," says former reporter and journalism Professor Mary Arnold-

Interest in Journalism Decreased

Twice as many journalism students decided not to become journalists in the past 10 years as decided to join the profession, according to university instructors surveyed in 1995.

Did the number of would-be journalists increase or decrease?

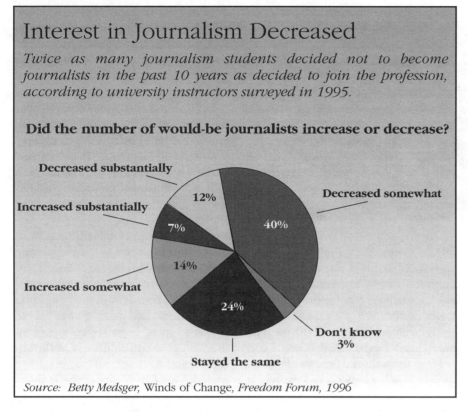

Decreased substantially 12%

Increased substantially 7%

Increased somewhat 14%

Stayed the same 24%

Decreased somewhat 40%

Don't know 3%

Source: Betty Medsger, Winds of Change, *Freedom Forum, 1996*

Hemlinger, who now develops minority journalism programs for the Newspaper Association of America. In Washington, only one high school in the entire city has published more than one issue of its newspaper this year. *(See story, p. 54.)*

At the other end of the spectrum are schools like Carmel High School in Indiana. Students turn out the *Carmel HiLite* — a hard-hitting, full-color tabloid — every week, along with a sophisticated online version. The paper's adviser, Tony Willis, has a degree in journalism and experience as a reporter, rare in a field where fewer than one-third of high school journalism teachers and advisers are certified to teach the subject.

For college students interested in journalism, there are hundreds of programs to choose from, and almost as many ideas about what should be taught, and how. For decades, college-level journalism education has been undergoing a profound and controversial transformation. Many journalism programs no longer stress a broad, liberal arts education backed up with core skills courses such as reporting and news writing. Instead, many programs focus on mass-communications theory, examining how mass media work in society. Such programs prepare students not only for traditional journalism but also for careers in advertising, marketing and public relations, as well as academia.

The rapid emergence of new communications technologies has pushed journalism education in an unexpected direction. New alliances between journalism/mass communications programs and engineering/computer-science departments reflect the powerful interest in preparing students for work in cyberspace. Columbia University's School of Journalism, for example, has linked up with Columbia's engineering department to develop technologies for its new-media courses.

"High-technology is where the students see the exciting jobs," says Bill Dickinson, resident professional at the University of Kansas' William Allen White School of Journalism and Mass Communication. "The kids feel the future is on the Web." [6]

Some journalists and educators worry that the new interest in technology will deflect attention away from teaching traditional journalism techniques. Others believe the new technologies will force journalism schools to return to the basics, as journalists become conduits for ever-increasing floods of information.

"The pendulum has begun to swing back, to recognize that at the heart of all the new communication industries is journalism: how to gather, organize and prepare information," says Robert H. Giles, executive director of the Freedom Forum's Media Studies Center.

Not surprisingly, many working journalists deride much journalism education as inadequate and irrelevant. "Many of the people we get are lacking the basics," said Linda Green, city editor at *The Californian,* in Salinas. "They don't know a lead from a nut graph." [7]

As journalists and journalism educators face the challenges of the new millennium, these are some of the questions they are asking:

Are students and administrators becoming less tolerant of free speech in the student press?

In a 1997 survey of attitudes toward the First Amendment, 54 percent of Americans disagreed with the following statement: "High school students should be allowed to report controversial issues in their student newspaper without approval of school authorities." [8]

School administrators in Frederick, Md., relied on the *Hazelwood* decision when they established a review board for the newspaper at Governor Thomas

Johnson High School. The board reviews articles and advertisements that "may be offensive to the school community," and was established after Principal Joseph Heidel barred distribution of the 1997 year-end edition of the newspaper because he feared a headline might be libelous.

Before *Hazelwood*, students' First Amendment rights were protected in the Supreme Court's *Tinker v. Des Moines Independent Community School District* decision, which overturned the suspensions of several students for wearing black armbands to protest the Vietnam War. The 1969 ruling was subsequently interpreted to give broad free-speech rights to student journalists. As a result, journalism advisers used it to encourage students to cover more controversial areas of concern to young people.

"I think when I was working on my high school paper, the most controversial story I wrote was about whether Madras plaid will bleed when you wash it," Arnold-Hemlinger quips. High school newspapers now tackle edgy topics such as racial prejudice, AIDS, drug abuse, teen pregnancy, body piercing and youth violence.

Student journalists and their advisers say that censorship today often seems more a matter of whim than policy, with lines drawn in unpredictable places. Journalism adviser Cindy Dixon says she had her principal's full support when students

at Alabama's Greensboro East High School asked for permission to survey other students for a story on safe-sex practices. But when the School Board learned of a planned story criticizing the cafeteria's food, "They axed it," Dixon says. "We are getting to be very quiet, hoping they won't get wind of things ahead of time."

To stay out of trouble, advisers advise: "Don't criticize coaches or cafete-

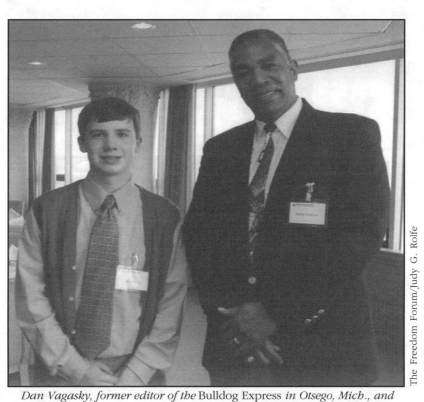

Dan Vagasky, former editor of the Bulldog Express *in Otsego, Mich., and Phillip F. Gainous, principal of Montgomery Blair High School, Silver Spring, Md., received Courage in Student Journalism Awards in April from the Newseum for their efforts on behalf of student-press freedom.*

ria food, and don't try to be funny."

"Humor is hard to do," says Rebecca Sipos, the journalism adviser at McLean High School in Northern Virginia. "We don't all find the same things funny, and these students are just finding their voices as writers."

Humor presents pitfalls for college journalists as well, as they negotiate the tricky political terrain of campuses where students often align

themselves with groups based on race, ethnicity, gender, religion and sexual orientation. Students at The George Washington University in Washington, D.C., have asked the student association to stop funding *Protest THIS!*, a newspaper of student humor that has "satirized domestic violence and rape and lampooned such events as the schoolyard shootings in Jonesboro, Ark." [9]

The paper sparked a protest rally attended by about 80 students when it ran mock advertisements for "Masta-Card" ("Helping Whitey Keep Us Down") and the "Asian Student Alliance," including five photos of the same young Asian man, each with a different name. ("We all look the same," said the caption.)

"I don't think the university should fund it," says James Allen Jr., head of the university's Black People's Union, "and if they keep publishing what they're publishing, I don't think it should exist."

Humorous or serious, campus coverage of race provokes intense reactions. In the mid-1990s, Eric Stern, then-editor of the *Daily Northwestern* at Northwestern University, Evanston, Ill., described the tense relations between the campus paper and minority students. Matters came to a head in October 1996, when a black student organization attempted to bar the newspaper from covering an appearance by black advocate Sister Souljah. The group had been angered by the *Daily's* coverage of her appear-

Majority of Teachers Favor Press Restrictions

Among public high school teachers, more than twice as many teachers of non-journalism courses as teachers of journalism favored the Supreme Court's 1988 Hazelwood *ruling increasing principals' authority to censor student publications. The general public was much more likely than journalism teachers to agree with the decision.*

Was *Hazlewood v. Kuhlmeier* a good or bad ruling?

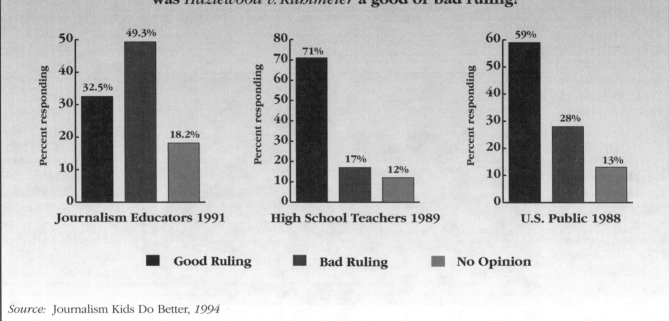

Source: Journalism Kids Do Better, *1994*

ance on campus three years earlier, when her anti-Semitic comments sparked several negative editorials. A reporter who managed to get into the event was denounced to the crowd as "another example of white supremacism." [10]

"Taking newspapers hostage is intended as a statement to the campus media that coverage needs to reach beyond white perspectives," Stern wrote. "It's also meant to raise awareness of legitimate complaints by black student groups about biased coverage and careless mistakes."

Administrators vary in their response to attacks on campus newspapers. At Cornell, university officials have argued that because the Review is distributed free, and because an entire press run was never burned, there is nothing to punish. "We support the right of news-

papers to publish and the right for people to protest what newspapers publish," said Jacqueline Powers, a Cornell spokeswoman. [11]

First Amendment advocate Nat Hentoff blasted Cornell, arguing that "so prestigious a university might have been expected to tell the revengeful students that the best antidote to bad speech is more speech — not a match." [12]

Other institutions have responded more forcefully. Last year, for example, a student suspected of burning 1,000 copies of the *Tiger Weekly*, a conservative student paper at Louisiana State University, was charged with suspicion of theft and criminal mischief.

Student governments, frequently critical of students' coverage of their activities, occasionally cut off funding for campus publications. Last October, the student government at the State

University of New York, Plattsburg, abruptly stopped payments to the local newspaper that prints the student paper in an attempt to block the distribution of a story that named a student suspected of setting fire to a campus dormitory. The local newspaper printed the edition for free.

Administrative censorship of college newspapers is relatively uncommon, however. "In general, there is very little oversight of college papers," says Kansas' Dickinson. "Universities in many cases have washed their hands of student newspapers."

And courts often have been willing to give college media considerable leeway. In February, the Virginia Supreme Court upheld the dismissal of an $850,000 defamation lawsuit filed against the *Collegiate Times* of Virginia Polytechnic University by Sharon Yeagle, a school administrator.

She had sued the newspaper in 1996 over a picture of her accompanied by a derisive, mock title. The court acknowledged that the title was "disgusting, offensive and in extremely bad taste," but said it could not be considered defamatory because no reader would believe it to be accurate. [13]

The Internet has opened up a new field for student journalism — and censorship. Hundreds of college and high school newspapers are now available online to a worldwide audience. Many observers worry that such access places school districts on shaky legal ground. "My sense is school officials are more inclined to censor online publications than traditional print publications," Goodman says. "Students are facing a lot more headaches and burdens online."

Wheeling High School in Illinois began publishing its *Spokesman On-Line* about three years ago. But administrators worry that the use of names and photos could expose students to hate mail for expressing unpopular views, or even to sexual predators who see their picture on the Internet. They are considering a proposal that would allow the full names of students to be used in reports about organized activities, such as athletic events or student competitions, because parents already know that their students are involved. But quotes from students on any other topic would require parental permission before they could be included on the Web site. And no students would be identified in photo cutlines. "I would

be devastated if a student at Wheeling was harmed by something on our site, but I do think we're being overly cautious," said newspaper adviser Susan Hathaway Tantillo. [14]

In addition to giving student journalism worldwide reach, Internet publishing quickly blurs the lines between school and non-school publications. "I think the move online may open up a whole new realm in *Hazelwood* we haven't thought through," says *Carmel HiLite* adviser Willis. "The Web site is not actually a publication of the school, so it isn't

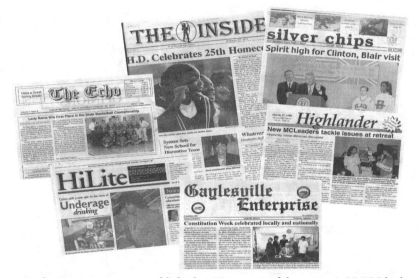

Student newspapers are published at 79 percent of the nation's 22,785 high schools, including, clockwise from lower left, Carmel (Indiana) H.S.; Suitland H.S., Forestville, Md.; H.D. Woodson H.S., Washington, D.C.; Montgomery Blair H.S., Silver Spring, Md.; McLean (Virginia) H.S.; and Gaylesville (Alabama) H.S., which serves as a community newspaper.

clear if *Hazelwood* applies."

Candace Perkins Bowen, coordinator of the Scholastic Media Program at Kent State University, advises school administrators not to worry too much over the perceived dangers of Internet publishing. "Part of the U.S. Supreme Court's 1997 ruling on the Communications Decency Act indicated that content on the Internet is legally equivalent to the printed word, and ought to be protected in a similar way," Bowen writes. "If the

student newspaper serves as an open forum for exploring problems and issues in a responsible manner, students should be entitled to reach the wider audience that's available through the Internet." [15]

Should high schools teach journalism, and if so how?

English teacher Carol Lange holds a Kit Kat bar in one hand and a chocolate Easter bunny in the other. "What are the similarities?" Lange asks. "They're both made of chocolate," a student offers. "Right, and how might we characterize that?" Lange asks. "Are we talking about style or content?"

The students are in Lange's intensive journalistic writing (IJW) course at Thomas Jefferson High School for Science and Technology in Alexandria, Va. The candy exercise serves as a mental warm-up for comparing style and content in passages from Jane Austen and Charles Dickens. Lange's students make the leap from Kit Kat to *Pride and Prejudice* effortlessly, near the end of an academic year that ranged through literature, advertising and newspaper and magazine writing.

With no newspaper to put out, there is no scramble to meet production deadlines, no worry about offending sensitive administrators. Lange uses a tightly focused, academic approach to journalistic writing to prepare her students for the advanced placement (AP) exam in English language and composition.

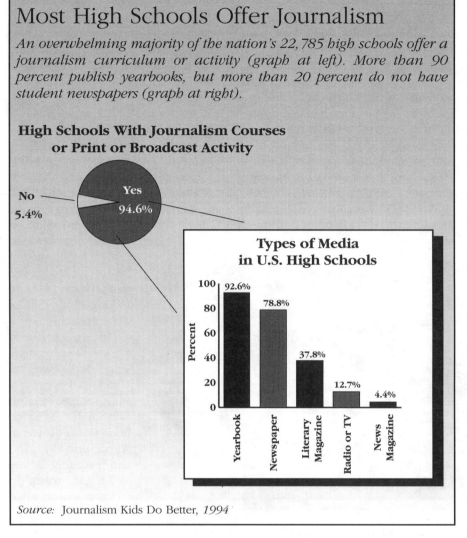

Most High Schools Offer Journalism

An overwhelming majority of the nation's 22,785 high schools offer a journalism curriculum or activity (graph at left). More than 90 percent publish yearbooks, but more than 20 percent do not have student newspapers (graph at right).

High Schools With Journalism Courses or Print or Broadcast Activity

No
5.4%

Yes
94.6%

Types of Media in U.S. High Schools

Yearbook 92.6%
Newspaper 78.8%
Literary Magazine 37.8%
Radio or TV 12.7%
News Magazine 4.4%

Source: Journalism Kids Do Better, *1994*

something that newspaper production classes often have difficulty doing.

Still, there are many who feel that newspapers are the heart of high school journalism. "Putting out a high school newspaper raises First Amendment issues in a kind of in-your-face way that teaches students a lot," says former newspaper publisher Loren Ghiglione, chairman of the fledgling journalism program at Emory University in Atlanta. "It involves teamwork, it involves assuming responsibility, often for a budget, certainly for ideas and language. It's a real-world experience."

But there is little evidence that this view is widely shared by the public, by high school teachers or by school administrators.

"I have had peers, my fellow English teachers, pass the newspaper out to their classes and say, 'Your assignment is to find 50 mistakes in here.' That is really not very supportive," says Pat Graff, a longtime newspaper adviser in New Mexico who serves as the liaison between the JEA and the National Council of Teachers of English.

While few school administrators are openly hostile to journalism classes or school newspapers, current trends in curriculum development have tended to push journalism to the edge of the high school universe. Increasing the number of required English, foreign language, science and math courses leaves little room for other courses.

Even when English credit is given for a journalism course, many colleges will not accept it. The National Collegiate Athletic Association (NCAA) has been keeping journalism advisers up nights with its refusal to recognize even highly academic journalism classes as contributing toward its requirement that college athletes complete four years of high school English. "I have a very academic program," says journalism adviser Sipos. "I think my students learn how to write better than they do in English

The approach has been growing, although slowly, since the Dow Jones Newspaper Fund first pioneered the IJW curriculum a decade ago. It is a key way that high school journalism has moved to align itself more closely with English and language arts.

"We have a lot of journalism teachers who are not certified to teach English," says Homer Hall, president of the Journalism Education Association (JEA). "That's been a problem. We don't want to offend those teachers, many of whom are doing a great job. Still, I believe it would be best if we could all agree that journalism is English." Hall believes lack of training is a major fac-

tor in the short lifespan of most journalism advisers. "The turnover is incredible, something like three years," he says. "The best programs are the ones with advisers who have had time to build a program."

By using journalism to teach writing and analytical skills, IJW serves the needs and interests of Lange's technology-oriented students at the nationally recognized magnet school. She estimates that less than 10 of her students are considering careers in journalism. By successfully preparing them for the AP exam, Lange proves conclusively, year after year, that her course meets its academic goals, classes. The NCAA doesn't agree; it seems to think that it's a blow-off course."*

Ten years ago, New Mexico began requiring high school students to take at least a year of communications skills. "We went and said to the state Board of Education, 'Journalism should count as communication skills,' " Graff recalls. "They said 'No, the students write, but they don't talk.' I said, 'Well, how do you suppose they know what to write about? They interview people.' I didn't get anywhere."

In poor urban districts, there isn't anything to debate, journalism is so far down on the wish-list. "I haven't even tried to get money from the school system," says Dorothy Gilliam, a former *Washington Post* columnist who heads the paper's effort to cultivate minority student journalists in the District of Columbia. *(See story, p. 54.)* "My understanding is this would not be a priority."

Students in Charmaine Turner's journalism class at H.D. Woodson High School in Washington, D.C., receive elective English credit, one credit per semester, with a maximum of two credits over their high school careers. "My students this year won't get credit if they want to do the paper next year," Turner says. "They'll have to work during lunch or after school. For them to get credit, we'd need to have an advanced journalism class. There is no such class in the system — there's no money."

Academic credit is certainly not the only, or even the best, motivator of high school journalists. Some simply seek the feeling described by Brian Yolles, editor-in-chief of the *Carmel HiLite*. "When the paper comes out, I stand in the hallway and watch people picking it up. I look to see what they read first, what they

---

*The NCAA says it is planning to change its procedures, and accept English credit for journalism courses if the high school gives it.

react to — that's the dream for print journalists." Others find working on the school paper a way to establish an identity among their peers. "It's how I got my name around the school; I'm always taking pictures," says Woodson student Patrick Scott. "People say, 'Hey, take my picture, take my picture.' "

Still, the wide differences in how high schools make room for journalism reflects what journalism researcher Jack Dvorak calls "the fragility" of journalism programs. "A program is going to be just as good as its teacher/adviser," says Dvorak, a former journalism teacher. "For journalism, that's usually just one person. When you have a great person, everything is great. Then something happens, and the program falls apart."

Co-author of the 1994 book *Journalism Kids Do Better,* Dvorak has researched how well-designed journalism courses can mesh with a language-arts curriculum.

In a 1994 study, Dvorak found that at-risk Native Alaskan high school students who studied journalism and produced a newspaper as part of their English instruction showed significant gains in standardized vocabulary tests and writing skills. Early this year, Dvorak published research examining how students who took IJW courses fared on the AP English Language and Composition Examination. In May 1997, fewer than 900 IJW students took the exam, compared with about 66,500 students who had taken traditional English composition courses. The journalism students had a 72.7 percent pass rate, compared with just over 65 percent for the students who took traditional composition courses.

Supporters argue that journalism is particularly well-suited to meeting the goals of high school reform, as identified in a series of reports over the past decade. "We say we want schools that teach children to be problem-solvers, to be critical thinkers, help-

ing them to gain insight into the world," Dvorak says. "All the things we give lip service to are happening in high school journalism."

High school reform "should prepare students to succeed in a fast-paced, technologically sophisticated setting," wrote Rima Shore in a Carnegie Foundation report. "At the same time, it should foster the kind of work habits, including the ability to sustain focus and to approach new challenges, that will hold students in good stead as they move through many different work settings in their lifetimes. High school should nurture in students the habit of engagement in a broader community, preparing them for active, thoughtful participation in the democratic process, and helping them to think through ethical standards for themselves and society." [16]

But many advisers say that to meet its potential, journalism must raise the standard of teaching and advising, which will require support from school administrators. "I often say to principals, 'You would never hire a football coach who had never played the game,' " says New Mexico's Graff. " 'You would never hire a chemistry teacher who had never studied chemistry. But you're always handing over the single, most high-profile products of your school, the newspaper and the yearbook to someone who doesn't know anything about it. And then you wonder why you have problems.' "

Indeed, all too often the job of school newspaper adviser is handed to a newly hired English teacher without the clout to refuse. Sometimes, the result is serendipity. Woodson's Turner has logged 11 years as the journalism adviser, keeping her program alive in one of the most demoralized school districts in the nation. "The principal wanted a newspaper, and I didn't know how to say no," is how she got into the job. Dixon of Alabama's Greenboro East had the same experience, and found herself "bitten by the journalism bug."

Spreading the Word in Rural Alabama

Not surprisingly, when the First Baptist Church welcomed a new pastor in January, the story was front-page news in the *Notasulga Times*. And in another rural Alabama community, when local students fared poorly on the SAT and ACT tests, the *South Barbour News* also carried the story on page one.

What is surprising is that both papers are staffed and run by high school students. They are among 25 community monthlies serving small towns in Alabama, all started within the last five years with help from the University of Alabama's Program for Rural Services and Research. Most turn modest profits, which are reinvested in technology to improve the papers. And most are the only newspapers offering regular coverage of their communities.

"I think Notasulga had the *Universalist Herald*, back in the 1800s," says Notasulga High School Principal Robert Anderson. "The newspaper has really brought the community together, and closed a gap between the school and some people in the town, especially older people."

"The idea from the beginning was to become a real newspaper, to publish on schedule, on newsprint," says the university's Jim Rye, one of the originators of the project. "The papers cover the Town Council, the police. And they've had an impact."

It was coverage by the *Gaylesville Enterprise*, for example, which led the Town Council to adopt street names and house numbers, so the community could have 911 emergency service. "For 14- and 15-year-olds to be able to effect positive change in their communities through the newspaper, that's really something," Rye says. "That's what newspapers are all about."

The papers are not polished, especially those established within the past year. They have their share of typos and awkward sentences.

Still, Rye contends that the newspapers "have become the best writing labs you can imagine. Student work becomes public work, and it really raises the bar for the students. Having an audience has a tremendous impact on how students perceive the importance of their work."

According to a spring 1997 survey of the participating schools, the newspaper staffs represent 7 percent of the schools' enrollment, with 341 students involved overall. The newspaper staffs are 58 percent female and 53 percent African-American. Staffers report that participation in the newspaper project improved their computer skills and made them more likely to consider going on to college.

Brandon Tubbs, a freshman journalism major at the University of Alabama, is the former editor-in-chief of *The Oakman Times*, one of the first papers produced by the project. The Times "was the one thing I learned the most from, and that includes the classes I'm taking now at the university," he says. "I'm taking stuff now, and I think, I've been there and done that."

Tubbs, whose career plans in high school originally had him heading to veterinary school, now plans to graduate from Alabama "with the best grades possible, go on out in the real world and work my way up the ranks in the profession, and be an editor and publisher of a newspaper in the South."

Like several graduates of the newspaper project, Tubbs now works at the rural services office at the University of Alabama while pursuing his journalism studies. One of his jobs is to help new high schools joining the project get their newspapers up and running.

At first, Rye says, administrators at the various high schools needed some convincing to sign on to the project. "Alabama is really looking to the standardized tests, to the Stanford 9, that's what schools are judged by," Rye says. "In that climate, when you tell a principal, 'You're going to publish a community newspaper,' they tend to say, 'No, our test scores are down, we have to hit the books.' "

But now, he says, most administrators are supportive. When the English teacher in Notasulga retired, Rye says, "The principal told me, 'I'm not hiring an English teacher, I'm hiring a newspaper teacher who also is going to teach English.' Kind of a twist on the old Alabama joke, 'I'm hiring a football coach who also teaches social studies.' "

"What it has done for writing skills in the school is beautiful," Anderson says.

Rye is hoping the Alabama project can be expanded to other areas of the rural South. "The newspapers have blurred the boundaries between the schools and their communities. They have become powerful demonstrations of the capacities of the students — they are economically viable, they are incredibly important for the town and they've had tremendous impact on the schools."

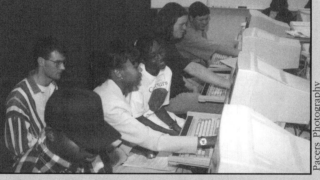

The University of Alabama's Program for Rural Services and Research brings journalism to small communities.

Pacers Photography

But for every Dixon or Turner, there are uncounted other advisers who never get "bitten." "There are some teachers who just don't want to cause trouble, and they produce boring things," Arnold-Hemlinger says. "And then there are the ones who are too hands-off, and that's dangerous, like handing the kids the keys to the car without giving them a driving lesson."

Several states, notably Indiana and Ohio, have fairly stiff requirements for journalism teachers — and turn out some of the best high school journalism in the country. But in Ohio, the certification requirements are being eliminated. The new system will allow teachers holding language-arts licenses to teach journalism, speech, theater or traditional English. Education students seeking the license will have to take a course in press law, but no other journalism courses will be required. Hall of the JEA believes broad language-arts licensure will eventually become a nationwide standard. "We need to make sure we don't get left behind," he says.

Is journalism education keeping pace with new technologies?

Five years ago, American University integrated computer skills into every level of journalism instruction. A state-of-the-art computer lab was constructed, with Internet access at every terminal. That was the easy part.

"Suddenly, the faculty had to learn computer skills, and use them. It created a real division," says Wendy Williams, an assistant journalism professor. "When I came to AU nine years ago, I was the first faculty member to come from a newspaper with a computer system. Some of the older members decided they'd rather not make that change, and they went into retirement a little earlier."

Even those who embraced new technology have struggled to keep up, Williams says. Sometimes, they must even ask their students for help. "I had to tell my students, 'I'm not very adept with Quark,' " Williams says. "Two or three of the students in the class are adept, and I pulled them aside, and said, 'For this part of the course, you are the teachers.' Most students feel empowered. But some faculty have trouble with it."

Williams sees AU's emphasis on computer skills — from how to dig in a database to designing a home page — as crucial to students, especially given the tight journalism job market. "A lot of our graduates are getting jobs because they have higher-level computer skills than people inside the news organizations," Williams says. "We give them the basic journalistic skills, but the computer skills are often what gets them in the door."

According to a 1996 survey by the Roper Center at the University of Connecticut, 75 percent of newsroom recruiters and supervisors rated computer-research skills as "somewhat" or "very important." Among journalists hired within the last 10 years, 86 percent said it was "very important" for journalism-education programs to teach students how to use computers for communication and research. Yet highlighting the conflicting attitudes toward new technologies, 56 percent of the journalists surveyed described themselves as "enthusiastic" about the technological changes in the industry, while 54 percent described themselves as feeling "threatened" by them. [17]

Journalism educators at the college level share the combination of enthusiasm and fear. "We're in a trap," says Professor Maurine Beasley of the University of Maryland, College Park. "We want to teach students to think critically, to gather information, to analyze it, to write well. But employers say they want people who know software, who can design a Web page, who can use databases. Most journalism programs are not set up to do that."

The number of online daily newspapers has tripled in the past year, to about 175. Just two years ago, researchers Gerald M. Kosicki of Ohio State University and Lee Becker of the University of Georgia found that among 1996 graduates of journalism and mass-communications programs, 20 students, or just under 1 percent, took jobs in online publishing. Kosicki and Becker note that the number, while small, represents a fourfold increase over the five graduates who reported taking such jobs in 1995. [18] By now, given the explosion of Web-related journalism products, high-tech jobs are probably grabbing a much bigger share of freshly minted J-school grads.

"The kids feel the future is on the Web, that news isn't going to be written the same way," says Dickinson of the University of Kansas. "The inverted pyramid, objectivity — these things are all being discredited by cyberspace geeks."

But many educators worry that poor and minority students may find themselves handicapped at the college level by lack of computer experience. According to a recent report in *Science* magazine, 73 percent of white students in the United States have home computers, compared with 32 percent of black students. The study also found that white students without a home computer are more likely than black students to go elsewhere to access the Internet. [19]

Barbara Hines, a journalism professor at predominantly black Howard University, says that many entering students, including those from the inner city, have considerable computer skills. "We're seeing kids who have had access in high school, middle school even elementary school," Howard says. "Some people are saying that particularly in the inner-city communities, young people don't have the access to new technology. But we are also seeing all kinds of programs to address that."

"I think a lot of people in journalism education are worried about technology, but I see it as an opportunity," says John Pavlik, director of the Center for New Media at Columbia. "Journalism education has an opportunity to take a leadership role. After all, the Web got its start in academia. We led the way, but a lot of us were asleep at the wheel when it came to seeing how it might be used by everybody else."

Pavlik argues that students, unhampered by the one-medium-at-a-time mentality that divides journalism into print, radio and broadcast, are the perfect guides to take the industry into the era of "convergence," when technology allows reporters to tell stories using text, graphics, still photos and video all at once, while providing links to related stories and information, giving consumers the freedom to explore just the aspects of a story that interest them.

"We don't need to be hamstrung by the constraints of the old technologies," Pavlik says. "We can go back to the basics of good storytelling." ■

BACKGROUND

Educating Journalists

Three men are generally considered the "fathers" of journalism education: Willard G. Bleyer, who launched journalism education at the University of Wisconsin; Walter Williams, who established the University of Missouri School of Journalism; and Joseph Pulitzer, who endowed the School of Journalism at Columbia University in New York City. [20]

All three "looked beyond the immediate goal of educating journalists and improving newspapers. The larger goal to which they aspired was to produce a more-informed citizenry through better journalism," writes journalism educator Betty Medsger. [21]

But improving the image of journalists, then considered an unruly, poorly educated lot, was also part of the program. Pulitzer initially had wanted to start his program at Harvard University, but college officials felt it would attract too many undesirables.

The first college-level program for aspiring journalists was established in 1869 at Washington College, now Washington and Lee University, in Lexington, Va. "We look upon this action as a very important step toward raising American journalism from the slough of venality, corruption and party subserviency into which it has too notoriously fallen to the high position it should occupy," wrote John Plaxton, a member of the Nashville Typographical Union, at the time.

Bleyer was an early supporter of accreditation for journalism programs and the guiding force behind what is now the Accrediting Council on Education in Journalism and Mass Communications. To many observers, its birth in 1947 marked the rise of journalism as an academic discipline.

Mass-Communications Studies

In the 1950s, the emergence of mass-communications studies created another new turning point for journalism education. Wilbur Schramm, who headed the journalism program at the University of Iowa shortly after World War II, went on to establish institutes of communication research at the University of Illinois and Stanford University. It was Schramm who brokered what Medsger terms "an institutional marriage" between journalism and mass-communications studies, a development seen by some as terribly misguided, and by others as inevitable.

Schramm and his followers, seeking the academic respectability bestowed by a doctoral degree, pushed journalism education away from the practical aspects of the craft and toward a social-science view of mass communications. Writing in 1943, Schramm described the traditional journalism school as "a group of teachers and students, sitting on the periphery of the university, playing with their toys, putting together the picture of who, what, where and when in the first paragraph." Schramm's goal, in contrast, was to study how mass-media institutions function in society, and how they affect people.

Gradually, the requirement that doctoral students in communication studies have journalism experience, preferably in newspapers, was dropped. As a result, such experience is no longer a prerequisite for teaching in journalism programs. Some 17 percent of faculty members in journalism programs today do not have professional journalism experience.

Working journalists tend to dismiss doctorate-holding professors who have never scrambled to nail down a late-breaking story. That attitude can create skepticism on the part of hiring editors and recruiters as to how well-trained J-school graduates really are. Journalism graduates are "absolutely not" better prepared than other recent college graduates, says Sheila Rule, senior manager of reporter recruiting for *The New York Times*.

Stanley Allison, hiring editor and internship director at the *Los Angeles Times,* says of recent interns from journalism programs, "I don't know if these kids always know how to handle a quote. Some of them think if it has slang, or might embarrass a person, then you need to clean that up. Or you can just say what you think they meant, as a quote."

Despite the doubts, journalism

Chronology

1700s The student press debuts early in the new nation's history.

1777
The first student newspaper in the United States, Students' Gazette, is published on June 11 at the William Penn Charter School in Philadelphia.

1860s Journalism joins academia.

1869
The first college-level program for would-be journalists is established at Washington College, now Washington and Lee University, in Lexington, Va. The move is hailed as a step toward "raising American journalism from the slough of venality, corruption and party subserviency."

1920s Scholastic journalism gets organized.

1921
National Scholastic Press Association established in Minneapolis, Minn.

1924
The Journalism Education Association is founded to represent journalism teachers and advisers nationwide, while the Columbia Scholastic Press Association is launched in the New York metropolitan area.

1926
The Quill and Scroll Society is established by Gallup Poll founder George H. Gallup to recognize individual student achievement in scholastic journalism.

1960s-1970s The Supreme Court recognizes free-speech rights for public school students, and student journalists respond with coverage of controversial issues.

1969
The Supreme Court rules in Tinker v. Des Moines Independent Community School District that the constitutional rights of students in Des Moines, Iowa, had been violated when they were suspended for wearing black armbands to protest the Vietnam War.

1974
The Commission of Inquiry into High School Journalism finds that despite the protections of the Tinker decision, student journalists still face high levels of censorship. In the same year, the Student Press Law Center is founded to educate high school and college students about their First Amendment rights.

1978
The American Society of Newspaper Editors (ASNE) finds that only 4 percent of the journalists at daily papers are members of ethnic minorities and pledges to increase minority newsroom staffing to equal the U.S. minority population level by the year 2000.

1980s Student free-speech rights are sharply limited by the Supreme Court. High school journalism struggles to move beyond its trade-school image.

1984
The National Council of Teachers of English passes a resolution in favor of schools granting English credit for appropriately ???designed journalism classes.

Jan. 13, 1988
The Supreme Court rules in Hazelwood School District v. Kuhlmeier that school officials can censor student expression when such censorship is "reasonably related to legitimate pedagogical concerns."

1990s The impact of the Hazelwood decision begins to be debated.

Nov. 14, 1997
Kentucky District Judge Joseph M. Hood relies heavily on the Supreme Court's 1988 Hazelwood ruling in upholding Kentucky State University administrators who refused to release the school's 1994 yearbook.

February 1998
Virginia Supreme Court upholds the dismissal of an $850,000 defamation suit against Virginia Polytechnic University's Collegiate Times by a school administrator.

October 1998
The ASNE is expected to discuss adopting a new, scaled-down diversity goal of 20 percent minority representation by 2010.

The Long Road to Newsroom Diversity

Twenty years ago, the American Society of Newspaper Editors (ASNE) looked out into the nation's newsrooms and saw a sea of white faces: Only 4 percent of the journalists at daily newspapers were members of ethnic minorities — just 1,700 out of 43,000 newsroom employees.

Following that first-ever annual newsroom employment census, the ASNE in 1978 adopted what then seemed an ambitious but reachable goal: to increase minority staffing in newsrooms to a level equivalent to the U.S. minority population by the year 2000.

But as the self-imposed deadline approaches, ASNE is preparing to acknowledge that the goal is unattainable. The organization's 1998 census found that the minority newsroom work force is only 11.5 percent. While that's an improvement over 1978, it is less than half the minority population of the U.S., which is estimated at about 26 percent. About 6,300 U.S. journalists at daily newspapers are members of ethnic minorities, out of a total newsroom work force of 54,700.

Not only has progress been slower than the organization had hoped, but the nation's ethnic makeup has been changing more rapidly than the ASNE expected. In 1978, ASNE estimated that minorities would make up 15 percent of the nation's population by the year 2000, not 26 percent.

So in October, when ASNE's board members meet in Miami, they will discuss adopting a new, scaled-down diversity goal of 20 percent minority representation by 2010, with a secondary goal of achieving "parity with local communities as soon as possible."

The proposal will certainly encounter opposition. A. Stephen Monteil, president of the Maynard Institute for Journalism Education, is part of a group of ASNE members who will push for a more ambitious set of goals. "There's a widespread sense of diversity fatigue," Monteil said. "The need is for the passion or the will to be reignited." But Rick Rodriguez, managing editor of the *Sacramento Bee* and a member of ASNE's board, warned that "an unrealistic goal is a disincentive to editors and publishers."[1]

Here is the ASNE's draft statement on diversity:

"Newsroom diversity is essential to the newspaper's responsibility in a democratic society and success in the marketplace. To accurately and sensitively cover the community, newsroom staffs must reflect society as a whole. The newsroom should be a place in which all employees contribute their full potential, regardless of their race, ethnicity, color, age, gender, sexual orientation, physical disability or other defining characteristic.

"To drive the quest for diversity and inclusion in the workplace, the American Society of Newspaper Editors will:

• Commit a significant portion of the Society's energy and resources to fostering newsroom diversity.

• Advocate diversity in content as a journalistic core value.

• Encourage and assist all newspapers to have minority journalists representation, to increase representation of journalists of color to reach 20 percent industrywide by 2010, and to achieve parity with local communities as soon as possible.

Monitor year by year the employment of Asian Americans, blacks, Native Americans and Hispanics in the newsroom.

Encourage collaboration on diversity among various groups."

---

[1] Quoted in *The New York Times*, April 6, 1998

---

seems safely ensconced in academia. The number of journalism and mass-communications programs grew from 394 in 1988 to 449 in 1996, when total enrollment was almost 150,000 students, the highest number since 1991.

High School Struggles

At the high school level, however, journalism often struggles at the margins. "High school journalism started in the vocational programs," notes the NAA's Arnold-Hemlinger. "The kids learned how to set type. Then it became the typing teacher's job. Because it has always been tied to a technology, high school journalism has always had that dual mission, and that dual identity, to overcome."

When Arnold-Hemlinger first taught high school journalism, "I was all fired up," she says. "I thought I'd get the best and the brightest. I was teaching at a small high school in Minnesota, and the kids I was getting were barely literate. I asked the prin- cipal, and he told me, 'We always put the kids who flunked out of English into journalism.'"

The uneven quality of journalism programs makes it harder for even the best programs to win academic respectability. "In a nationwide survey, we found only 28 percent of teachers had state certification to teach journalism," Dvorak says. "If the situation were the same in math or science, we'd have an uproar from parents and communities." What exactly that 28 percent of certified teachers knows about journalism is also far from clear, since almost half of the states do not require journalism educators to take any journalism courses.

High school journalism teachers find different ways to meet the dual burden of teaching and producing a publication. At Carmel High School, students must take a two-semester introductory journalism class before they can work on the newspaper. That means that adviser Tony Willis is not teaching the basics of the inverted pyramid while trying to get the paper out. With 21 news staffers out of a student body of 3,000, he can be sure that his staff is interested in journalism. "The school is very academically oriented," says Willis. "There are a lot of excellent programs here across the board, a real culture of excellence. No newspaper staff wants to do less than the previous year."

But for poor inner-city schools, just getting the paper out can become overwhelming. Carol Merrill, an English teacher at West Philadelphia High School, struggled for five years to help her students put out *Quest*, a student-produced community newspaper.

Merrill still believes in the project. "For one student in particular, this was his saving grace. He learned to speak to people, to develop an idea, to write. It changed how he viewed himself." But Merrill is tired, and this year she took a break.

"When we started, most of the students were college-bound, and they were interested in the paper," Merrill says. Then the school was reorganized in small learning communities, and Merrill had to draw her staff from a population of students not necessarily inclined toward journalism. "The last three years, my students had problems with reading and writing," she says. "It was good exposure for them, but it was harder." The number of annual issues dropped from four to three, and now, with a new adviser, to one.

"It's a Catch-22," says Bowen of the struggle to strengthen journalism programs. "We need good, viable pro-

Few Minorities Attracted to Journalism

Most high school journalism students and advisers are white. Only about 12 percent of the nation's Hispanic and African-American students participate in journalism.

Percentage of:	All Students	Journalists	Advisers
White	72.6%	80.6%	90%
Hispanic	10	6.5	2.1
African-American	10	5.6	1.2
Asian-American	4.6	5.3	1.5
Native American	1.6	1	1

Note: Numbers do not total 100 percent due to rounding or no answer given.

Source: Death By Cheeseburger: High School Journalism in the 1990s and Beyond, *1994; Journalism Education Association, 1992*

grams, so we can convince state departments of education that it's important. Then we have to convince the universities to train the teachers, so we can have good viable programs."

Supreme Court Action

The idea that the free-speech protections embodied by the Bill of Rights should be extended, within limits, to high school students did not become case law until 1969, when the Supreme Court ruled in *Tinker v. Des Moines Independent Community School District*. The court held that school officials could only censor student expression when "material and substantial disruption of school activities or invasion of the rights of other students" could be proven. "Neither students nor teachers shed their constitutional rights to freedom of speech or expression at the schoolhouse gate," wrote Justice Abe Fortas.

From 1969-88, Tinker factored into several lower-court decisions involving high school publications. But in 1988, a reconstituted court gave public school administrators greater censorship power in *Hazelwood School District v. Kuhlmeier*. In May 1983, Principal Robert Reynolds decided that a story about three Hazelwood East High School students who became pregnant was inappropriate, and that the girls' identities had not been adequately protected. Reynolds also felt that a story on the impact of divorce on students was unfair because it quoted a student's criticism of her father but failed to include a response from the father. To eliminate the offending articles, Reynolds excised two full pages of the newspaper, eliminating four other articles on the pages along with the censored articles.

It took the case five years to reach the Supreme Court. In its 5-3 decision, the high court cited Fortas' "schoolhouse gate" comment but modified it with reference to a 1986 case, *Bethel School District No. 403 v. Fraser*, in which the court upheld the district's right to suspend a student for making a lewd campaign speech. The court ruled in *Bethel* that "A school need not tolerate student speech that is inconsistent with its basic educational mission."

The *Hazelwood* decision empowered schools to censor any forms of expression deemed "ungrammatical, poorly written, inadequately researched, biased or prejudiced, vulgar or profane, or unsuitable for immature audiences," or any expression that advocated "conduct otherwise inconsistent with the shared values of a civilized social order."

High school advisers today, while generally professing a preference for the good, old, *Tinker* days, often report that when *Hazelwood* is applied in the context of a consistent policy rather than at an administrator's whim, it does not interfere with the development of a strong newspaper.

Meanwhile, college media are wondering if the strictures of *Hazelwood* are about to "trickle up" to campus newspapers and radio stations, which have long operated within the free-speech culture enjoyed by the mainstream press. On Nov. 14, 1997, Judge Hood upheld the university officials who had confiscated the 1994 KSU yearbook.

The yearbook editor and another student sued, claiming the administration had abridged their First Amendment right to free speech. Hood's decision quoted from *Hazelwood*: "A school must be able to set high standards for the student speech that is disseminated under its auspices, and may refuse to disseminate student speech that does not meet those standards." ∎

CURRENT SITUATION

State, Local Efforts

Five states give student journalists press freedoms modeled on the earlier *Tinker* decision: California, Massa-

chusetts, Iowa, Colorado and Kansas. California's law predates *Hazelwood*; the others were passed following the 1988 decision. A number of local school districts also have adopted policies that are more liberal than the standard set by *Hazelwood*.

However, a recent effort to pass such a law in Illinois failed late last year after last-minute lobbying by the School Management Alliance, a coalition of school boards and school administrators. The bill had passed both houses of the Illinois General Assembly, and a veto by Republican Gov. Jim Edgar had been overridden by the House. But a Senate override vote was canceled at the last minute, after polling indicated the override would fail as senators' support wavered under an avalanche of alliance faxes and phone calls.

In Kansas, no action was taken this session on a bill in the Senate to amend the state's Freedom of Student Expression law to give school officials new censorship power. "It wouldn't be *Hazelwood*, but it would be a trimming back from what they have now," says JEA President Hall, a newspaper adviser at Kirkwood High School in Missouri.

At the school-district level, strong support of student free-speech rights can collapse in the face of controversy. In Montgomery County, Md., an 18-month-old battle over a student-produced television program that included a panel discussion of same-sex marriage resulted in a new county policy that makes it easier for administrators to censor student TV productions and publications.

After *Hazelwood*, says the Student Press Law Center's Goodman, the momentum to strengthen student press rights at the state level "was very strong, but it has diminished somewhat." Still, he believes that student journalists soon may benefit from a broader political alliance working in their favor.

"This was initially perceived as a liberal-conservative issue," Goodman says. "That's ludicrous. As conservatives see their perspectives being silenced in the scholastic press, this is slowly becoming something more bipartisan."

Meanwhile in Missouri, home of the *Hazelwood* case, Hall of the JEA takes part in an annual ritual: drumming up support for a long-shot bill to give back to Missouri students the rights they lost in 1988. "I think we're making some headway," Hall says. "*The Post-Dispatch* and the *Kansas City Star* have come out editorially in favor — at least there's progress there."

Dismal Economics

The fundamental issues facing college journalism programs are clearly evident in the dismal economics facing journalism graduates. In 1995, the average starting salary for journalists was $20,154, making new journalists the lowest-paid college-educated people entering the work force. More than 20 percent of all new journalists under age 25 earned below $15,000. Perhaps most disturbing, at least for journalism educators, is the finding that holders of undergraduate journalism degrees are more likely than other new newsroom employees to earn less than $20,000 a year. [22]

"There are so many small dailies and weeklies in this country that are still paying just above the minimum wage," says Howard University's Hines. "These kids want to know where the dollars are. They hear the number $20,000, and they laugh, especially when they have classmates in advertising who are hearing the number $33,000, plus $3,000 hiring bonus, plus we'll pay you to move.'"

"For reporters, part of the pay is supposed to be the psychic reward of the byline," Gilliam says. "So there's an additional issue for minori-

At Issue:

Should would-be journalists pursue undergraduate degrees in journalism?

DEAN MILLS

Dean, University of Missouri School of Journalism

WRITTEN FOR THE CQ RESEARCHER, MAY 1998

yes

do you need a journalism education to become a journalist? No, as thousands of successful journalists have shown. Will a good journalism education help you become a good journalist? Of course, as thousands of other journalists have shown — many of whom might not have entered the field without the encouragement and support they got from dedicated journalism faculty.

Some of the sillier, but alas persistent, critics of journalism education cherish a false dichotomy. They argue that students should get a "good liberal arts education" instead of taking a journalism degree. They are wrong, whether the degree in question is a bachelor's degree or a professional master's degree.

A bachelor's degree in journalism at all accredited schools is not something chosen instead of a liberal arts degree. It is a liberal arts degree, and one of the best. Journalism students take 75 percent of their course work outside the journalism school. And that non-journalism course work is often more coherently structured and more rigorous than that required of students in other liberal arts fields. What's more, most journalism courses require students to find, analyze, organize and communicate information and ideas.

Journalism students in a rigorous program spend more time on core, liberal learning activities than students in any other major. Other journalism courses, whether about the history, law or institutions of journalism, deepen students' understanding of one of the most powerful forces in the modern world, an understanding that could benefit any citizen.

Journalism education serves the cause of democracy as well as the students it educates, attracting a wide range of students into the field. The world's democracies need skilled, thoughtful journalists from a wide spectrum of economic, ethnic and social backgrounds. Good journalism schools recruit and educate just such people.

The master's degree in journalism has also never prevented a student from getting "a good liberal arts education." The master's adds work in journalism to an educational portfolio that already includes four years of liberal arts and sciences. It is an efficient way for the degree holder to learn the skills, traditions and ethics of the craft.

Bachelor's and master's programs are also beneficial when graduates apply for jobs. Smaller news organizations — where most recent graduates get their first jobs — hire people who can do the job. Journalism graduates can, and do.

DOUG RAMSEY

Senior Vice President, Foundation for American Communications; former newspaper and broadcast journalist

WRITTEN FOR THE CQ RESEARCHER, MAY 1998

no

undergraduates should major in substantive fields that will equip them with analytical minds they can employ to help people understand issues that affect their lives. It does not take four years to obtain the craft skills of journalism.

Journalism schools respond to what they think their market demands. They see their market as editors and news directors who want a steady supply of young people trained in the processes of newspapers or broadcasting. Their true market is the consumer of news, the reader, viewer and listener who wants to understand the issues that influence his life. The training in craft and process that fills the curricula of most undergraduate schools of journalism or communications does little to prepare a student to analyze, understand and report on those issues.

Undergraduate journalism schools should be abolished or absorbed into institutions teaching bodies of academic knowledge that shape minds into critical instruments able to handle complex problems. The rigors of education in history, philosophy, science or economics shape a mind for analytical thinking. An understanding of page layout or videotape editing does not. If students learn to think, writing well for publication or air will follow with a reasonable amount of guidance.

Technology is delivering floods of information at increasing rates. A journalist must be able to examine a mass of information, absorb it, analyze it, subject it to critical examination and ask himself and his sources the right questions. He may then be able to tell with clarity what it means, making the information useful to his audience. Too often, journalists do not ask the right questions because, apart from how intelligent they may be, they do not have the intellectual tools to understand the story they are reporting.

If schools teach production and process techniques, they should keep them at a minimum. The basic principles of accuracy, fairness and balance do not require a four-year curriculum. A reasonably intelligent person can learn the nuts and bolts of journalism in about six weeks. Among the best reporters I ever hired were a lawyer, a medical doctor and a historian. None had journalism experience, but each had a keen, critical intelligence and a passion for issues and public affairs. After a few weeks of on-the-job training and a certain amount of fumbling around, each became a superb reporter.

The Washington Post Lends a Hand

Patrick Scott ponders a blackboard crammed with story and photo assignments for *The Insider*, the school newspaper at Washington's H.D. Woodson High School. "We're not shooting baseball because they're not sure they're going to have a season," Scott says. It's a familiar problem at Woodson. A few months ago, the paper ran a front-page story about the school's struggling swim team, which hopes to survive despite having no pool, no funds and no meets.

Scott and other Woodson journalism students are familiar with the problem: Last year, *The Insider* didn't publish a single issue, for similar reasons: no funds, no camera, no film, not enough computers. "We wrote stories, but they didn't get published," says Mirena Heigh, 17. But this year, the newspaper is having a fine season: With substantial financial and volunteer assistance from *The Washington Post, The Insider* is publishing five issues — four more than any other high school in the financially strapped city.

The Insider is one beneficiary of a high-profile new commitment by the Post to finding and nurturing local journalism talent among minority teenagers in the region. Nationally, newspapers offer varying levels of assistance to high school journalists. Many run regular youth pages, made up of articles written by local teens. Youth editors sometimes work closely with the writers. Some papers, like the Post, offer free or reduced-price printing to high school publications, and some welcome high school advisers into their newsrooms for training. But there is general agreement that the industry doesn't do enough. "Newspapers are starting to pay attention, but it may be too little too late," says Mary Arnold-Hemlinger, who helps the Newspaper Association of American set up scholastic journalism projects for minorities.

Dorothy Gilliam, a reporter and columnist at the Post for more than 20 years, is now working full time to direct its new Young Journalists' Development Project. At Woodson, the Post has donated photographic equipment, computers, a fax machine and other materials to *The Insider*. The newspaper also matched a $2,500 grant from the American Society of Newspaper Editors (ASNE) and the Freedom Forum to purchase printers and software. And 60 newsroom employees have volunteered to work with the students on putting out the newspaper.

"We're keeping an eye out for six to eight bright kids to put into the University of Maryland 'boot camp' this summer," Gilliam says. The two-week session for high school students is sponsored by the university and the National Association of Black Journalists. "Some will go on to college, some will go back to their high school newspaper," she says. "We're hoping it will give us a way to keep in touch with bright, local students." The long-term goal is to help a few of those students eventually make it to the Post.

Woodson was selected for the project in large part because of Charmaine Turner, Woodson's veteran journalism adviser. For Turner, the newspaper is both a way for her to find and nurture special students, and an important voice for the school community. "Every year, there's always at least one talented student who gets motivated by the paper," Turner says.

But if Gilliam and the Post are looking for future interns, Turner has more modest goals. Almost 60 percent of Woodson students tested below average in reading on the spring 1997 Stanford 9 Achievement Test, and more than 98 percent tested below basic in math. "Yes, journalism is a way to teach writing," Turner says. "But first you need advanced grammar and experience with other kinds of writing. Our kids don't get that. I have kids who can't write a sentence come to me and want to be on the paper, and I take them. Because I won't close my door on anybody."

The Insider has published stories on a student father who is raising his young daughter, a recent shooting outside the school and persistent problems with broken escalators, bathrooms and lockers. But it has also celebrated school life with front-page spreads on homecoming week, athletic victories and a 25th reunion for alumni.

The Post is printing *The Insider* and papers at two other suburban Maryland schools free this academic year. Students from all three newspapers attended a four-hour workshop at the newspaper in January.

Gilliam says the transition from columnist to director of the development project was made easier by her own strong feelings about the sorry state of high school journalism in the nation's capital. "As we were beginning to put this together, I was continuing to write my column, and doing the research for this project with my left hand — and I was getting more and more outraged. So when the time came to switch full time to this, I was ready."

The Young Journalists Development Project has other facets. The Post is providing primary financial aid for two-dozen high school journalists who have been attending Saturday workshops sponsored by the Washington Association of Black Journalists. At the college level, *The Washington Post* Semester will be offered in fall 1998 at the University of Maryland, and then in spring 1999 at Howard University. Post reporters, editors, photographers and others will team-teach a for-credit course for upper-level undergraduate and graduate students.

"Newspapers are not doing enough to bring in and retain minorities," Gilliam says. "Having a full-time director represents a substantial commitment by the Post. It's the first time they have done something like this."

ties, in that given the coverage of their communities, the reality is that in many minority communities journalism has a negative value, so that psychic payoff isn't there."

However, the Roper survey found that minorities entering journalism are faring better in some regards than whites. For example, 29 percent of the new ethnic-minority journalists, defined as those entering the profession within the past 10 years, work at large dailies, which offer the highest-paying entry-level jobs in the industry. Among new journalists at large dailies, 37 percent are ethnic minorities. And a larger percentage of new minority journalists are making more money than whites: 7 percent of whites make less than $15,000 a year, but only 1 percent of minorities earn at that level; and while 9 percent of whites make more than $50,000, 21 percent of ethnic minorities earn above that amount. [23]

Despite the generally low pay, the number of journalism programs is growing. Giles of the Media Studies Center says that the current roster of 105 accredited journalism programs has grown by 20 in the past few years. "There is a real unevenness in the quality of schools," says Giles, who is also president of the accrediting council. "In my view, some of the accredited schools don't represent a quality program. We should be able to guarantee quality."

In 1997, journalism programs awarded 32,150 undergraduate degrees and 3,600 graduate degrees. But only 20 percent of the new grads wound up at newspapers, magazines, radio or television stations; about 12 percent landed in public relations and advertising. [24]

At many J-schools, including highly regarded Medill at Northwestern, courses in marketing, public relations and advertising now draw more students than journalism. "The question is whether you will see [only] a few

traditional schools, like Columbia, Missouri and, I trust, Maryland, that stand alone from the trend toward consolidation with the communication department," Beasley says. ■

OUTLOOK

Impact of Internet

The rise of the Internet is opening the door to a creative explosion among high school and college newspapers, with the best online student papers exceeding professional standards.

Some observers are hoping that as computers with Internet links become universally available in schools one of the constant killers of publications in poor schools — the high cost of printing — will gradually be eliminated. In a 1993 survey of 19 schools where newspapers ceased production, 10 cited a lack of funds for production as a primary reason. Printing expenses often eat up about 50 percent of the annual budget for high school papers. [25]

By fall 1997, 78 percent of U.S. public schools were connected to the Internet. Among schools in low-income areas or with more than 50 percent minority enrollment, 63 percent had Internet access, according to the Department of Education. The agency projects that by 2000 fully 95 percent of all schools — including 91 percent of poor and minority schools — will be, hooked up to the Web. [26]

But according to Richard Holden of the Dow Jones Newspaper Fund, these figures are misleading. "You go to some high schools, in Newark or Camden [N.J.], and they may be wired," he says, "but it's all in a locked room open one hour a day. The students aren't getting

the same exposure as the ones who have computers at home."

Nevertheless, computers are already luring students to newspaper staffs who ordinarily wouldn't be interested. Terrance Dennis, a sophomore at Woodson, has learned to use Quark Express, a popular publishing program, as part of the newspaper project at Woodson. "That's why I like it. I like computers," says Dennis. "I don't have one at home. I have two or three years here to really get good at it." "One wonderful thing about a computer is, it doesn't see what color you are," says Howard's Hines. "Kids can go out on the Web and develop their voice." The opportunity may exist to make the newspaper a truly interdisciplinary, community-building project, bringing together the computer geeks and the campus newshounds, the shutter-bugs and the writerly recluses.

But such an optimistic vision will require a much deeper commitment from the news industry toward supporting the student press. "The industry really hasn't done enough," Hines says. "It's a relatively recent phenomenon that they are starting to do stuff for kids, particularly minorities."

If there is a bright spot for minority students, it's that talented, young, minority journalists are targeted early and have no trouble landing internships at top newspapers, Holden says. The problem comes in the second tier of newspapers, and the second tier of students. "A lot of editors are eager to have minority interns," he says. "So they hire one, and the intern winds up in some small town with no other minorities, and they might have a great experience and learn a lot, but they're not going to go back there to work. It's a difficult issue to resolve."

The newspaper fund is trying to deepen the pool of available minority talent. "Out of 117 [historically black colleges and universities], 105 offer journalism programs," Holden says. Below the top tier of schools like Howard and Grambling, "There's an issue of quality. Even if they have good students, quite honestly, they don't have the faculty. The students might have more talent than the professors. We've had an increase in applications, but the test scores are so low."

Holden says the news industry needs to do more to improve the journalism programs at historically black institutions. "A lot of people in the industry seem to think they can send someone to a campus for a week to teach a little seminar, and that's going to make a difference. That's unrealistic," Holden says. "You need at least a semester to raise the level of language skills. But no [newspaper] wants to let someone go for that long." ■

Notes

[1] Quoted in *The Kalamazoo Gazette,* Jan. 19, 1998.
[2] *Student Press Law Center Report,* fall 1997.
[3] *SPLC News Flash,* June 27, 1997.
[4] *SPLC Report, op. cit.*
[5] Quoted in Eric Stern, "Black Students vs. Campus Newspapers," *American Journalism Review,* May 1997, p. 14.
[6] For background, see "High-Tech Labor Shortage," *The CQ Researcher,* April 24, 1998, pp. 361-384, and "Jobs in the '90s," *The CQ Researcher,* Feb. 28, 1992, pp. 181-204.
[7] Quoted in Betty Medsger, *Winds of Change: Challenges Confronting Journalism Education* (1996), p. 160.
[8] Student Press Law Center Web site, "Support for a Free Press," Jan. 19, 1998.
[9] *The Washington Post,* May 17, 1998.
[10] Stern, op. cit., p. 14.
[11] Quoted in Nat Hentoff, "Students Burning Newspapers (Again)," *The Washington Post,* March 7, 1998.
[12] *Ibid.*
[13] Larry O'Dell, "Va. Court Clears Student Newspaper," The Associated Press, Feb. 28, 1998.

[14] Quoted in Candace Perkins Bowen, "What Are Your Students Publishing on the Web," *The School Administrator,* April 1998.
[15] *Ibid.*
[16] Rima Shore, "The Current State of High School Reform," A Report to the Carnegie Corporation of New York, 1996, p. 7.
[17] Medsger, *op. cit.*
[18] Lee B. Becker and Gerald M. Kosicki, "Annual Survey of Enrollment and Degrees Awarded," *Journalism and Mass Communication Educator,* autumn 1997, pp. 63-74.
[19] D.L. Hoffman and T.P. Novak, "Information Access: Bridging the Racial Divide on the Internet," *Science,* April 17, 1998.
[20] Unless otherwise noted, information in

this section is from Medsger, *op. cit.*
[21] Medsger, *ibid.,* p. 54. Medsger is a former newspaper reporter and former journalism professor at San Francisco State University.
[22] Medsger, *op. cit.,* p. 29.
[23] Medsger, *op. cit.,* pp. 111-112.
[24] James Ledbetter, "The Slow, Sad Sellout of Journalism School," *Rolling Stone,* Oct. 16, 1997, p. 78.
[25] *Death by Cheeseburger: High School Journalism in the 1990s and Beyond* (1994), p. 68.
[26] Adam Clayton Powell III, "78 percent of public schools Net-connected, new study shows," *The Freedom Forum On-Line,* March 9, 1998. For background, see "Networking the Classroom," *The CQ Researcher,* Oct. 20, 1995, pp. 921-944.

FOR MORE INFORMATION

Journalism Education Association, Kansas State University, 103 Kedzie Hall, Manhattan, Kan. 66506-1505; (785) 532-5532; www.jea.org. The 1,800-member JEA is the only independent national scholastic journalism organization for teachers and advisers.

The Freedom Forum, 1101 Wilson Blvd., Arlington, Va. 22209; (703) 284-2876; news@freedomforum.org. An international foundation dedicated to "free press, free speech and free spirit."

Columbia Scholastic Press Association, Mail code 5711, New York, N.Y. 10027-6902; (212) 854-9400; www.columbia.edu/cu/cspa. The CSPA publishes the monthly *Student Press Review* and holds an annual convention for high school journalists in New York City. It also offers critiques of student publications and gives awards.

National Scholastic Press Association/Associated Collegiate Press, 2221 Univ Ave SE Suite 121, Minneapolis, Minn. 55414; (612) 625-8335; www.studentpress.org. These two nonprofit organizations devoted to high school and college journalism provide a critique service for publications and hold national contests and workshops.

Association for Education in Journalism and Mass Communication, 234 Outlet Pointe Blvd., Columbia, S.C. 29210-5667; (803) 798-0271; www.aejmc.org. The AEJMC is the primary organization for faculty and administrators of college journalism and mass-communications programs. It publishes the *Journalism & Mass Communication Educator* and the *AEJMC News.*

Student Press Law Center, 1815 Fort Myer Dr., Ste 900, Arlington, Va 22209; (703) 807-1904; www.splc.org. The SPLC offers free educational materials and legal advice to high school and college journalists facing problems with access to information or censorship. Mark Goodman is the executive director.

Bibliography
Selected Sources Used

Books

Dvorak, Jack, Larry Lain and Tom Dickson, *Journalism Kids Do Better: What Research Tells Us about High School Journalism,* **Eric Clearinghouse on Reading, English, and Communication, 1994.**

The authors provide a comprehensive report for and about high school journalism editors, including innumerable charts and graphs.

Articles

Bowen, Candace Perkins, "What Are Your Students Publishing on the Web?" *The School Administrator,* **April 1998.**

Bowen, a former high school journalism teacher who now coordinates the Scholastic Media Program at Kent State University, reviews some of the concerns of high school administrators worried about liability and other issues connected with giving students access to the World Wide Web.

Hentoff, Nat, "Students Learning to Burn Newspapers," *The Washington Post,* **Aug. 16, 1997.**

Hentoff takes Cornell University administrators to task for failing to condemn black students who burned copies of the *Cornell Review* to protest offensive articles.

Kushner, David, "Young Editors Speak Up and Out," *The New York Times,* **Feb. 26, 1998.**

Kushner looks at the founding of *Bolt Reporter,* an online site for teenagers that features a regular section on stories that have been banned from high school papers.

Ledbetter, James, "The Slow, Sad Sellout of Journalism School," *Rolling Stone,* **Oct. 16, 1997.**

Ledbetter looks at the journalism/mass-communications model of journalism education, and doesn't find much to like. The impact of marketing and public relations courses on journalism programs, the low pay and tight job market faced by graduates and the lack of consensus on what students need to know are all reviewed here.

Parker, Rosemare, "In Otsego: Student keeps up fight for press rights; Administrators take editorial control of formerly award-winning school paper." *The Detroit News,* **Jan. 19, 1998.**

Parker looks at the chain of events surrounding the shutdown of the award-winning middle school newspaper, *The Bulldog Express,* following the editor's efforts to publish a story about a shoplifting incident.

Powell, Adam Clayton III, "78% of public schools Net-connected, new study shows," *Free! — The Freedom Forum Online,* **March 3, 1998.**

Powell reviews findings of a fall, 1997 study conducted by the U.S. Department of Education and released by the National Center for Statistics. The study found that most public schools have Internet access, with small-town schools leading the way, and urban schools trailing.

Stepp, Carl Sessions, "The New Journalist," *American Journalism Review,* **March 10, 1998.**

Stepp looks at the skills and qualities online publishers are looking for in the people they hire and suggests ways in which the new technologies may change journalism.

Reports

Dvorak, Jack, "High School Journalism Student Performance on the Advanced Placement English Language and Composition Examination," Jan. 17, 1998. A research paper presented at the midwinter meeting of the Association for Education in Journalism and Mass Communication.

Dvorak presents evidence that students in Intensive Journalism Writing courses fare better on the Advanced Placement exam in English Language and Composition than students who prepare for the test by taking a traditional AP English class.

The Freedom Forum, *Death By Cheeseburger: High School Journalism in the 1990s and Beyond,* **February 1994.**

This report, drawing on hundreds of interviews and an analysis of hundreds of high school newspapers, presents a clear picture of the the situation facing high school journalists and their teachers. The report finishes with 12 recommendations, including a call for every high school to publish a newspaper at least once a month.

Betty Medsger, *Winds of Change: Challenges Confronting Journalism Education,* **The Freedom Forum, 1996.**

Based on surveys and interviews with industry professionals, recent journalism school graduates and journalism educators, Medsger's report paints a bleak picture of journalism education as deeply divided and unsure of its mission. Medsger recommends the development of graduate programs focussed more clearly on journalism as opposed to communications; and stronger relationships between journalism education and the news industry.

Rima Shore, *The Current State of High School Reform,* **a Report to the Carnegie Foundation of New York, 1996.**

Shore summarizes current thinking on the goals of high school reform efforts, and the barriers to achieving them, such as the low percentage of high school students graduating with proficient writing skills.

4 School Choice Debate

For Rachgina Jeff and Brenda Ewart of Cleveland, Ohio, school choice is more than a matter of public policy. It's personal.

State-funded tuition vouchers enable Jeff's son Charles and Ewart's son Brandon to attend St. Adalbert's Roman Catholic elementary school.

"Charles already has two strikes against him — living in the inner city and being an African-American male," Jeff says. "I just wanted to give him a chance to get a decent education." To Jeff, that means keeping Charles out of the neighborhood public school.

"With the drugs, the gangs and the violence, it's hard for kids to learn in that environment," Ewart adds.

At St. Adalbert's, with its emphasis on core curricula, discipline and parental involvement, kids learn.

"Charles is really doing well there," Jeff says, noting that he recently scored in the 99th percentile on a standardized test.

Jeff and Ewart also are pleased that their children are receiving religious and moral instruction. "They're reinforcing the values I teach at home," Ewart says.

But St. Adalbert's is more than just a good school — it is affordable.

"The voucher is a blessing," says Jeff, a full-time student at Case Western Reserve University. "I would have to get a second job" without it, says Ewart, who works in a bank.

For school choice advocates, there are too few such success stories. Milwaukee is the only other city that offers publicly funded tuition vouchers. As pilot projects, however, the Cleveland and Milwaukee programs only offer assistance to a few thousand students. Moreover, the state laws that created the programs are being chal-

From *The CQ Researcher*,
July 18, 1997.

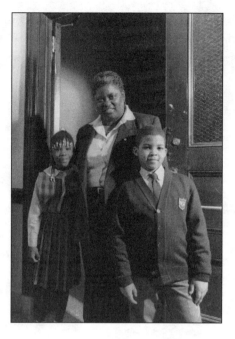

lenged and may not survive judicial scrutiny. (*See story, p. 62.*)

Still, school choice proponents say that support for vouchers has been rising and will continue to increase as more and more Americans come to believe that public schools, especially in low-income areas, are failing. As evidence, they point to a Gallup Poll showing that 36 percent of Americans favored school choice in 1996, compared with 24 percent in 1993. [1]

In addition, voucher advocates say, school choice, over the last decade, has been transformed from a fringe issue dear to some conservatives and religious groups into a major part of the national education debate. For instance, vouchers were a major plank in Republican Bob Dole's 1996 presidential campaign.

Proponents say that vouchers are getting more attention because they make sense, especially for inner-city children like Charles and Brandon.

First and foremost, they argue, vouchers empower parents by giving them the freedom to choose what they believe to be the best school for

their children. The power of choice, they say, would especially benefit the poor, who unlike Americans in higher income brackets often have no alternative but to send their children to the local public school.

"Choice is already in the hands of parents with money," says Nina Shokraii, an education policy analyst at the Heritage Foundation. "We have to extend that choice to parents without money."

Proponents also argue that vouchers will ultimately make the public schools better by injecting a healthy dose of competition into what is currently a stagnant and monopolistic system. Under the existing system, they say, public schools have no incentive to undertake real reform measures because, no matter what they do, their budgets won't shrink. But allowing parents to remove their children — as well as some of the money allotted to educate them — will force public schools to stop taking their students for granted, voucher advocates say.

Opponents of vouchers agree that as an issue, school choice is more visible than it once was. But that is where agreement ends between the two sides in the debate. And, they point out, a solid majority of Americans still oppose vouchers, a fact borne out by more than just polls. For instance, they say, every time school choice has come before voters in state referenda, it has been rejected, usually by overwhelming majorities.

As for the growing attention vouchers are getting, opponents say, it is due in part to legitimate anger over the inadequacy of public education in some areas. In particular, they say, school choice supporters are gaining ground by exploiting the frustrations of poor and minority parents, like Jeff and Ewart, who feel that neighborhood public schools are inadequate.

School Choice Debate   59

States Where School Choice Is Being Considered

School choice programs have been considered, or are being considered, by lawmakers in at least 20 states, but only two legislatures — in Wisconsin and Ohio — have actually enacted voucher programs.

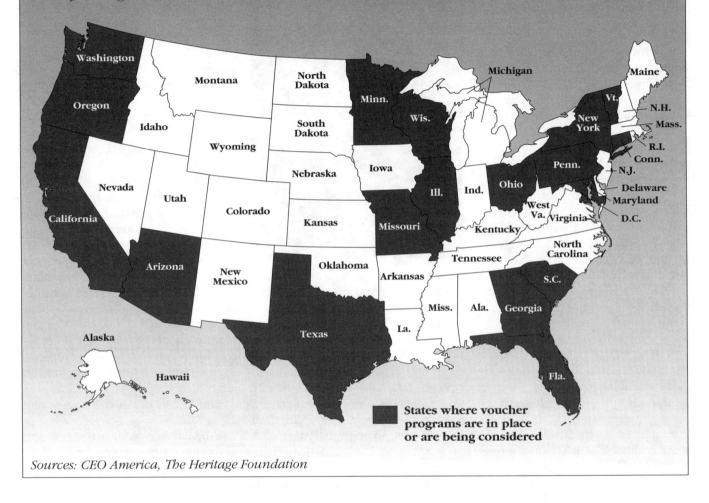

States where voucher programs are in place or are being considered

Sources: CEO America, The Heritage Foundation

"For them to say to poor people that [vouchers are] the answer is unfortunate because of course people in difficult situations are going to be more likely to listen," says Bob Chase, president of the National Education Association (NEA), the nation's largest teachers' union.

But Chase and other opponents say that school choice offers little more than a false, cruel hope to desperate parents. Vouchers, they point out, rarely amount to more than a few thousand dollars, not nearly enough to pay tuition at most top private schools.

"No one's going to go to Sidwell Friends," Chase says, referring to the expensive private school Chelsea Clinton began attending in Washington, D.C., after Bill Clinton won the presidency in 1992.

In addition, Chase and others argue, school choice actually will make public education worse, not better. For one thing, they say, instituting a voucher plan will take resources away from public school systems that in many cases are already desperately in need of additional funds. In addition,

presenting vouchers as the solution to a school district's problems will only help to delay needed reforms.

"Where there are dysfunctional [school] systems, we need to correct those systems — expeditiously," Chase says, adding that the solution isn't to divert money to private schools.

Moreover, opponents say, it would still be the public schools that ultimately would have to educate the vast majority of the nation's children, even if vouchers were initiated nationwide. It's simply a question of size, they say. The public school

School Choice Battles Embroil Many States

Voucher programs have only been instituted in a few places, but battles over school choice have touched many states. Proposals have been considered in at least 20 state legislatures over the years, and since 1990 vouchers have been the subject of referenda in California, Oregon, Colorado and Washington state.

The most recent vote occurred last November in Washington, where citizens decisively rejected a proposal to allow parents to receive tuition scholarships for non-religious private schools.

The fight over vouchers in Washington was typical of recent school choice campaigns. Both sides spent significant sums of money — about $2 million each — to get their message to the voters. The debate was contentious and at times even rancorous, with each side accusing the other of distorting the truth and representing interests other than educational improvement. By the time voters went to the polls, Initiative 173 was receiving almost as much attention in the state as the contest for president and governor. [1]

Voters in Washington rejected the initiative by a sizable majority, as they did in the other three states where referenda were held recently. For example, California's widely watched 1993 ballot initiative (Proposition 174) was defeated by a 2-1 margin. [2]

Voucher opponents say that the results in the recent referenda are further evidence of public opposition to school choice. "When voters have had the opportunity to vote on it, they've rejected it every time because they understand that it's counterproductive," says Bob Chase, president of the National Education Association, the nation's largest teachers' union.

But voucher proponents argue that the results are a testament to the power of groups like the NEA. For example, they claim, in California, opponents outspent supporters of school choice by 10-1.

And, the advocates say, the cause for vouchers has fared much better in state legislatures. Wisconsin and Ohio have voucher plans up and running. Other states, among them Iowa, have created tax credits that parents can use for educational expenses, including private school tuition.

The most recent legislative success for voucher advocates has come in Arizona, where on April 7 Republican Gov. Fife Symington signed into law a measure that allows residents to take a tax deduction of up to $500 for contributions to nonprofit foundations that provide scholarships to send children to private schools. [3]

The bill's sponsor, Republican state Rep. Mark Anderson, considers it a step toward a full voucher program. [4] Quentin L. Quade, director of the Blum Center for Parental Freedom in Education at Marquette University in Milwaukee, agrees: "This is a uniquely and distinctly important development."

Voucher proponents also are buoyed by recent events in Minnesota. On June 4, Republican Gov. Arne Carlson vetoed an education spending bill because it did not contain his proposal to give low- and middle-income families a $1,000 per child educational tax credit. Carlson has pledged to veto any new school spending bills that do not contain the tax credit provision.

School choice opponents also have had recent successes at the state level. In addition to their victory in the Washington referendum, they have beaten back a variety of tuition tax credit and voucher proposals in legislatures in Louisiana, Connecticut, Texas, New Jersey, New York and California.

In California, voters defeated a proposal that would have given vouchers to students scoring in the lowest 5 percent on state standardized tests. The plan passed the Republican-controlled Assembly only to stall in the Democratic-controlled Senate.

Both sides say that the real battle over vouchers will continue to be at the state level. "It's the states that really count," Quade says. "After all, 94 percent of all education spending comes from the states."

---

[1] Kerry A. White, "Choice Plans Face Big Statewide Test in Wash.," *Education Week*, Oct. 30, 1996.

[2] Barbara Kantrowitz, "Take the Money and Run," *Newsweek*, Oct. 11, 1993.

[3] From "Educational Freedom Report," Quentin L. Quade (ed.), April 25, 1997.

[4] *Ibid.*

---

system is almost eight times larger than its private counterpart, and vouchers would not be able to help more than a small percentage of public school students to attend private schools.

Finally, opponents say, even if vouchers are good education policy, they are barred by the Establishment Clause of the U.S. Constitution, which prohibits state support for religion. [2] They point out that courts in Wisconsin and Ohio have recognized that school choice leads to massive state subsidies for religious institutions, because the vast majority of private schools are sectarian. In Cleveland, for instance, 31 of the 48 schools participating in the voucher program are Roman Catholic. [3]

But school choice supporters argue that vouchers do not violate the Constitution because the funds go to the parents of the children, not directly to the schools. They also point out that the federal government and the states already are supporting

Key Voucher Cases in the Courts

The U.S. Supreme Court has yet to consider the constitutionality of using publicly funded vouchers to send children to private, sectarian schools. At the state level, however, several school choice cases are working their way through the courts. Any one of these cases could form the basis for a future Supreme Court ruling. Here are the main voucher cases currently before state courts:

Wisconsin — The state Supreme Court deadlocked when it first considered Wisconsin's 1995 law expanding Milwaukee's existing voucher program to include religious schools. The 3-3 decision, which was handed down on March 29, 1996, was only possible because the court's seventh justice had recused herself from the case, citing a conflict of interest. [1]

The case was remanded back to the trial court, which ruled on Jan. 15, 1997, that including religious schools in the voucher program violated the state constitution's prohibition on government support of sectarian institutions. The law expanding the program to include sectarian schools has not been implemented. [2]

The trial court decision has been appealed and is once again before the state Supreme Court. Although only six judges will rule on the case, leaving open the possibility for another tie vote, voucher supporters are heartened by the recent retirement of one of three justices who voted against their position the first time. The new justice was appointed by Republican Gov. Tommy G. Thompson, an ardent supporter of vouchers.

Ohio — Cleveland's one-year experiment with school choice was put on hold on May 1, when Ohio's 10th District Court of Appeals ruled that the program violated the federal and state constitutions, which prohibit direct government support for religion. The case has been appealed to the state Supreme Court, which has yet to decide on the issue.

Even though the law in question allows parents to use vouchers to send their children to any private school participating in the choice program, the district court was troubled by the fact that 80 percent of these schools were sectarian. "The only real choice available to most parents is between sending their children to a sectarian school and having their child remain in the troubled Cleveland city school district," wrote Judge John C. Young. Hence the voucher program essentially provided assistance to religious schools, the judge concluded. [3]

The appeals court decision followed a trial court ruling the year before that allowed the voucher law to be implemented. In this earlier decision, Judge Lisa L. Sadler wrote that the vouchers were constitutional because the benefit to religious schools flowed through the parents (who choose how to use the voucher) and hence was indirect.

Vermont — The school board of tiny Chittenden, Vt., has filed a lawsuit against the state. The conflict centers around Chittenden's intention to pay tuition for 15 high school students to attend a local Roman Catholic school. The practice, known as "tuitioning," is common in Vermont, where many rural towns have no high school. All of Chittenden's 100 high school-age children are sent to outside public and private schools. The town pays the cost of tuition.

Citing a 1961 Vermont Supreme Court ruling outlawing tuitioning at sectarian schools, the state has threatened to deny Chittenden its share of education funding if it pays for students to attend the parochial school.

The town has sued the state, citing a 1994 Vermont Supreme Court decision allowing tuition reimbursement for parents who send their children to sectarian schools. Chittenden, and its attorneys at the Washington-based Institute for Justice argue that the more recent decision essentially overturns the earlier ruling.

---

[1] Mark Walsh, "Court Deadlocks on Vouchers," *Teacher*, May/June, 1996.

[2] Rene Sanchez, "In Wisconsin, Vouchers for Religious Schools are Handed Legal Setback," *The Washington Post*, Jan. 15, 1997.

[3] Paul Souhrada, "Court: Cleveland Vouchers Program Unconstitutional," The Associated Press, May 2, 1997.

---

thousands of religiously affiliated organizations such as hospitals, universities and social service providers with billions of dollars each year. Much of the state money assists K-12 students in parochial schools by providing them with textbooks, standardized tests, transportation and remedial education.

In addition, supporters say, recent Supreme Court decisions, including *Agostini v. Felton,* handed down in June (*see p. 66*), have steadily expanded the definition of what is permissible when it comes to government assistance for religious schools. These decisions, supporters argue, clearly indicate that vouchers will be adjudged constitutional by the Supreme Court.

As lawmakers, policy-makers, educators and parents continue to debate school choice, these are some of the questions being asked:

Does a voucher program that includes religious schools violate the constitutional separation of church and state?

The First Amendment states that "Congress shall make no law respecting the establishment of religion, or prohibiting the free exercise thereof. . . ." On its face, the Establishment Clause is clear: The state cannot support one denomination or faith over others; nor can it inhibit citizens' practice of their religion.

But, like many parts of the Constitution, the Establishment Clause can be interpreted in a variety of ways when applied to more narrowly tailored, practical situations.

According to many legal scholars, the question of state support for religious schools has been especially perplexing because the Supreme Court has produced what some say are a host of confusing and contradictory decisions.

The question is simple: How far can the state go in supporting schools that are religiously affiliated? Some assistance is clearly allowed. For example, state governments have long been permitted to provide transportation and textbooks to students who attend parochial schools. The logic is that the assistance is going directly to the student, not the school, and hence is not supporting religion.

But the question becomes harder to answer when the assistance benefits the school more directly. While the Supreme Court has never ruled on the constitutionality of vouchers, it has looked at other schemes aimed at helping parents with educational expenses.

In 1973, for example, the court ruled in *Committee for Public Education and Religious Liberty v. Nyquist* that a New York state law granting parents reimbursements and tax credits for private school tuition was unconstitutional. The court said that even though the law was neutral on its face (allowing the benefit for any kind of private school tuition), it had the effect of subsidizing religious education because roughly three-quarters of parents receiving the reimburse-

ments or credits sent their children to sectarian schools. Hence, regardless of its intent, the law resulted in advancing religious education and violated the Establishment Clause.

But over the next two decades, the court handed down several rulings that many regard as contradictory, including *Mueller v. Allen* in 1983. The court ruled in *Mueller* that an Ohio law offering a parental tax deduction for educational expenses was consti-

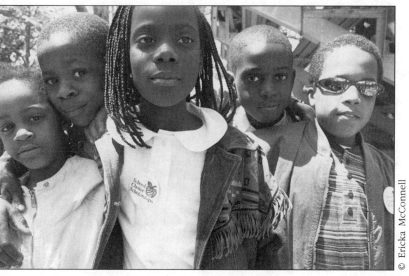

The privately funded School Choice Scholarships program in New York City awarded 1,300 three-year tuition grants to enable poor children to attend private schools.

© Ericka McConnell

tutional even though 93 percent of those claiming the deduction had children in religious schools. The court distinguished this case from *Nyquist* because the tax deduction also was available to parents with children in public schools. In addition, the justices argued that the deduction was a much less direct subsidy of religious schools than were the tuition reimbursements available under the New York law struck down in *Nyquist*.[4]

In other cases in the 1980s and early '90s, the Supreme Court allowed various forms of state assistance for students enrolled in religious schools. For example, in *Zobrest v. Catalina Foothills School District* the court ruled in

1993 that a state could provide a sign language interpreter for a deaf student in parochial school, even when that student was in religion class.

And on June 23, in *Agostini,* the court ruled that remedial education teachers supplied by New York state could assist parochial school children on school property. Previously, such teachers had worked in buses parked off the grounds of the religious schools as a result of a 1985 Supreme Court ruling, *Aquilar v. Felton.* Voucher supporters were heartened by the fact that in *Agostini* the court reversed itself, overturning *Aguilar v. Felton.*[5]

Supporters of vouchers see cases like *Mueller, Zobrest* and *Agostini* as part of a trend within the Supreme Court away from what they say is the more restrictive view of the Establishment Clause put forth in *Nyquist.*

"This is just the court's way of moving from one position to another without actually admitting that they are changing the law," says Michael McConnell, a professor at the University of Utah's College of Law and an expert on the Establishment Clause.

According to McConnell, the court's shift is long overdue. "*Nyquist* was the product of the kind of separationist thinking that is really disguised hostility toward religion," he says. McConnell and others contend that there are a host of reasons why voucher programs would be constitutional.

First, they argue, the benefits go to the parents and children who receive them, not the school. "It's up to the parents to decide whether they want

Privately Funded Vouchers Aid Students in 18 States

When the School Choice Scholarships Foundation offered tuition vouchers to 1,300 low-income children in New York City early this year, the response was an unanticipated — and overwhelming — 16,000 applications.

"It shows that the perception of need for the program is high," said Bruce Kovner, chairman of Caxton Corp., a New York investment firm, and head of the foundation.[1]

Kovner and other New York businessmen have already raised $7 million, enough to guarantee the recipients of the vouchers (who were chosen by lottery) up to $1,400 a year for three years. Kovner hopes to raise another $3 million in the near future in order to increase the number of scholarships and begin making a dent in the waiting list, which has swelled to 23,000 hopefuls.[2]

Amid the hoopla over publicly funded vouchers, efforts to privately finance school choice have gone almost unnoticed. But New York is just the latest in what has become a long list of cities where private philanthropists, usually in the business community, are establishing charities to pay for tuition vouchers.

The first privately financed voucher program was created in Indianapolis in April 1991 by J. Patrick Rooney, then-chairman of the Golden Rule Insurance Co., who put up $1.2 million for 746 vouchers.

The following year, Jim Leininger a physician and businessman in San Antonio, Texas, decided to duplicate Rooney's efforts in his hometown. At roughly the same time, programs were being established in Atlanta, Milwaukee and Battle Creek, Mich.

Today, there are at least 30 programs in 18 states, including Dallas, Buffalo, N.Y., and Oakland, Calif. Some of the programs have just a few benefactors. Others are supported by large groups of well-to-do individuals. A few, like the group in Milwaukee, solicit funds from the general public.

The smallest group, in Midland, Texas, spent $6,000 on four students during the 1996-97 school year. The largest program is in Milwaukee, where $4.2 million provided vouchers for 4,127 children during the same period. Currently, all of the programs combined are serving 13,648 students,

more than twice the number receiving privately funded vouchers two years ago.

"As time has gone on, this idea has really grown," says Fritz Steiger, president of Children's Educational Opportunity (CEO) of America, a group that supports local efforts to privately finance vouchers.

Founded in 1992, CEO America offers information and training to people interested in creating an organization to provide privately funded vouchers. In 1994, Steiger's group received a $2 million grant from the Walton Family Foundation. The money was used to help start nine programs. "We've gone in and said, "We'll give you $50,000 [for each of three years] if you can raise $50,000 to get the program started," Steiger says.

One reason these programs have proliferated so quickly, Steiger says, is that they can be relatively inexpensive to establish. The average voucher totals about $1,100, so a program can often serve 100 students with an annual budget of little more than $100,000.

Not surprisingly, new programs are being established each year. According to Steiger, new organizations have been or are being founded in San Francisco, Chicago, New Orleans, Miami, Baltimore and other cities.

"I think that by the year 2000, we'll have 60 programs and 30,000-40,000 students," he says.

But those who are starting these groups are not trying to build permanent charities. "The people who are funding this are not in it for the long haul," Steiger says. "These are transitional organizations that are models for public policy."

The hope, Steiger says, is to show politicians and the public at large how vouchers work and what they can do.

And what if the Supreme Court eventually rules that taxpayers' money cannot be used to finance vouchers that send children to religious schools? "Then many of these groups might become permanent," Steiger says.

Cities With Private Voucher Programs

The number of voucher programs funded by nonprofit business and citizen groups has grown steadily since the first program was started in Indianapolis in 1991.

Year	Programs
1991	1
1992	5
1993	12
1994	17
1995	23
1996	29

Source: CEO America

---

[1] Jeff Archer, "16,000 N.Y.C. Parents Apply for 1,300 Vouchers to Private Schools," *Education Week*, April 30, 1997.

[2] Susan Lee and Christine Foster, "Trustbusters," *Forbes*, June 2, 1997.

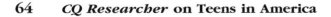

to send their child to a religious school or not," says Nicole Garnett, a staff attorney at the Institute for Justice, a public advocacy law firm that has assisted voucher supporters in a number of school choice cases. "If an unemployment check winds up in a church collection plate, does that matter?" she asks. No, Garnett and other supporters answer, because the recipients of the benefit can spend it any way they please.

Advocates also point out that the federal government already supports religious institutions in a variety of ways. For instance, each year, tens of thousands of students use Pell grants and GI Bill benefits to attend religious colleges and universities. "You could use your Pell grant to go to a university where there is a prayer before every class," Garnett says, adding that this is no different than a voucher.

Howard Fuller, Milwaukee's school superintendent from 1991-95, agrees. "I find it strange that we are able to do it with higher education," he says, "but when that logic is applied to K-12, people start coming up with reasons why that can't be."

But opponents of school choice see big differences between Pell grants and vouchers. For one thing, they argue that children are more easily influenced by religious teaching than adults in college or graduate school, a fact recognized by the Supreme Court.

The court's "concern over [government] endorsement [of religion] is especially acute in the area of primary and secondary education, where many of the citizens perceiving the governmental message are children in their formative years," writes Steven K. Green, legal director of Americans United for the Separation of Church and State. [6]

In addition, Green and others argue, unlike primary and secondary schools, most colleges and universities with a religious affiliation are not overtly reli-

gious. "Let's face it, there's a big difference," he says.

School choice opponents also dismiss the argument that vouchers benefit parents and children and not religious schools. "They say [voucher laws] are neutral because they are based on the independent choices of the parents," says Bob Chanin, general counsel of the NEA. But, Chanin argues, in Milwaukee and Cleveland, which have voucher programs, "75-80 percent of [private] schools are sectarian." Hence, giving parents public money to send their children to private school amounts to a de facto subsidy for religious schools, he says.

Green agrees. "You cannot wash money through the hands of a third party when it is basically going to an entity that wouldn't get the money otherwise."

Opponents also dispute the idea that the legal winds of change are blowing against them. According to Chanin, *Nyquist* clearly invalidates current voucher schemes since it struck down tuition reimbursements, which are not a direct subsidy for religious schools. In addition, he says, despite what McConnell and others say about a trend toward allowing similar types of state aid in subsequent decisions like *Mueller, Nyquist* has not been overruled. "In fact, in *Mueller* the court specifically said it was not overturning *Nyquist,*" he says.

Finally, those against vouchers dismiss the recent hoopla over the recent *Agostini* decision. "To imply that this is opening the door to vouchers is a misreading of this decision," says NEA President Chase. "They made very careful distinctions in this case, saying that the [public] money could only be used for public school teachers and for remedial education." In other words, Chase explains, *Agostini* is not a sign that the court is about to allow states to pay private school teachers to teach subjects like religion.

Can vouchers really offer poor children better educational opportunities?

A recent poll commissioned by the American Education Reform Foundation found that 61 percent of all low-income residents of Washington, D.C., would send their children to private school if money were not an issue.

According to school choice advocates, the poll and others like it show that regardless of what many educators and scholars say, poorer Americans favor choice for their children. "Of course they do," Fuller says. "It's in the best interests of parents and children to have the widest range of options available when it comes to education."

Fuller and others say that having options is especially important when children are caught in poorly functioning school systems that fail to provide even basic remedial skills.

"Kids at the bottom are almost guaranteed to go to the scrap heap," says Diane Ravitch, a senior fellow at the Brookings Institution and an assistant secretary of Education in the Bush administration. "They need another option."

Voucher advocates argue that having options would provide a host of benefits for poor children. First, it would empower parents to get more involved in their child's school. [7] "There's this myth that low-income parents don't care about their kids' education," says Shokraii of the Heritage Foundation. She argues that private schools, and especially parochial schools, generally are more successful at tapping into parental concerns than public schools. "They do a better job of attracting parents and keeping them engaged in their kids' education," she says.

In addition, supporters of school choice say, many of the private schools that would take children with vouchers have a better track record of succeeding with poor students than their public counterparts, particularly Catholic schools in inner-city areas. For proof, they point to a 1990 RAND Corporation report showing that 95 percent of all students who attended Catholic schools in New York City graduated. Many of these students were from disadvantaged backgrounds. By contrast, only 25 percent of New York's public school students received their high school diploma. [8]

Various reasons are given for the success of Catholic and other parochial schools. Some voucher supporters acknowledge that private schools can be selective when it comes to whom they choose to admit.

But advocates also say that other more important factors lie behind the success. "Catholic schools . . . never went through the rights revolution of the 1960s, which eroded the order-keeping authority of schools and discouraged teachers and principals from disciplining disruptive students by establishing elaborate due-process procedures," writes Sol Stern. [9] Others point to parochial schools' emphasis on core curriculum and parental involvement.

Many of those who oppose school choice agree that some children in public schools might do better in a private school. "But you can't just help a few kids at the expense of everyone else," Green says.

In addition, Green and others say, it is counterproductive to compare public schools with their private counterparts. "If [public schools] could pick and choose the students who do not have discipline problems or special needs," Green says, "you'd see real improvement there."

James Coomer, a political science professor at Mercer University in Macon, Ga., agrees. "The public schools are asked to do too much," he says. "They are asked to take students who don't want to learn, students with disabilities and students who are disruptive."

Opponents of school choice also

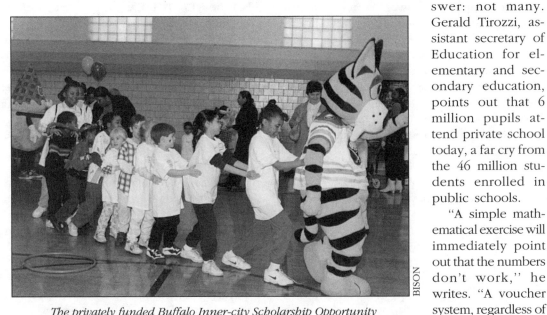

The privately funded Buffalo Inner-city Scholarship Opportunity Network (BISON) enabled more than 200 children from low-income families in Buffalo, N.Y., to attend private school last year.

worry that vouchers might be used to subsidize private school tuition for those who can already afford it. In Cleveland, for example, 27 percent of the first vouchers awarded by the city went to students already enrolled in private schools.

Moreover, opponents say, existing and proposed voucher programs do not offer enough money to give poor parents much of a choice outside of the public system. In Cleveland, vouchers provide up to $2,250 per pupil per year. And the school choice plan put forth by Dole during last year's election campaign would have offered students a maximum of $1,500.

"Many [poor families] would not be able to afford the extra tuition,

transportation and related costs of using a voucher," says Kweisi Mfume, president of the NAACP, which opposes vouchers. [10]

In addition, opponents ask: How many students can actually be accommodated in a private school, even if every child in America were eligible to receive a voucher? The answer: not many. Gerald Tirozzi, assistant secretary of Education for elementary and secondary education, points out that 6 million pupils attend private school today, a far cry from the 46 million students enrolled in public schools.

"A simple mathematical exercise will immediately point out that the numbers don't work," he writes. "A voucher system, regardless of the amount of money provided, can only accommodate a minimal number of public school students." [11]

Given the very limited and brief use of vouchers in the United States so far, it is too soon to tell whether school choice will benefit students, poor or otherwise, who transfer from public to private school. Still, both sides in the debate have pointed to studies indicating that vouchers either do or don't make a difference in the performance of the students who use them.

According to voucher opponents, a series of studies of students in Milwaukee concludes that those who used vouchers performed no better on standardized tests than public school students. The state-sponsored studies by University of Wisconsin Professor John Witte focused on test scores from 1991-1995.[12]

But another evaluation of the same test data by Paul E. Peterson and Jiangtao Du of Harvard University and Jay P. Greene of the University of Houston discovered that voucher students performed better in key subjects than children who had applied for but had not been given vouchers. The voucher students scored 3-5 percent higher in reading and 5-12 percent higher in math, the researchers found.[13]

Different methodologies could explain why the two studies differed. For example, while Witte compared voucher students with all children in the same grades, Peterson and his colleagues used only those who had tried unsuccessfully to get a voucher.

Many experts believe that neither study should be used as a rationale for making decisions on school choice. "It's going to take a lot more analysis than this to figure out what's going on in these choice programs," says Richard Elmore, a professor of education at Harvard.[14]

Will vouchers lead to increased educational competition and improve the public schools?

In a sense, voucher advocates say, public schools are like the automobile industry in the 1970s. Like Detroit's Big Three automakers 25 years ago, public schools today can afford to put out a shoddy education product because they have a virtual lock on the market.

"The auto industry was arrogant until it lost 25 percent of the market to the Japanese," Fuller says.

Fuller and others believe that like the auto industry or any other business, public education will only improve if it is subjected to outside competition. "When there is a captive audience," Ravitch says, "there is no incentive to change anything."

The idea is to unshackle that audience by giving them the option of taking some or all of the public money spent on their education with them to another school. "If children can get vouchers, public schools will begin treating them like customers," says Heritage's Shokraii.

Joe McTighe, executive director of the Council for American Private Education, agrees. "The opportunity to take your business someplace else is a powerful inducement to improve," he says.

As evidence, Shokraii, McTighe and others point to actions taken in those school districts that have had limited voucher programs. In Milwaukee, McTighe says, educators have opened a charter school and given principals in all schools more autonomy since vouchers were made available in 1990. According to McTighe, these innovations were a response to the competition posed by the new school choice program.[15]

But opponents of vouchers say that it is not school choice that is nudging public schools to make necessary reforms. "Those things happening in Milwaukee are going on all over the country," says Deanna Duby, director of education policy at People for the American Way, a First Amendment rights advocacy group. Duby argues that charter schools, principal autonomy and other innovations are part of a broad nationwide reform movement that has nothing to do with vouchers.

Instead, Duby and others argue, vouchers would simply take away money from already underfunded public school systems, especially in poor, inner-city areas. "You would drain badly needed money from public schools that already can't do what they need to," she says, adding that unlike a private institution, which can select the students it wants to admit, public schools must admit all children, including those who are disruptive or have special needs.

In addition, opponents argue, vouchers take more than much-needed money away from public schools. "The choice system is a system of segregation because it removes the most motivated kids and parents from the public system and puts them in private schools," says Richard Rothstein, a research associate at the Economic Policy Institute. Highly motivated parents would take a large share of any vouchers offered, he says, because they "are the most interested in their child's education" and thus more likely to take advantage of new opportunities. The resulting exodus, he says, would be disastrous for the students left behind, because these more-committed parents are often the impetus for positive change. "Everybody who has been involved in a public school knows that if you have a teacher who is not doing well, it only takes one or two parents in that classroom to complain to the principal to get a change," he says.

Opponents also dismiss the idea that you can treat a school district like a business and parents like consumers. "This market theory of competition assumes that people have good information on the choices they are making," Rothstein says, "but we really don't have any information on school quality. So if parents don't know what schools are good, there's no reason to believe they will choose the best school."

In addition, opponents say, there really is a difference between business and government. "To assume that market modalities will have an impact in the government sector is wrong," Green says. "What's good for selling cars is not necessarily good for schools."

But Fuller dismisses the argument that schools are unique institutions. "They are organizations just like any other," he argues, "and many of the principles that apply to business will apply to them." For example, Fuller says, the important issues in school districts, as in businesses, revolve around money. "People know that for all of the yakking, the key is how to allocate resources," he says.

In addition, voucher supporters say, private schools don't always just take the best students.

"We take the low achievers," says Lydia Harris, principal of St. Adalbert's, which has 47 voucher students. "It's a myth that we only take the cream of the crop," she says, adding: "We put our own cream on the crop."

Choice advocates also challenge the notion that vouchers will drain needed money from public schools. "There would not be a net loss of per-pupil funding because the fewer students you have the less it's going to cost," McTighe says.

In fact, McTighe and others say, most proposed vouchers are worth much less than the per-pupil amount spent by the school district. For example, in Cleveland, vouchers are worth a maximum of $2,500 per year, less than half of what the city spends for every pupil in public school. "So [the public school] actually does better [financially] with this," McTighe says.

But voucher opponents argue that the overall cost of education won't necessarily drop every time a student leaves the school system. "A lot of the cost of having the student in the school would still be there," Duby says. For example, she points out, the building would still need to be maintained and the teachers paid. "If a third of the students left an elementary school, almost all of the costs would remain," she says. ∎

BACKGROUND

Rise of Public Schools

The proper role of government in education has been debated for more than 200 years. But public schools, as they exist today, are a relatively new phenomenon.

During the Enlightenment, thinkers like Thomas Jefferson, called for increased taxation to support a public school system that would educate "common people." Jefferson believed that only through education could citizens understand and exercise their rights. Indeed, he said, an educated populous was essential to the functioning of the new American republic. [16]

But others were more wary of using the public purse to finance education. Scottish economist Adam Smith, whose landmark work, *The Wealth of Nations,* was published the same year as Jefferson's Declaration of Independence, believed that the "invisible hand" of the market could not adequately provide enough incentives for universal education. But the father of laissez-faire economics also said that an educational system administered by the government would be inefficient and would fail to create a literate population.

By the early 19th century, the debate over public education had become one of the most important social questions in the United States. Trade unions and other advocates for workers' rights said that universal education was needed to fight social injustice and poverty. But business leaders in the North and slaveholders in the South worried that universal literacy could stoke the fires of revolution among the lower classes. [17]

The nation's leading proponent of public education was Horace Mann, secretary of the Massachusetts Board of Education and one of the most well-known social reformers of the last century. Mann argued that a public school system would inculcate the native-born poor and newly arrived immigrants with "American values." [18]

Over time, Mann's idea that education could mold disparate social and ethnic groups into good citizens gained currency around the country. By the time the Civil War broke out,

most states had public elementary schools. And yet, while free, they were not compulsory. Moreover, public high schools were rare and would remain so throughout the 19th century. In fact, as late as 1920, only one-third of all eligible Americans attended high school. [19]

During the first half of the 20th century, public school attendance and respect for the nation's educational institutions grew at a rapid pace. By the 1950s, most American children were in school and, according to polls of their parents' attitudes, were receiving quality educations.

It was at this time, nonetheless, that the case for vouchers was first put forward. In 1955, libertarian economist Milton Friedman published an influential essay proposing vouchers as a way to give parents greater flexibility in choosing their child's school as well as an antidote for what he said was an increasingly inefficient and ineffective public education system.

Friedman advanced what has become the classic school choice argument: Vouchers will allow parents more choice when it comes to their children's education, which will in turn improve all schools, public and private, by injecting competition into the system. Friedman argued that this scheme would prove especially beneficial for the poor, who have no choice but to send their children to the local public school, even if it offers an inferior education. [20]

Friedman might have seemed an alarmist in the 1950s, but his ideas made sense to many more people two decades later. By the 1970s, the national consensus on public education had changed, with most Americans believing that public schools were failing. Statistics seemed to bear them out. In one key measure of education quality, SAT scores dropped steadily from the mid-1960s to the early '80s. [21]

Chronology

1950s-1980s

The perception that public schools are inadequate in many parts of the country gathers momentum, giving birth to the school choice movement.

1955
Libertarian economist Milton Friedman publishes an essay proposing tuition vouchers as a means to expand educational opportunity and improve public schools.

1973
The U.S. Supreme Court strikes down a New York state law granting parents reimbursements and tax credits for the cost of private school tuition.

1979
The Department of Education is created.

1980
Studies show a steady decline in Scholastic Aptitude Tests (SATs) over the previous 15 years.

1983
The Education Department's *A Nation At Risk* report charts what it sees as a decline in discipline and standards in the country's public schools.

———— • ————

1990s *The push for school choice is transformed into a national movement. The first voucher plans are created on a small scale.*

April 1990
Wisconsin establishes a voucher program to allow students in Milwaukee to go to non-sectarian private schools.

April 1991
The nation's first privately financed voucher program is created in Indianapolis, by J. Patrick Rooney, chairman of the Golden Rule Insurance Co. Rooney's action sparks dozens of similr programs in cities around the country.

September 1993
A pilot voucher plan is signed into law in Puerto Rico, and more than 1,800 vouchers are awarded.

November 1993
Voters in California overwhelmingly reject Proposition 174, which would have entitled every student enrolled in public or private school to a tuition voucher equal to half of the state's per pupil spending, or about $2,600.

November 1994
Puerto Rico's Supreme Court strikes down the commonwealth's voucher law, ruling that it violates a constitutional ban on transferring public funds to private schools.

June 1995
Ohio creates a pilot voucher program for the Cleveland public school system. Under the plan, vouchers can be used in both sectarian and non-sectarian private schools.

July 1995
Wisconsin legislators expand the Milwaukee voucher program to include religious schools.

February 1996
A proposal creating a $5 million voucher program for the District of Columbia is defeated in the Senate.

May 1996
The 10th District Court of Appeals for the State of Ohio strikes down the voucher plan in Cleveland on the grounds that the program violates federal and state constitutional Establishment clauses. The case is appealed to the state Supreme Court.

July 1996
Republican presidential candidate Bob Dole announces a proposal to spend $2.5 billion annually to fund a nationwide voucher program.

November 1996
Voters in Washington state reject Initiative 173, which would have created tuition vouchers for non-religious private schools.

January 1997
A Wisconsin trial court rules that state efforts to expand the Milwaukee voucher program to include sectarian institutions violates the Establishment Clause in the state's Constitution.

June 1997
In *Agostini v. Felton,* the U.S. Supreme Court overturns a 1985 ruling that barred public school remedial education teachers from entering parochial schools to help students there.

Teachers' Choice

In cities throughout the country, a large percentage of public school teachers whose household income is $35,000-$70,000 opt for private school for their own children, though teachers' groups uniformly oppose school choice.

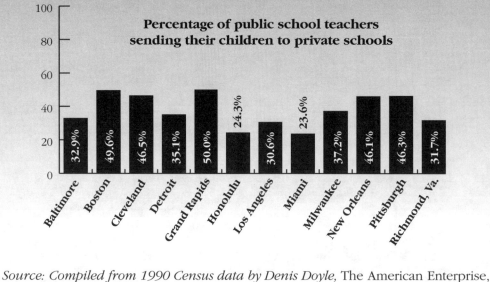

Percentage of public school teachers sending their children to private schools

City	Percentage
Baltimore	32.9%
Boston	49.6%
Cleveland	46.5%
Detroit	35.1%
Grand Rapids	50.0%
Honolulu	24.3%
Los Angeles	30.6%
Miami	23.6%
Milwaukee	37.2%
New Orleans	46.1%
Pittsburgh	46.3%
Richmond, Va.	31.7%

Source: Compiled from 1990 Census data by Denis Doyle, The American Enterprise, *September/October 1996*

In 1983, an influential Department of Education report seemed to confirm the public's worst fears. Commissioned by Education Secretary Terrel H. Bell, *A Nation at Risk* painted a bleak picture of the state of learning in America. Among other things, it criticized schools for a marked decline in discipline and academic standards. [22]

When *A Nation at Risk* was published, the school choice movement already had a dedicated following in conservative circles. Over the next decade, the choice movement broadened its base of support significantly. Today, vouchers are still largely rejected by the Democratic Party and most liberal groups. But school choice has substantial support among a growing number of African-American political leaders and others who are normally identified with the left, though the NAACP remains opposed to choice,

in large part, voucher proponents say, because of its traditional alliance with labor unions.

Voucher Programs

School choice has never been established on a grand scale. Voucher plans have been carried out as pilot programs and have impacted very few students. The most significant school choice plan to date was created in Milwaukee in 1990, where the state provides up to $3,209 to some 1,100 mostly low-income children. The vouchers can only be used to send students to non-religious private schools. [23]

In the summer of 1995, the Wisconsin Legislature voted to include religious schools in the voucher program. The law also expanded the

current program significantly, increasing the number of eligible students to 7,000 in 1996 and 15,000 the following year. But the expansion has not been carried out due to a court challenge filed by the state affiliates of the NEA and the American Civil Liberties Union (ACLU). [24]

Although the voucher program in Milwaukee has received the lion's share of national media attention, it does not represent the first or most recent attempt to experiment with school choice.

Indeed, since 1869, Vermont has allowed parents in sparsely populated districts without a high school to send their children to a public or private alternative at state expense. Until 1961, "tuitioning, as the practice is known," included parochial schools. That year, the state Supreme Court ruled that using government funds to pay tuition at parochial schools, in this case three Catholic schools, violated Vermont's Constitution.

An attempt last year to send 15 Vermont students from tiny Chittenden to a nearby Roman Catholic high school has reopened the debate over religious schools. Although the Chittenden case has not yet reached the state Supreme Court, a 1994 high court ruling allowing tuition reimbursement for a man who sent his son to a sectarian school is an indication that the tribunal may be willing to overturn its 1961 decision. [25]

Puerto Rico has also experimented, albeit briefly, with school choice. In 1993, the commonwealth's legislature created a pilot voucher program for children whose parents earn less than $18,000 per year. The program offered students up to $1,500 toward tuition at the school of their choice, including religious institutions. One year and 1,181 vouchers later, the commonwealth's Supreme Court struck down the program on the grounds that the Puerto Rican Constitution prohibits the use of public funds to support private schools, sectarian or otherwise.

Almost two years after vouchers were struck down in Puerto Rico, a similar school choice plan was instituted in Cleveland. The program, which began in September 1996, allows up to 2,000 elementary-age students to receive up to $2,500 annually to attend the school of their choice. As in Puerto Rico, a challenge to the plan is pending before the Ohio Supreme Court. ∎

CURRENT SITUATION

Politics of Choice

During the 1996 presidential campaign, school choice became a major issue for the first time in a national election. The issue rose to prominence after Republican nominee Bob Dole announced a plan to spend $2.5 billion annually to give lower-income children vouchers. Dole's plan offered students up to $1,000 a year for elementary school and $1,500 for high school.

On Oct. 6, in the first of Dole's two debates with President Clinton, Clinton came out against vouchers.

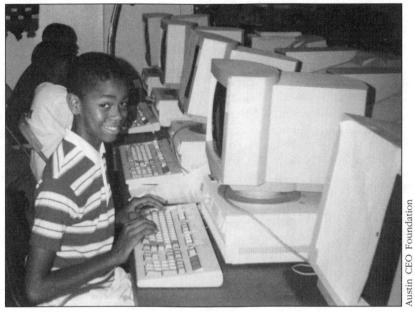

Scholarships to private schools in Austin, Texas, are provided by the private Austin Children's Educational Opportunity Foundation.

Clinton's victory a month later assured that school choice would likely be off the White House agenda until at least the year 2000.

Still, voucher advocates say, the fact that school choice was in the spotlight during the campaign is evidence that the issue has now become an integral part of the national debate on education.

"When Bob Dole started talking about school choice and took on the teachers' unions ... we realized that it had become a mainstream issue," says Fritz Steiger, president of Children's Educational Opportunity of America (CEO America), which helps private groups that raise money to fund tuition vouchers.

Indeed, vouchers have become a top priority for many Republican politicians, who are supported by many religious groups and some education reformers.

On Capitol Hill, Republicans and a few Democrats have made frequent and concerted efforts since the early 1990s to create pilot voucher programs.

Last year, for instance, an attempt to establish a $5 million voucher program in the District of Columbia failed after Democrats in the Senate blocked action on the D.C. spending bill to which the proposal was attached. [26]

This year, a number of voucher plans are pending before Congress. A proposal sponsored by Sen. Paul Coverdell, R-Ga., would authorize $50 million in fiscal 1998 to establish school choice demonstration projects in 20-30 school districts.

Another measure, sponsored in the House by Majority Leader Dick Armey, R-Texas, and in the Senate by Daniel R. Coats, R-Ind., would authorize $7 million in fiscal 1998 to provide vouchers of up to $3,200 for 2,000 poor children in Washington, D.C.

Leading the charge against these and other attempts to create school choice programs are several labor and civil rights groups. By far the most powerful and notable of these organizations is the NEA. Other important players include the American Federation of Teachers (AFT), the NAACP, People for the American Way and the ACLU.

These and other groups claim that proponents of vouchers are not interested in finding new ways to provide a better education for poor children. Instead, they say, they are interested in subsidizing children already attending private schools at the expense of public education. Some even suggest that many school choice advocates, especially religious groups, want to do away with public schools entirely. "Their goal is to end public education," Chase says.

Supporters of school choice, among them the Institute for Justice, the Heritage Foundation and the Christian Coalition, contend that teachers' unions are only interested in protecting their members' jobs, regardless of performance or qualifications. "They protect teachers who have no business being with children," Fuller says.

Choice advocates also say that opposition by civil liberties groups actually reflects a thinly disguised fear of religion as much as an effort to guard constitutional principles.

"Their primary concern is what they take to be the undue influence of religion, in particular the Roman Catholic Church," says Quentin L. Quade, director of the Blum Center for Parental Freedom in Education at Marquette University in Milwaukee. ∎

OUTLOOK

Momentum Building?

Proponents of vouchers believe that, despite recent setbacks in state courts, overall momentum is with them.

"This issue is on a roll because the alternatives have been tried for years and are failing," McTighe says.

Ravitch agrees, adding: "There's a growing interest because there's a growing sense of desperation, especially in the black community."

Indeed, choice advocates can point to a number of recent converts to the cause, among them Rep. Floyd H. Flake, D-N.Y., and *Washington Post* columnist William Raspberry, who are not only national figures with impeccable liberal credentials but also African-Americans.

But while well-known black voucher advocates are important to the school choice movement, it is at the grass-roots level where African-Americans are having the greatest impact.

For instance, proponents say, black community leaders and parents have been the driving force behind the school choice movements in Cleveland and Milwaukee. "The battle for parental choice [in Milwaukee] began in the church basements and meeting halls of the Near North Side," writes scholar Daniel McGroarty in his recent book *Break These Chains: The Battle for School Choice*. McGroarty, a fellow at the Institute for Contemporary Studies, says that the language used to advance school choice was reminiscent of the civil rights movement. "Their rhetoric was more redolent of Martin Luther King than the free-market pronouncements favored by conservative voucher proponents," he says. [27]

What McGroarty says is happening in Milwaukee and Cleveland is spreading to more and more cities and towns around the country, choice proponents say. Some of these movements are sure to succeed in bringing school choice to their communities, they say.

"I think it's going to start happening soon in the states," Steiger says. "In five years, we'll see three or four significant choice programs, and in 10 years a significant number of states will have vouchers."

Opponents of school choice concede that the movement has built up a head of steam. "There's a certain amount of momentum," says Duby of People for the American Way. But, she argues, the movement reflects parents' legitimate frustration, not necessarily the validity of vouchers as a public policy. "I understand when people say, 'I don't care about everyone else, I need to get my kid out of these schools,'" she says.

Duby and others fear that frustration may lead people to embrace choice as a panacea while avoiding more concrete reform efforts. "I think we could do a lot of damage with school choice," she says, adding that "if nothing else, choice could delay the work we need to do."

Chase agrees, saying that the NEA and other groups need to educate people adequately so that they understand that private school is not a "magic bullet." Still, Chase disputes the notion that there is a grass-roots groundswell for vouchers all over the country.

"This is not something that is being seriously discussed in most school districts," he says. "There is such a thing as the public good, and for [the American people] the public good means public schools for all children."

Chase and other voucher opponents, including many African-Americans, also reject the notion that school choice is akin to the fight for civil rights, noting that organizations like the NAACP firmly oppose choice.

In fact, they point out, many black leaders think that school choice will be a huge step backward, and not only in education. "Choice is a subterfuge for segregation" as it existed in the South before the civil rights movement, says Felmers Chaney, head of the Milwaukee NAACP. [28]

Supreme Court to Rule?

But whether school choice is embraced as a policy initiative or not, it may not be the most important immediate question facing those on both sides of the debate. Many supporters and some opponents of vouchers predict that the Supreme Court is likely to rule on the issue in the next two or three years.

At Issue:

Is meaningful school choice possible within the public school system?

RICHARD W. RILEY
Secretary of Education

WRITTEN FOR *THE CQ RESEARCHER*

*a*s changes in our economy expand and transform our educational needs, America's public schools must become more flexible and offer students and parents more choices with higher standards and accountability. School districts are responding by creating new types of schools — charter schools, magnet schools, "schools within schools." They are letting parents pick among schools from across the district, even the entire state. This growing menu of choices is improving education by creating new models for learning, and we must do more to promote such advancements.

The Clinton administration is encouraging this trend with a significant effort to expand charter schools. Charter schools are public schools operated by teachers, parents or others in the community who enter into an agreement with the school district or another chartering agency authorized by the state. Since start-up capital is the primary obstacle to starting a charter school, President Clinton requested $100 million in his fiscal 1998 budget to provide seed money for up to 1,100 charter schools.

The progress achieved by charter schools and other innovations is threatened, however, by those who seek to funnel public tax dollars to private schools. More than any public institution, public schools unite citizens from all walks of life and pass on our democratic ideals to each generation. Any voucher program for private schools would drain much-needed resources from public schools and accommodate a limited number of students. Further, private school vouchers would make parochial schools less parochial and private schools less private, subjecting them to public supervision and compromising their independence.

There are several reasons for keeping publicly financed school choice within the public school domain. A public school is held in the public trust by local voters who select the 16,000 local boards that govern their schools. A private school is not required to be open to all students that live within a district, which means that it can choose to turn away students. A successful public school offers the potential to serve as a model that can be replicated elsewhere, while a school that fails to create a quality learning environment can be held accountable to the public and closed if necessary.

The nation's public schools educate close to 90 percent of America's 52 million schoolchildren. At a time of increasing enrollments and growing demands on the public schools, our limited resources should be focused on giving students and parents as many high-quality options as possible within the schools that serve the vast majority of America's students.

JOE MCTIGHE
Executive Director, Council for American Private Education

WRITTEN FOR *THE CQ RESEARCHER*

*a*s beauty is in the eye of the beholder, meaningful choice is in the mind of the selector. When it comes to schools, the selectors, of course, are parents, a child's primary educators. For many parents, the options already at play within public education constitute meaningful choice, but others can find such choice only outside the realm of public schools.

A growing number of parents, for example, desperately desire schools whose primary purpose is to provide youngsters with a sound moral and spiritual education — schools that touch the soul and call children to a life of love. Private schools are the only schools we have that can address the religious development of children — a sphere beyond the proper reach of public education.

And then there are the parents whose children are trapped in chronically failing and sometimes unsafe schools. They don't have the money to move to communities where the schools are better, and they don't have the time to see if the latest promise of improvement proves any more trustworthy than its predecessors. For those parents, an immediate alternative would be neighborhood private schools where high expectations, caring communities and remarkable records of success are the rule.

The same rationale that drives proposals for tax reductions, Pell grants and Hope scholarships to help low- and middle-income students attend the public, private or religious college of their choice applies to K-12 education. How can one argue that aid to the parents of a 12th-grader is taboo while the same aid a year later is laudable? We need a unified plan of parent aid in America — one that guarantees meaningful choice to needy parents across all grade levels.

There are some who say that choice within the public school system is sufficient. They consider such choice the silver bullet of school reform. But let's face it: The difference between the P.S. 8 and P.S. 9 is often inconsequential. And while some charter schools offer parents genuine alternatives, the truth is that many are nothing more than standard public school clones in a prettied-up package.

A single system of government schooling cannot possibly meet everyone's needs. Fortunately, our country is blessed by a rich diversity of schools that collectively serve a noble purpose: the education of our nation's children. Why not a comprehensive program of school choice that truly respects and promotes the right of all parents to choose the kind of education their children shall receive?

FOR MORE INFORMATION

Americans United for the Separation of Church and State, 518 C St., N.E., Washington, D.C. 20002; (202) 466-3234; www.au.org. The group opposes federal or state aid to parochial schools and other religious institutions.

Council for American Private Education, 13107 Wisteria Dr., Suite 457, Germantown, Md. 20874; (301) 916-8460; www.capenet.org. The council is a coalition of private-school associations that seeks greater access to private schools for American families.

Institute for Justice, 1717 Pennsylvania Ave. N.W., Suite 200S, Washington, D.C. 20006; (202) 955-1300; www.ij.org. The institute is a conservative public interest law firm that litigates cases involving parental school choice.

National Education Association, 1201 16th St. N.W., Washington, D.C. 20036; (202) 833-4000; www.nea.org. The NEA is the nation's largest teachers' union with more than 2 million members. It is opposed to vouchers and works to defeat school choice proposals through lobbying and litigation.

"Without a question, the Ohio case will go to the U.S. Supreme Court," Quade says, referring to the Cleveland voucher case currently working its way through the state court system. Duby at People for the American Way agrees. "At some point in the next five years, we will have a voucher case before the Supreme Court," she says.

But others are not so sure about the Ohio case, or any other for that matter, making it to the nation's highest court. According to the NEA's Chanin, if voucher proponents lose the Ohio or another state case based on the court's reading of the state's constitution, there will be no grounds for an appeal to the Supreme Court because there will be no federal constitutional issue to decide

Still, if a voucher case does reach the nation's highest court, school choice supporters are confident the justices will rule that publicly financed tuition vouchers do not violate the Establishment Clause.

"In the long run, the Supreme Court will uphold a properly drafted voucher program," says the Institute for Justice's Garnet, citing *Mueller* and the other cases that school choice supporters say shrink Establishment

Clause restrictions on government support for religion.

But Chanin thinks otherwise. "I'm confident we would win," he says, adding that the Supreme Court has gone out of its way not to overturn *Nyquist,* which is the closest existing case on the voucher question.

Either way, a high court decision would have a tremendous and possibly decisive impact on the school choice debate. A ruling in favor of allowing vouchers would undoubtedly give a huge boost to school choice advocates and lead to a frenzy of new activity on federal, state and local levels.

But if the court struck down a school choice law, the drive for publicly funded vouchers could diminish and even die. With the exception of funding from private sources, says CEO America's Steiger, "there would be no alternatives." ∎

Notes

[1] Richard Lacayo, "Parochial Politics," *Time,* Sept. 23, 1996. See "Attack on Public Schools," *The CQ Researcher,* July 26, 1996, pp. 649-672.
[2] For background, see "Religion in Schools," *The CQ Researcher,* Jan. 7, 1994, pp. 145-168.
[3] *Ibid.*
[4] Lawrence H. Tribe, *American Constitutional Law* (1988), pp. 1217-1218.
[5] Linda Greenhouse, "Court Eases Curb on Providing Aid in Church Schools," *The New York Times,* June 24, 1997.
[6] Steven K. Green, "The Legal Argument Against Private School Choice," *University of Cincinnati Law Review,* summer 1993. Green is quoting *Grand Rapids School District v. Ball.*
[7] For background, see "Parents and Schools," *The CQ Researcher,* Jan. 20, 1995, pp. 66-89.
[8] Sol Stern, "The Invisible Miracle of Catholic Schools," *City Journal,* summer 1996, published by the Manhattan Institute.
[9] *Ibid.* Stern is a *City Journal* contributing editor.
[10] Quoted in a recent letter to NAACP members.
[11] Gerald Tirozzi, "Vouchers: A Questionable Answer to an Unasked Question," *Education Week,* April 23, 1997.
[12] Lynn Olson, "New Studies on Private Choice Contradict Each Other," *Education Week,* Sept. 4, 1996.
[13] Jay P. Greene, Paul E. Peterson and Jiangtao Du, "The Effectiveness of School Choice in Milwaukee: A Secondary Analysis of Data from the Program's Evaluation," Aug. 14, 1996, p. 3.
[14] Olson, *op. cit.*
[15] For background, see "Private Management of Public Schools," *The CQ Researcher,* March 25, 1994, pp. 265-288.
[16] Bernard Mayo (ed.), *Jefferson Himself* (1942), p. 89.
[17] Peter Carrol and David Noble, *The Restless Centuries* (1979), pp. 220-221.
[18] *Ibid.*
[19] Daniel J. Boorstin, *The Americans: The Democratic Experience* (1973), p. 500.
[20] Milton Friedman, "The Role of Government in Education," in Robert A. Solo (ed.), *Economics and the Public Interest* (1955), pp. 127-134.
[21] John E. Chubb and Terry M. Moe, *Politics, Markets and America's Schools* (1990), p. 8.
[22] *Ibid.,* pp. 9-10.
[23] Mark Walsh, "Court Deadlocks on Vouchers," *Teacher,* May/June 1996.
[24] Dorothy B. Hanks, "School Choice Programs: What's Happening in the States," Heritage Foundation, 1997.
[25] Sally Johnson, "Vermont Parents Ask State to Pay Catholic School Tuition," *The New York Times,* Oct. 30, 1996.
[26] David A. Vise, "In a Win for Teachers Unions, Senate Rejects D.C. Tuition Vouchers; City Budget Stalled," *The Washington Post,* Feb. 28, 1996.
[27] Daniel McGroarty, *Break These Chains: The Battle for School Choice* (1996), p. 73.
[28] Nina Shokraii, "Free at Last: Black America Signs Up for School Choice," *Policy Review,* November/December 1996.

Bibliography
Selected Sources Used

Books

Lieberman, Myron, *Privatization and Educational Choice*, St. Martin's Press, 1989.
  Lieberman, an education policy consultant, covers the entire sweep of the school choice debate, from the effect of competition to the constitutionality of vouchers. He also examines the political landscape, describing the groups and interests lined up on both sides of the issue.

McGroarty, Daniel, *Breaking These Chains: The Battle for School Choice*, Prima Publishing, 1996.
  McGroarty, a fellow at the Institute for Contemporary Studies, chronicles the efforts of parents and community leaders in inner-city Milwaukee to establish and sustain a voucher program. McGroarty argues that for many of these mostly black residents, the fight for school choice is akin to the civil rights battles of the 1960s.

Moe, Terry M., and John E. Chubb, *Politics, Markets and America's Schools*, The Brookings Institution, 1990.
  Moe and Chubb look at the recent history of education and education reform in the United States and the problems that have plagued America's schools in the last three decades. The authors come to the conclusion that the institutions governing the nation's schools hamstring them and prevent real reform from taking hold. Moe and Chubb argue that vouchers are a way to break this institutional vise grip.

Articles

Goldberg, Bruce, "A Liberal Argument for School Choice," *The American Enterprise*, September/October, 1996.
  Goldberg criticizes public schools in the United States, arguing that they are "fundamentally at war with individuality." Only by allowing families to be education consumers will the public schools begin to respond to their needs, he says.

Green, Steven, "The Legal Argument Against Private School Choice," *University of Cincinnati Law Review*, summer 1993.
  Green, legal director for Americans United for Church and State, examines Establishment Clause case law. He concludes that optimism on the part of school choice advocates over recent Supreme Court decisions is misplaced. Green points out that the high court has never considered the constitutionality of vouchers and that many legal questions remain unanswered.

Hawley, Willis D., "The Predictable Consequences of School Choice," *Education Week*, April 10, 1996.
  Hawley, dean of the College of Education at the University of Maryland, argues that among other things, school choice will drive up the tuition at private schools and reduce diversity and funding at public institutions.

Lacayo, Richard, "Parochial Politics," *Time*, Sept. 23, 1996.
  Lacayo gives a good overview of the current school choice debate, focusing on the voucher program in Cleveland, Ohio.

Peterson, Bob, "Teacher of the Year Gives Vouchers a Failing Grade," *The Progressive*, April 1997.
  Peterson, a teacher in the Milwaukee public school system, says that in his hometown school choice has been a failure. Among the problems that followed the issuance of vouchers was massive fraud on the part of some private schools that participated in the program.

Tirozzi, Gerald, "Vouchers: A Questionable Answer to an Unasked Question," *Education Week*, April 23, 1997.
  Tirozzi, assistant secretary of Education for elementary and secondary education, picks apart the arguments for vouchers and concludes that they are specious. Among other things, Tirozzi says that even if they were effective, vouchers would not impact more than a small fraction of the students currently enrolled in public schools because the private school system is just not big enough to accommodate many more students.

Reports

Hanks, Dorothy B., *School Choice Programs: What's Happening in the States*, The Heritage Foundation, 1997.
  The report gives an exhaustive state-by-state rundown of existing and proposed school choice programs and related news.

5 Liberal Arts Education

DAVID MASCI

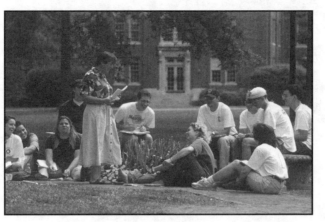

Michael J. Collins maneuvers between two students in the first row of his Shakespeare class at Georgetown University and stops abruptly. He is all energy and enthusiasm.

In his left hand Collins holds aloft the bard's epic tragedy, "Hamlet." His right is raised above his head, motionless, almost as if he were using it to balance himself.

Two students have just performed the pivotal scene in which the play's troubled heroine, Ophelia, and her father, Polonius, argue about her relationship with Hamlet. Now Collins is looking for feedback.

"Why is Polonius angry?" he asks.

Silence. No one wants to be the first to speak up. Finally, a young woman begins, slowly, to explain the source of Polonius' anger. Another offers her impressions of Ophelia's predicament.

Similar discussions take place daily in college classrooms around the country. The liberal arts tradition, embracing not only Shakespeare, but the Civil War, biology, Langston Hughes and myriad other topics, lives on, sustained by teachers like Collins.

The liberal arts have been taught since ancient times. In fact, until the 20th century, liberal arts was just about the only form of higher education available in the United States, or anyplace else. Today, the humanities, social sciences and natural sciences — the three foundations of a contemporary liberal arts education — still form the core of most college and university programs.

But much has changed in the last century. A large number of students no longer focus on the liberal arts. At many colleges and universities, busi-

From *The CQ Researcher,* April 10, 1998.

ness, communications, education and engineering programs are much more popular than, say, history or English. According to the U.S. Department of Education, 234,323 undergraduates earned bachelor's degrees in business-oriented subjects in 1995. By comparison, only 128,154 students earned bachelor's degrees in the social sciences, and only 51,901 received English degrees. [1]

Many liberal arts professors and others involved in education argue that colleges and universities are doing students a great disservice by allowing them to devote most of their time to the study of career-oriented subjects like business. Some go so far as to say that non-vocational schools should largely or wholly eliminate professionally oriented programs for undergraduates. "If a student wants to study business, let him do it at the graduate level," says Kenneth Pennington, a professor of medieval history at Syracuse University.

Pennington and others say that a real undergraduate education should entail immersion in liberal arts subjects like history, literature, philosophy and the natural sciences. They believe that students should spend their undergraduate years reading, talking and thinking about ideas, not the finer points of marketing or journalism. *(See story, p. 84.)*

Others agree in part, arguing that career-oriented programs for undergraduates are acceptable so long as they are accompanied by a solid grounding in the liberal arts. "I don't begrudge someone the opportunity of getting a more vocational education," says Glenn Ricketts, public affairs director at the National Association of Scholars (NAS), in Princeton, N.J. which favors tougher academic standards. "But you need to know something about things like our political system, about history, philosophy and how to express yourself."

But many say that Pennington and even Ricketts are elitists, as well as unrealistic. "They believe they know what's best for the individual, and they simply don't," says Omer Waddles, president of the Career College Association, representing schools with career-oriented programs.

Waddles and others argue that students, not faculty, should decide what kind of education they will receive. After all, he says, students and their families are paying for their schooling, and the choice should be theirs, not some academic's.

But if students choose liberal arts or something in-between, what should they be required to study? What books should they read, and what history should they learn? A century ago, those questions would have been easy to answer. Students immersed themselves in the culture of the West, including the great classical civilizations of Greece and Rome, the Judeo-Christian tradition and the artists and thinkers of the Middle Ages, the Renaissance, the Enlightenment and the early modern period.

For many scholars, the Western tradition is still the foundation of any good education. Americans, regardless of their

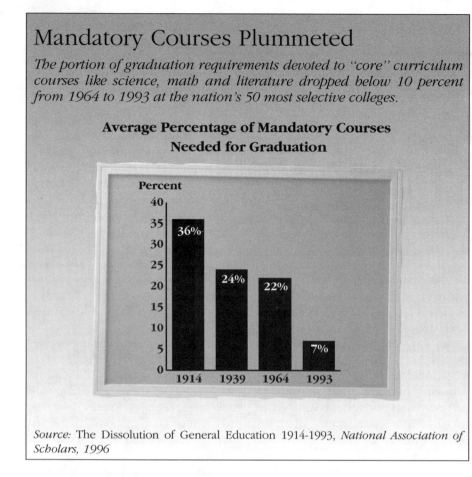

Mandatory Courses Plummeted

The portion of graduation requirements devoted to "core" curriculum courses like science, math and literature dropped below 10 percent from 1964 to 1993 at the nation's 50 most selective colleges.

Average Percentage of Mandatory Courses Needed for Graduation

Percent

Year	Percent
1914	36%
1939	24%
1964	22%
1993	7%

Source: The Dissolution of General Education 1914-1993, *National Association of Scholars, 1996*

ethnic origin, live in a Western country, governed by Western ideas in politics, economics and the world of science and technology, they say. Hence, they cannot understand their society without a grounding in the Western culture, these scholars maintain.

In addition, many argue, the intellectual achievements of the West far surpass those of all other cultures. For instance, they say, almost all scientific and political advances have taken place in the West. Even in less quantifiable disciplines, like literature or philosophy, the size and historical impact of the Western canon far outweigh those of, say, Asia or Africa. "There just isn't much in the other traditions," says Alvin Schmidt, a professor of sociology at Illinois College in Jacksonville, Ill.

But other scholars say that focusing on the primacy of Western tradition is misguided. Non-Western cultures also have rich traditions that any student could and should benefit from, they claim. In fact, people steeped only in the art and ideas of Europe cannot consider themselves well-educated, they say.

Just as important, these scholars argue, the curriculum needs to reflect trends in our world and our country. Revolutions in transportation and communications have brought the planet much closer together. In this new global society, they say, students need some understanding of all traditions, not just that of the West.

"In today's global environment, learning about other cultures is vital for everyone," says Yolanda Moses, president of the City College of New York.

In addition, immigration and other factors are transforming the United States from a nation peopled largely by the descendants of Western Europeans into a multiethnic society.

"We need to prepare students for living in a diverse democracy," says Carol Schneider, president of the Association of American Colleges and Universities. Focusing only on the West won't accomplish that, she says.

The debates over the primacy of the Western tradition or the utility of a liberal arts education are not new. Indeed, academics have argued and deliberated over the question, in one form or another, for decades.

A more recent controversy has involved the growing concern among some educators about how colleges and universities treat their students. The problem stems from student attitudes. "Students want to be entertained," Ricketts says, largely blaming television and computers.

But the bigger problem, many say, is that administrations and faculty are laboring to comply. They point out that in the last decade more and more universities have squandered precious resources on plush dorms, fitness centers and other amenities in an effort to keep students happy.

Even more disturbing, they say, many professors spend their time trying to be diverting and entertaining instead of instructive. "Affability and the one-liners often seem to be all that land with students," wrote Mark Edmundson, a professor of literature at the University of Virginia. [2] Edmundson also charges that many professors don't openly challenge or vigorously question students for fear of offending them or being seen as insensitive.

Others disagree and applaud new attempts on the part of many institutions to be more accountable to undergraduates' needs. "We need to take students much more seriously," says Caryn McTighe Musil, a senior research associate at the Association of American Colleges and Universities.

The real problem, Musil says, isn't

oversensitive or spoiled students but arrogant professors who themselves are pampered and inattentive to the needs of those in their classes. Pennington agrees, but adds that the biggest reason students are neglected is that universities require professors to devote most of their time to research and not teaching. "It's a big problem," he says.

The needs of students — what they should learn and how they should learn it — have long concerned educators. But the arguments over the liberal arts have never been more insistent. Indeed, many educators predict a resurgence in liberal education as liberal arts degrees become more, not less, important in the coming decades *(see p. 92)*. These educators believe that as people try to prepare for living and working in an increasingly fast-paced and mobile society, they will need basic skills like writing and analytical thinking, more than specific professional training.

As professors and others look to the future of liberal education, these are some of the questions they are asking:

Should a liberal arts education primarily entail the study of Western civilization?

If the so-called "culture wars" have a Lexington and Concord, it is the 1987 publication of Allen Bloom's *The Closing of the American Mind: How Higher Education Has Failed Democracy and Impoverished the Souls of Today's Students.* The surprise best-seller was literally a shot heard 'round the world of academia.

Within months of publication, it had sold more than 1 million copies. A year later it was still on the best-seller list. And Bloom, until then a respected but little known philosophy professor, had became a media superstar.

Bloom traced what he deemed to be the precipitous decline of higher learning. He concluded that students, even at the nation's best universities, were being fed a diet devoid of intellectual and spiritual nourishment. To restore proper university education, Bloom recommended, among

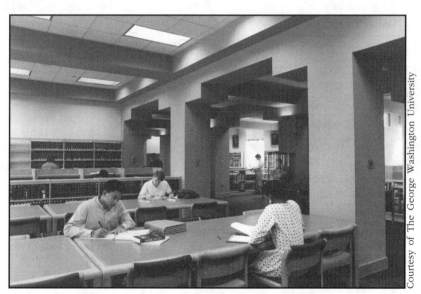

The term liberal arts comes from the Latin phrase "liberales artes" (that which should be known by a free man).

other things, a return to key texts and ideas of the Western tradition. [3]

Bloom brought the debate on the primacy of Western civilization — previously confined to campuses — into the open. A few months after his book appeared, civil rights leader Jesse Jackson and a group of students at Stanford University made headlines by marching against the school's core curriculum, which focused on the Western tradition. "Hey, hey, ho, ho, Western culture's got to go," they chanted. [4] Later that year, Stanford's Western-oriented core curriculum was replaced with a new program titled "Cultures, Ideas and Values," which offered students more choice and included non-Western authors.

Similar headlines were made at other universities. And everyone from professors to pundits weighed in on the debate with a barrage of books and articles that continues to this day.

On one side of the divide are the many who say that it is undemocratic and just plain narrow-minded to expose students solely or largely to Western culture and a Western point of view. Those who focus only on the traditions of the West, they argue, are missing out on the tremendous richness offered by cultures in Asia, Africa and Latin America. "These other traditions are also important," Moses says, "and we need to make sure students are taught them, too."

Moses further argues that it is hubris to presume that all or most of "the answers" are contained in the Western canon, a view shared by Musil. "This notion that the West did it all alone is a fallacy," she says. "Take the Greeks, for instance. They were influenced by the rich cultures of the Mediterranean and Africa."

In fact, Martha Nussbaum, a professor of law and ethics at the University of Chicago, argues that the ancient Greeks — the very pillars of Western tradition — rejected the idea that people should focus on one tradition. In her 1997 book *Cultivating Humanity: A Classical Defense of Reform in Liberal Education*, she writes, "Plato ... alludes frequently to the study of other cultures, especially

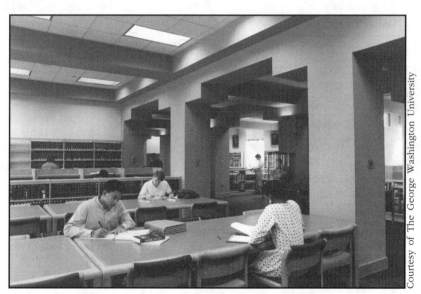

vertical text on right side of image: Courtesy of The George Washington University

Few Schools Require Core Courses

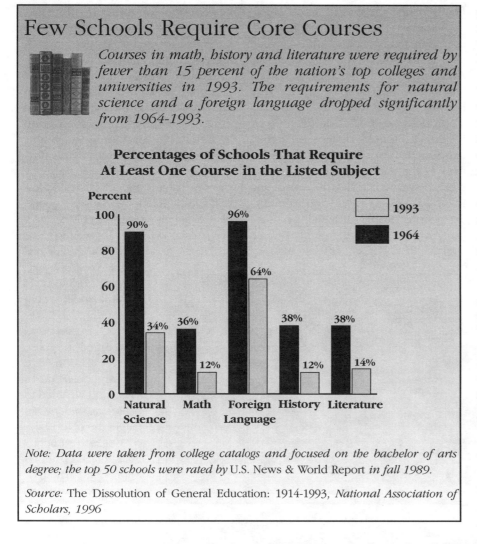

Courses in math, history and literature were required by fewer than 15 percent of the nation's top colleges and universities in 1993. The requirements for natural science and a foreign language dropped significantly from 1964-1993.

Percentages of Schools That Require At Least One Course in the Listed Subject

Percent

1993
1964

	Natural Science	Math	Foreign Language	History	Literature
1964	90%	36%	96%	38%	38%
1993	34%	12%	64%	12%	14%

Note: Data were taken from college catalogs and focused on the bachelor of arts degree; the top 50 schools were rated by U.S. News & World Report in fall 1989.

Source: The Dissolution of General Education: 1914-1993, National Association of Scholars, 1996

those of Sparta, Crete and Egypt." [5]

Advocates of a broader curriculum also argue that a change away from the West makes sense in light of the growing diversity of American students. "The demographics today are very different," says Robert Orrill, executive director of The College Board, a New York City-based association of colleges and universities. "Until recently, a large number of students were of Western European origin, and that is no longer true."

As a result, Orrill and others say, the curriculum should be broadened to reflect other "points of view." Such inclusion — known today as multiculturalism — is among the foundations of an open and free society, they argue. "With greater [student] diversity there needs to be greater cultural diversity," Orrill says. "That's how it is in a democracy."

And, Orrill and others say, broadening the curricula to include non-Western cultures should not be limited to non-white students. "We are interconnected to the rest of the world, economically and in other ways," Musil says. She and others argue that students, regardless of their color or ethnicity, cannot properly prepare to live in an increasingly global society without having at least some understanding of a broad range of cultures. "We are in a transnational world, and we need to be exposed to these other cultures, period," says Peter Magrath, president of the Association of State Universities and Land Grant Colleges.

But proponents of the Western tradition argue that while they favor teaching students about other cultures, the core of any required curriculum should still focus primarily on the writers, ideas and achievements of the West.

To begin with, they say, Americans, regardless of their heritage, live in the West, with Western traditions, institutions and culture. "We live in a Western society, whether we know it or not," says the NAS' Ricketts.

As a result, Ricketts says, students in the United States need a grounding in the Western tradition in order to understand their own society. For example, he and others point out, the Founding Fathers were heavily influenced by Greek and Roman culture as well as by Enlightenment philosophers like Rousseau and Locke. "Notions like equality before the law and democratic institutions come out of the Western tradition," he says.

But this tradition is more than just the foundation of American government. It encompasses every aspect of American life, Ricketts and others argue. "The Western tradition is our shared culture," says George Douglas, a professor of English at the University of Illinois, Champaign-Urbana. Douglas argues that it is important for all Americans to have "common cultural connections" to preserve national unity and cohesiveness. "There's something to be said for all of us reading the same things."

On the other hand, Douglas argues, multiculturalism destroys the idea of shared culture. "When you add a lot of different pieces without any connections, you lose that cohesiveness and the benefits that accrue to society with a shared tradition," he says.

Finally, some opponents of multiculturalism argue that the

achievements of the West far surpass those of any other cultural tradition. "The world is governed by Western models in science, government and other areas," says Schmidt of Illinois College. As a result, he says, the Western tradition is, to a large extent, a global tradition and not just important to Europeans and Americans.

Another problem with broadening the core curriculum, Schmidt and others say, is that many peoples, including American Indians and most sub-Saharan Africans, have not had a written tradition until recently. "What do we have from the American Indians that matches Shakespeare, Dante, Goethe or Sophocles?" he asks, adding: "People say I'm prejudiced, but I say, 'Show me the works.' They can't because [the other groups] don't have the literature available."

But opponents argue that multiculturalism is not an attempt to push Western ideas and history aside. "There is no either-or choice here," Magrath says. "I see no inconsistency in exposing a student to Plato and Aristotle and Confucius and Lao-tse at the same time."

sors who were tardy or did not teach what their young charges wanted could be fined or even fired by them. In a very real sense, the university, founded in the 11th century, was a business whose students were its customers.

Today's universities are different, of course. The faculty, overseen by an administration, sets academic policy on behalf of the students. But some professors and education-watchers are begin-

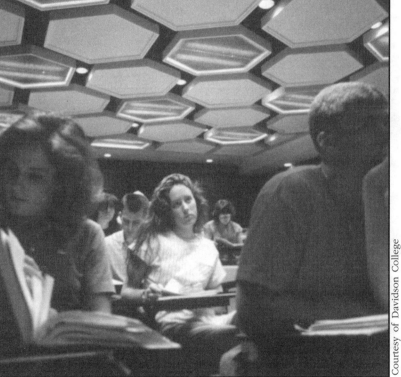

Since the turn of the century, colleges have offered more career-oriented programs like business and communications.

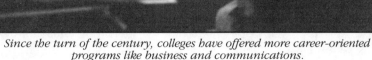

Courtesy of Davidson College

critics is the University of Virginia's Edmundson. In an article published in *Harper's* magazine in September 1997, Edmundson details what he sees as a transformation of the student body and the academy over the last few decades. Today, he writes, the "university culture, like American culture writ large, is, to put it crudely, ever more devoted to consumption and entertainment, to the using and using up of goods and images." [6] As a result, he and others say, learning and real critical thinking take a back seat to enjoyment.

The biggest impact of this trend, according to Edmundson, is that students now want to be entertained continually. Institutions meet some of these needs by spending ever-increasing sums on building plush new dorms, gyms, student centers and other facilities designed to make university life comfortable.

But even more disturbing, Edmundson and others say, is the pressure to please in the classroom. With a clientele that has grown up on television and the Internet, they argue, professors today feel compelled to use a variety of "tricks" to keep their students engaged. "I'm disturbed by the serene belief that my function — and, more important, Freud's or Shakespeare's or Blake's — is to divert, entertain and interest," Edmundson writes. [7]

Schmidt agrees. "We're teaching the "Sesame Street" kids, who have been taught to expect instant gratification —

Have universities become too consumer-driven, focusing on what students want as opposed to what they need in pursuing a liberal education?

The first modern university, in Bologna, Italy, was funded and largely administered by its students. Profes-

ning to complain that many institutions are pandering to their students and giving them too much control. What they call a growing "consumerism" on campus is degrading the quality of education that students receive because they are increasingly getting what they want instead of what they need.

One of the most outspoken of these

What Is a Liberal Education?

The term "liberal arts" is taken from the Latin phrase "liberales artes" (that which should be known by a free man). But the definition of liberal education has never been static.

The Greek philosopher Plato believed that education should focus primarily on civics and social responsibility in order to prepare the best and brightest for their role as leaders in society. Enlightenment thinker Jean Jacques Rousseau, on the other hand, argued that learning should protect a child from civilization's corrupting influences and seek to bring out his natural instincts.

Today, views on the purpose of a liberal arts education still range wide and far. For some educators, a good liberal education teaches how to see the world from a variety of viewpoints. "We need to give students the capacity to grapple with several competing versions of the truth," says Caryn McTighe Musil, a senior research associate at the Association of American Colleges and Universities. The purpose is not to turn students into relativists, or those who see all truth as variable, she argues. Instead, she says, it's about giving students the tools they need "to come to their own conclusions."

To Alvin Schmidt, a professor of sociology at Illinois College in Jacksonville, Ill., the aim of a good liberal education should be knowledge. "Education is about freeing and liberating the human mind from the shackles of ignorance," he says.

Schmidt is troubled by the thought that students can graduate without knowing a foreign language or acquiring a grounding in "core" subjects like philosophy, history and literature.

On the other hand, many educators are more focused on skills. "Students should be able to write and communicate in English," says Yolanda Moses, president of City College of New York. In addition, she says, "it is important that they are able to think analytically." Many educators share Moses' concern that too many students leave college unable to draft a proper letter or give a short speech.

Others, echoing Thomas Jefferson, argue that while knowledge and skills are important, liberal education should also concern itself with turning students into good citizens. "Education should prepare us to live in a democratic society," says Robert Orrill, executive director of The College Board, by focusing on citizenship and social responsibility.

Above all, says Kenneth Pennington, a professor of medieval history at Syracuse University, a liberal arts education must give students the tools they need to spend the rest of their lives learning and thinking. "Most of the time," he says, "teachers don't convey well enough to students that college is only the beginning."

and that learning is fun," he says. But, he says, a lot of learning is sometimes very painful. "For instance, many people don't like conjugating Latin verbs, but you have to do it if you want to learn Latin."

To Edmundson, working with students in the age of instant gratification pressures professors in a variety of ways. In his own case, it has resulted in a change in his style of teaching. For instance, he says, he often finds himself trying to be more funny and affable with students, all in an effort to engage them.

At the same time, Edmundson claims, he and many of his colleagues in the liberal arts are afraid to confront students or challenge them in class for fear of offending them. "Students frequently come to my office to tell me how intimidated they feel in class; the thought of being embarrassed in front of the group fills them with dread," he writes. [8] But, he and others argue, how can you learn if your views and opinions are always affirmed and never questioned?

Teachers also say they are pressured to give students high grades, whether they deserve them or not. "Many students today feel that they are entitled to good grades," says Joseph Scimecca, chairman of the department of sociology and anthropology at George Mason University in Fairfax, Va.

Some of these "offended" students get teachers in trouble by complaining to a receptive administration that believes faculty members must be sensitive to student needs. "Colleges have brought in hordes of counselors and deans to make sure that every-

thing is smooth, serene, unflustered and everyone has a good time," Edmundson writes. [9]

Tougher teachers are also kept in line with evaluations that students fill out at the end of a semester rating their professors' performance. "The bottom line is that if you're rigorous and demand a lot, you get a poor teacher evaluation and don't get tenure," Douglas says. "So you're always pressured to keep [students] happy."

But many other faculty members and education experts argue that most university faculty are not mindlessly pandering to every student whim. In fact, many say, the new consumerism is long overdue because the real problem is that professors and administrators don't listen enough to their students.

"At some point we lost sight of the

students because schools became too professor-oriented," says Musil of the Association of American Colleges and Universities. "There was this feeling that the students were just supposed to sit at the professors' feet and learn."

Syracuse's Pennington agrees. "The real problem is the teachers, who have spent too much time worrying about research," he says. As a result, Pennington and others say, undergraduates have often been ignored by their professors, even at good universities.

Indeed, they argue, teachers who complain about students are often the problem themselves. "In studies that we've done, we've found that faculty members who are effective as teachers are often perceived as effective in their teaching by their students," says Schneider of the Association of American Colleges and Universities. "Those who are not effective often do not like their students."

Hence, many educators argue, universities should spend more time listening to students. "To me, the whole purpose of universities is to focus on students," Magrath says. "We need to put students first."

In addition, he says, there is nothing wrong with treating students, to a certain extent, like customers. "I don't think consumer or customer is a dirty word," he says. The reason, Magrath and others argue, is simple: Students are investing a lot of money and time in their education, and it is unrealistic to think that they won't see universities as they do other businesses. "We are a consumer-driven, marketplace society," he says, "and universities have to keep that in mind when they provide services to students."

And if part of those services include changing long-held teaching methods in order to better relate to the students, then so be it, supporters of consumerism say. "I think the job of a teacher is to convey the information in as interesting and in as compelling a way as is possible," Pennington says. "We need to present material in a way that will arouse students."

Moses of City College agrees that professors shouldn't assume they are pandering when they try to connect with their students. "Learning is multi-

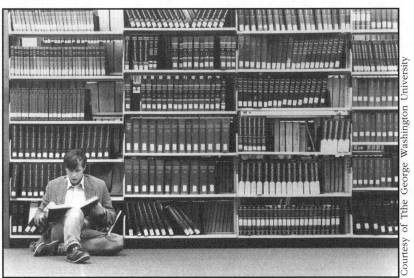

More undergraduates earned degrees in business-related fields in 1995 than in English or the social sciences.

dimensional, encompassing a lot of things," she says, "and you need to be flexible when you're teaching."

Is a liberal arts education the best way to prepare for the workplace?

A recent poll commissioned by Hobart and William Smith Colleges in Geneva, N.Y., found that 75 percent of all parents and 85 percent of their college-bound high-schoolers believe that the goal of higher education is to prepare students for a career. By contrast, only 37 percent of business executives questioned in the same survey felt that career should be the primary focus of education. They were much more supportive of "learning for learning's sake" than were parents or high-schoolers. [10]

Why the disparity between those who are preparing (or helping someone to prepare) for a career and those who will hire them? According to Richard Hersh, president of Hobart and William Smith, the high cost of higher education as well as the perception that the job market is extremely competitive have made parents and children very pragmatic when choosing schools and fields of study. "The smart choice, they say, is a professional program tailored to specific jobs in business, computer technology, engineering, law or medicine," he writes. [11]

By contrast, he says, business executives value employees who are prepared for a long-term career, not just their first job. "But to them [this] means the ability of higher education to produce people of strong character with generalized intellectual and social skills and capacity for lifelong learning." [12]

A century ago there was little argument over how to best take advantage of higher education. To begin with, few people — fewer than 3 percent of the population — actually attended college or university. In addition, 70 percent of those who did go attended liberal arts colleges

Aristotle and Plato Still Reign . . .

What is "natural?" Is something unnatural if it is the product of human labor or invention? Is a wooden table more a part of nature than a jumbo jet?

On a balmy evening recently in Annapolis, Md., 14 college students, sat around a large table and wrestled with such weighty questions, having just read selections from Aristotle's *Physics*.

As is the practice at St. John's College, the students did almost all of the talking. The two professors guiding the session, known as tutors, broke in only occasionally to pose a new question or nudge the inquiry in a new direction.

Such seminars reflect the approach to education at St. John's, "Where great books are the teachers." The college is dedicated to providing "a true liberal arts education" to 850 undergraduates on campuses in Annapolis and Santa Fe, N.M. In the process, it breaks many of the rules by which most institutions of higher education operate today.

The traditional class lecture — common at most colleges and universities in the United States — has largely been discarded at St. John's. Instead, students attend a series of seminars and tutorials each week, where

---

On the Great Books Shelf

St. John's College students study more than 100 works of literature, science and music, including the following:

First Year
Homer: *Illiad, Odyssey*
Sophocles: *Oedipus Rex, Antigone*
Plato: *Meno, The Republic, Apology, Phaedo, Symposium*
Aristotle: *Poetics, Metaphysics, Nicomachean Ethics*
Lucretius: *On the Nature of Things*
Lavoisier: *Elements of Chemistry*

Second Year
The Bible
Virgil : *Aeneid*
Tacitus : *Annals*
St. Augustine: *City of God, Confessions*
Dante: *Divine Comedy*
Machiavelli: *The Prince* **Shakespeare:** *Richard II, Henry IV, The Tempest, As You Like It* **Montaigne:** *Essays*
Bach: *St. Matthew Passion, Inventions*

---

their participation is emphasized, from discussing ideas to demonstrating mathematical principles. Moreover, the usual complement of midterm and final exams does not exist. Grades are given, but they are not shown to students unless they ask for them. And students are encouraged not to ask.

But the most unique thing about St. John's is its curriculum: a four-year tour of the great books and great ideas of the West. There are no majors or minors. And except for two nine-week elective seminars, everyone studies the same subjects.

The great-books curriculum is based on the idea that the issues addressed in the classics of literature, philosophy and science are just as important today as they were when they were written. "The heart of a liberal education is reading very good books, thinking very hard about them and talking about it," says Harvey Flaumenhaft, dean of the Annapolis campus.

Freshmen start with Homer, Plato, Sophocles and other Greek writers and work their way through the great authors of ancient Rome to James Joyce and Virginia Wolff in the 20th century — more than 100 novelists, philosophers and scientists in all. Many are still

---

where courses in subjects like business or journalism did not exist. [13]

Today, the situation could not be more different. Such factors as the expanding middle class and the GI Bill and other government-assistance programs have dramatically increased the number of people going to college. Currently, more than one-third of all high school graduates go on to college (although not all graduate) at one of the more than 3,500 institutions of higher learning around the country.

At the same time, the percentage of students who choose liberal arts has declined dramatically. In 1968, more than 21 percent of all bachelor's degrees were awarded in the hu-

manities. A quarter-century later the figure had dropped to 13 percent. [14]

Today, all but a few four-year colleges offer a wide range of career-oriented majors, from accounting to education to nursing. And the number of occupations that can be quantified and studied increases every year. Today, students can major in fields as diverse as advertising and theater design.

But many liberal arts faculty and some in the business world question whether colleges and universities are doing their students a service by allowing them to study pragmatic fields such as business, with often little or no exposure to the humani-

ties or sciences. Some, like Syracuse's Pennington, go so far as to say that universities should eliminate or largely eliminate professional schools at the undergraduate level and focus solely on the liberal arts.

"Many universities have rejected the idea that there's a core body of knowledge that every student should have, and that's wrong," he says. "When you graduate, you should know something about history, art, music and the great philosophical and religious traditions."

Pennington sees the modern emphasis on more practical fields of study as part of a movement toward what he calls "experiential" learning.

... At St. John's College

widely read like St. Thomas Aquinas, Montaigne, Goethe and Darwin. Others, like the Italian mathematician Evangelista Torricelli and the French statesman Lazare Carnot, are important, although no longer household names.

The great books are not just used to teach literature and philosophy. In the mathematics tutorial, for instance, students learn from Euclid, Ptolemy, Descartes and other giants in the field. The science readings combine the writings of great scientists like Newton and Niels Bohr with work in the laboratory. Rounding out the curriculum are languages (ancient Greek and French) and music.

Some have criticized St. John's for its focus on great books to the exclusion of everything else. "The kind of education you get there is very tight and structured, and the real world isn't like that," says Robert Orrill, executive director of The College Board.

But St. John's students don't feel constricted by the lack of choice. "I needed the structure they offer here," says sophomore Eowyn Levene. Classmate Buck Cooper agrees, adding that many students pursue outside intellectual interests by forming clubs and informal study groups. Indeed, extra groups tackle

---

On the Great Books Shelf

Third Year

Cervantes: *Don Quixote*
Galileo: *Two New Sciences*
Pascal: *Pensees*
Swift: *Gulliver's Travels*
Newton: *Principia Mathematica*
Rousseau: *Social Contract*
Mozart: *Don Giovanni*
Austen: *Pride and Prejudice, Emma*
Melville: *Billy Budd, Benito Cereno*

Fourth Year

Moliere: *The Misanthrope, Tartuffe*
Darwin: *Origin of Species*
Lincoln: *Selected Speeches*
Thoreau: *Walden*
Nietzsche: *Thus Spoke Zarathustra, Beyond Good and Evil*
Dostoevski: *Brothers Karamazov, The Possessed*
Jung: *Two Essays in Analytic Psychology*
Woolf: *To the Lighthouse*
Conrad: *Heart of Darkness*

---

everything from the Bible to the Chinese language.

The students also are not put off by the school's focus on the Western tradition. "There isn't some kind of belief that what we're reading is the only thing worth reading," says Cooper, who spent much of his free time last summer reading the classic texts of the East. And yet, Cooper and others argue, it's important to have an understanding of the works that shape our culture. "We live in the West, and there's no getting around that," says sophomore Marshall Hevrone.

In any event, the process seems to work. The college says that almost 75 percent of its graduates go on to graduate or professional school.

More important, the school generates great enthusiasm for learning. "You don't have to work to get them interested," Flaumenhaft says. Indeed, five minutes after it had begun, more than half the students at the seminar on Aristotle's *Physics* had spoken at least once. There were no pregnant pauses or silent moments as every comment elicited at least one response and usually a question. All the while, the tutors listened, saying almost nothing.

"This is the bane of education because it does not involve reading books or thinking about ideas."

Schmidt largely agrees with Pennington that undergraduate education should focus almost entirely on the liberal arts. "I might let them have a few [career-oriented] courses to whet their appetite," he says, but "the whole purpose of education is to stretch the mind, not train for a job."

In addition, Schmidt argues, narrowly focused training in a career-oriented major will probably give a student little practical knowledge because fields like business and technology change so rapidly. "By the time you finished, it would probably

be out of date," he says. By contrast, "the liberal arts are eternal. The *Odyssey, Crime and Punishment* and *The Aeneid* address concerns that never change."

George Mason's Scimecca sees another practical reason to favor liberal arts. "Look at business leaders: They feel like all their new hires with business degrees are not prepared," he says. "They want people who are literate and can think analytically, and that's what you get with a good liberal arts education."

But others say that the emphasis on liberal arts to the exclusion of everything else is both elitist and unrealistic. Those who favor solely

liberal arts "assume that the same shoe will fit everyone," says the Career College Association's Waddles. "That's a narrow-minded way of looking at things because many kids and their families choose a career-oriented form of study because they have to," he says, referring to students who are less well-off financially and must maximize career opportunities.

Waddles and others argue that some liberal arts supporters are longing for the days when an institution of higher learning "was like some great castle on a hill" guiding students through the halls of rarefied learning. "In the past, you went to college, and they told you what to take and when to take it," he says.

But today, students have much more influence over the direction of their course of study, "And that's a good thing," Waddles says. "People should have as many choices as they can." In other words, if a student wants an all-liberal arts education or one with only career-oriented courses, that's fine.

Colleges and universities embrace this philosophy and have restructured accordingly. "Colleges are simply responding to the demands of parents and students, who want to make sure that when they get a degree they are employable," says Sheldon Steinback, general counsel of the Business-Higher Education Forum.

And, Waddles and Steinback contend, being employable, especially in certain fields, often entails a professional degree. "Talk to employers today," Waddles says, "and they say the first thing they want is specific skills to do a specific job." After that, they look for other skills, like effective communication and analytical thinking, he adds.

Other observers take a more middle-of-the-road view. They favor choice in education, but with some conditions. "I think the best kind of education is one that combines liberal arts and professional study," says Magrath of the Association of State Universities and Land Grant Colleges. He and others argue that it is fine to study business or computer science so long as it offers exposure to the liberal arts as well. The two are not "as inconsistent or incompatible as many people think," Magrath says. ∎

BACKGROUND

Higher Ed Evolves

Although Harvard University and the College of William and Mary were founded before 1700, higher education in the American Colonies did not develop in earnest until the 18th century. Even then, progress was slow. By the time the United States declared independence, the 13 Colonies still had only 10 collegiate institutions.

Most early colleges, like Harvard and Yale, were founded to train ministers. Not surprisingly, their students spent the bulk of their time mastering theology and classical languages.

But there were a few exceptions, most notably the University of Pennsylvania. Founded in 1740, the university (under its first president, Benjamin Franklin) emphasized the natural and social sciences.

Through the 19th century, the number of institutions of higher learning grew at a rapid rate, keeping pace with an America expanding in both area and population. Like earlier colleges, many of the new institutions were founded by Christian denominations with an eye toward training clergy. But as the century progressed, more and more colleges and universities were created with a secular mission, often by state governments.

Before the Civil War, Maryland, Iowa and other states had already established public universities. But in 1862, efforts to create state institutions of higher learning were given a huge boost by congressional passage of the Morrill Act. The law made every state eligible to receive a grant of 30,000 acres of federal land for every senator and representative it had serving in Congress. The land, if accepted by the state, was to be used for the creation of vocational schools known as industrial colleges. [15]

The Morrill Act led to the founding of many so-called land-grant colleges and universities. Many states also allowed existing institutions, including Rutgers, the Massachusetts Institute of Technology and the University of Missouri, to use public property to expand.

The new schools quickly changed the U.S. higher-education landscape. In 1870, fewer than 15,000 Americans were enrolled in institutions of higher learning. By 1895, nearly 25,000 students were attending land-grant colleges and universities alone. [16]

The second half of the 19th century also produced great changes in curriculum. Until the Civil War, most institutions of higher education had no electives. Students followed a set course of study — emphasizing Greek and Latin, rhetoric, theology and mathematics — designed to give them a thorough grounding in the liberal arts.

But after the war, more colleges began deviating from the set curriculum to one that included a choice of disciplines and elective courses. The trend was spearheaded by Charles W. Eliot, president of Harvard from 1869-1909. Eliot believed that in the new, freer and more mobile society taking shape in America students should have greater freedom to choose what they wanted to learn than their more class-conscious counterparts in the Old World. [17]

By 1900, most liberal arts colleges were allowing students to meet the requirements for a bachelor's degree by focusing on one of a variety of disciplines ranging from history to chemistry. In addition, the number and types of courses offered had grown tremendously.

While Eliot was pushing for more choice within the liberal arts, others, particularly at institutions in less-settled parts of the country, began teaching more pragmatic subjects, like agriculture and engineering. At Kansas State University in 1875, for instance, students could take wagon-making, blacksmithing and carving. [18]

New Age, New Mission

During the 20th century, the role of colleges and universities

Chronology

1600s-1700s

American higher education develops slowly and is largely religiously based.

1636
Harvard College is founded near Boston to train ministers. It is the first institution of higher learning in America.

1693
The College of William and Mary is founded in Williamsburg, Va.

1740
The University of Pennsylvania is founded with an emphasis on the natural and social sciences rather than theology.

1795
The University of North Carolina is founded, becoming the first state university.

———— • ————

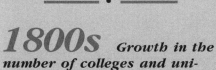

1800s

Growth in the number of colleges and universities accelerates, especially after the Civil War.

1862
Congress passes the Morrill Act, which grants property or money to states for the purpose of higher education and leads to the founding of scores of so-called land-grant colleges and universities.

1869
Charles W. Eliot becomes president of Harvard University and begins instituting reforms, such as elective courses, aimed at giving students more educational choice.

1870
Fewer than 15,000 Americans are enrolled in institutions of higher learning.

———— • ————

1900s

New debates over the purpose of liberal education emerge as the number of students entering college skyrockets, fed by the growth of the middle class and government aid programs.

1900
Institutions of higher education are attended by 238,000 people in the United States.

1915
The Association of American Colleges and Universities is founded to promote liberal education.

1930
The number of Americans enrolled in colleges and universities hits 1 million.

1936
The Higher Learning in America by University of Chicago President Robert Maynard Hutchins calls for education to be a search for great truths.

1937
Educator John Dewey criticizes Hutchins' ideas, sparking a debate between the "pragmatists" and the "idealists" over the purpose of liberal education.

1944
Congress passes the GI Bill of Rights, which provides returning soldiers with financial support for higher education.

1987
University of Chicago Professor Allan Bloom attacks relativism and other trends in higher education in his best-selling book *The Closing of the American Mind.*

1988
After heated debate, Stanford University replaces its "Great Books" requirement with "Cultures, Ideas and Values," a program designed to broaden the required curriculum by including non-Western works.

1995
The Department of Education grants the American Academy for Liberal Education the power to accredit liberal arts colleges.

1996
Brooklyn College announces that it will reorient its core curriculum, prompting a well-publicized debate over the role of general education.

1997
Martha Nussbaum publishes *Cultivating Humanity*, which argues that the concept of multiculturalism is supported by the great writers and thinkers of the classical world.

1998
The Virginia Association of Scholars accuses that state's colleges and universities of "dumbing down" core curricula and urges a back-to-basics approach.

Life at Medieval U. Was No Picnic

The Middle Ages may have been chaotic and violent at times, but they were anything but intellectually bleak. Many of the ideas, inventions and institutions that are fixtures of modern life came into existence then, including the modern university.

Higher learning did not begin in medieval Europe. Sophisticated centers of education had flourished in ancient Greek cities like Athens and Alexandria more than 1,500 years before the first university was founded. But the systematic approach to higher education that characterizes the modern college or university, hinging on formal curricula and exams, only came into being in the late 11th century.

The medieval university has its roots in Italy. For centuries, Italy's many independent or semi-independent towns and cities had grown rich through trade and industry. With economic success came a growing political sophistication that required the new city governments to establish an increasingly complicated legal structure. To seek guidance, administrators turned to the law of ancient Rome.

But few knew or understood Rome's ancient codes, leading to a chronic shortage of capable administrators. The first school, in Bologna, arose to fill that need. By the early 12th century, students from around Europe were flocking to the northern Italian city to study the Code of Justinian and other key Roman laws. By century's end, the school had expanded its curriculum to include rhetoric, canon law and medicine.

During the second half of the 12th century, two of Europe's other important universities were founded. The first, in Paris, was formed by scholars who had congregated around a school affiliated with the city's famed cathedral, Notre Dame. The second, at Oxford, was created by English scholars who had been studying in Paris and were forced to flee when one of the many wars between England and France began in 1167.[1]

These early universities were often loosely organized affairs with little physical or institutional structure. Typically, there were no lecture halls or dormitories. Instead, classes were held in rented rooms, and students were required to provide their own room and board.

Over the next three centuries, universities were founded in Cambridge, Padua, Naples, Heidelberg, Prague and other cities. By 1500, Europe boasted 80 universities, including many where the faculty and administration had become more permanent and structured.

The life of a medieval university student was in many ways harder than that of today's typical undergraduate. Students rose with the sun, often after spending the night in cold, cramped quarters. Each day was devoted largely to class attendance and study.

Lectures were not as free-wheeling as they often are today. Professors spoke *ex cathedra* (from the chair) about a specific text. Often, the teacher simply read the book to the students, who were expected to take copious notes on wax tablets, which were cheaper than parchment. Afterwards, they would neatly recopy their notes on paper.[2]

The language of students and professors (and literature) was Latin, and not only in class. Students were expected to speak only Latin to each other. Those caught conversing in Italian, French or some other vernacular tongue could be penalized.

Unlike today's students, undergraduates in the Middle Ages did not declare majors or take electives. All generally studied the same subjects, which allowed them to change universities (a common practice) without having to begin their studies again.[3]

A liberal arts education was comprised of seven subjects. The first three, known as the trivium, were rhetoric, grammar and logic. When a student had mastered the trivium, he became a bachelor of arts. Next, he moved onto the quadrivium: arithmetic, geometry, music and astronomy. Study of the last four subjects usually lasted five years or more, after which the student became a master of arts.[4]

Students who finished the liberal arts course of study had several options: They could teach at a university or go on to the medieval equivalent of graduate school to study law, medicine or theology. Those who pursued an advanced degree usually faced another four or more years of hard study.

Still, all was not books, writer's cramp and damp rooms. Contemporary accounts indicate that gambling, drunkenness and rowdiness were not uncommon among university students. *Plus ça change.*

---

[1] Brian Tierney and Sidney Painter, *Western Europe in the Middle Ages: 300-1475* (1983), pp. 405-406.

[2] James Powell, *The Civilization of the West* (1967), p. 177.

[3] *Ibid.* p. 178.

[4] Tierney and Painter, *op. cit.*, p. 408.

---

changed dramatically, as the trends that had begun after the Civil War accelerated greatly. The shift toward more practical fields of study continued as professions that had once been learned through apprenticeship were increasingly offered as courses of study.

Some American educators and philosophers, known as the pragmatists, applauded efforts to give higher learning more real-world applications. Led by philosopher and educator John Dewey, they argued that there were no universal truths and that knowledge should focus less on the abstract and more on solving real problems.

Others, who came to be known as the idealists, disagreed. Led by University of Chicago President Robert Maynard Hutchins and, later, philosopher Mortimer Adler, the idealists argued that a traditional liberal arts education based on the great ideas of Western thought was still important. [19] In 1936, Hutchins published *The Higher Learning in America*, which sparked a heated debate between the two schools that continues, in various forms, to this day.

After World War II, colleges and universities again changed. The GI Bill of Rights offered generous government assistance to any ex-serviceman who wanted to go to college. It was followed by student loans and other government programs designed to make higher education affordable to any American who qualified.

The resulting explosion of students seeking a higher education in the 1940s and '50s prompted the expansion of existing schools and the creation of many new ones. The GI Bill generation was followed by the maturing of the baby boomers in the 1960s and '70s. Many of the boomers, born just after World War II, were from newly minted middle-class families that could, for the first time, afford to send their sons and daughters to college.

As the number of students increased, the trend toward more prac-

tical fields of study continued, with schools of business, engineering, nursing, journalism and other professions cropping up on campuses all over America.

Within the liberal arts, big changes came as well, especially after 1960. The number of fields of study expanded tremendously to include so-called interdisciplinary studies, which knitted together a number of different academic areas. [20] For instance, American studies, an especially popular discipline, encompassed history, political science, lit-

erature and other fields.

Another trend in liberal education has been the movement to focus more on non-Western cultures. Before World War II, courses on Asia or Africa were rare, even at the best universities. By the 1970s, many schools were forming new departments to study the language, history and culture of non-Western peoples. ∎

CURRENT SITUATION

Curriculum Battles

In late 1996, Brooklyn College announced that it was going to "reorient" the institution's famed core curriculum. Instead of the existing 10 required courses — among them "The Classical Origins of Western Culture," "Knowledge, Existence and Values" and "Landmarks of Literature" — future students would fulfill graduation requirements by taking classes offered in a broad, new program called "Brooklyn Connections." The new, less rigid core curriculum would be organized around four "themes": Community Studies, Communications, Environmental Studies and Science Studies. [21]

By summer 1997, a growing number of faculty and alumni were demanding that the traditional curriculum not be replaced. Calling "Connections" a radical departure from the college's liberal arts mission, they argued it would give students only "skills and tactics, not bodies of knowledge." [22]

A letter released by a group of prominent alumni, including scholars Gertrude Himmelfarb and Eugene D.

Many educators want liberal education to focus on the Western tradition, but others say it should embrace all cultures.

Courtesy of Davidson College

Genovese, said implementation of the new scheme would be a "tragic mistake." [23] And a number of local newspaper articles portrayed the new plan in an unfavorable light.

But "Connections" had supporters as well. Many faculty members and administration officials argued that it was intended to expand the core curriculum to include issues — like environmental and community studies — that were closer to the real world and the everyday lives of Brooklyn's students.

Still, within months of the alumni letter, Brooklyn College President Vernon E. Lattin announced that "Connections" would in no way replace the core curriculum and that any impression to the contrary was due to confusion and misunderstanding.

Cuts to the 'Core'

Similar curriculum battles have taken place all over the country. And, according to a recent study of the nation's top 50 colleges and universities by the NAS, the advocates of change appear to be winning. It concluded that "during the last 30 years the general-education programs of most of our best institutions have ceased to demand that students become familiar with the basic facts of their country's history, political and economic systems, philosophic traditions and literary and artistic legacies that were once conveyed through mandated and preferred survey courses."- [24]

For instance, the NAS report states, the average number of required courses at the 50 schools surveyed dropped from 9.9 in 1914 to 6.9 in 1964 to 2.5 in 1993. More specifically,

90 percent of the institutions required students to take at least one course in the natural sciences in 1964, compared with 34 percent in 1993. The percentage of institutions with history requirements dropped during the same period from 38 percent to 12 percent. [25]

The NAS and other critics say that many universities have replaced general survey courses with no requirements at all or a broad range of often-unrelated classes that the student can

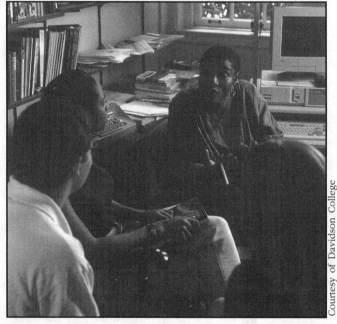

Liberal arts education is expected to become more popular in the future because it enhances career flexibility.

choose from. "A [selective] college like Dartmouth — or Harvard, Princeton, etc. — has requirements so broadly defined that almost anything goes," wrote Jeffrey Hart, who teaches English at Dartmouth. [26] At George Mason, for example, students can choose from 419 different classes to fulfill their four core requirements. [27]

Moreover, critics of the anti-core curricula trend argue, many of the classes students can choose to fulfill requirements are very specialized and of questionable value. A member of the Vir-

ginia Council on Higher Education recently noted that parents would be "flabbergasted" to learn that students at Virginia Polytechnic Institute could take a course in basic floral design to satisfy an art history requirement. [28]

Leaving basic curriculum choices to students is dangerous, the critics argue, because many are not qualified enough or mature enough to understand what their educational needs are. "Many students don't think a great deal about what they study," says the NAS' Ricketts, "which is why requirements are so important."

Without educational requirements, Ricketts and others say, students end up with few of the cultural reference points they need to be well-informed, well-educated people. "Educators always talk about concepts instead of facts today," says Schmidt of Illinois College. "But you can't understand the concept unless you know the facts behind it." For instance, he says, many students don't have even a rudimentary knowledge of the key players, places and dates of the American Revolution or the Civil War. "How can you truly know about the Civil War when you don't know when it occurred?" he asks.

But many educators say that people with Schmidt's point of view are alarmists who are clinging to an old way of learning by focusing too much on imprinting certain kinds of knowledge on students. They argue that schools can't just assume that if they've provided students with a broad survey of the humanities and sciences they will be educated.

"I don't want 'bingo' education, where you pick one course from

Courtesy of Davidson College

At Issue:

Should a liberal arts education primarily entail the study of Western civilization?

ALVIN J. SCHMIDT
Professor of sociology, Illinois College

WRITTEN FOR THE CQ RESEARCHER, APRIL 1998

*t*o be well-educated, students need to know and understand the underlying foundations of Western civilization. They also need to know the noteworthy contributions it has made to their nation and to much of the world. Here are a few key examples:

• From the Bible's portrayal of a rational God, Western thinkers concluded that human beings — the crown of creation — also were rational beings, capable of critical thinking, of discovering objective knowledge and truth, deductively and inductively. Without these premises, the world would still be in the pre-Industrial Age.

• In the Middle Ages, the monasteries of the Christian church created universities. Here knowledge was discovered and disseminated, giving rise to the seven liberal arts: grammar, rhetoric, logic, arithmetic, geometry, astronomy and music. All enriched human life.

• The brilliant Greek philosophers theorized, but because of their low view of manual labor they never tested their theories. With Christianity dignifying manual work, the West linked theory to practice, making it possible for modern science to appear.

• The Greco-Romans had no hospitals for their people. Hospitals were first built in the fourth century as Christians, moved by Christ's compassion, cared for the sick.

• The Athenians introduced a limited democracy. But England's Magna Carta and America's Declaration of Independence and Constitution made government by the people a reality. These documents often inspire nascent democracies today.

• At times, the West mimicked some of the evil practices of other cultures, such as its treatment of women and slavery. But it was the first to repent of these sins. It has elevated the rights of women, whereas in some non-Western societies women still have very few rights. Inspired by Christian leaders, the British were the first to outlaw slavery in the 1830s. Thirty years later America followed suit. In India, slavery existed until 1976, and African Sudan still has slavery.

We cannot afford to dilute or cut the lifeline of a liberal arts education — the study of Western civilization — because of a self-imposed guilt complex, prompted by the propaganda of anti-Western multiculturalists. Students have the right to see and understand how the knowledge, insights and contributions of Western civilization, unlike those of any other civilization, have benefited billions of people.

CAROL GEARY SCHNEIDER
President, Association of American Colleges and Universities

WRITTEN FOR THE CQ RESEARCHER, APRIL 1998

*o*ur current debates about societal diversity and multiculturalism are part of a continuing negotiation over the meaning and application of this nation's fundamental democratic principles. The Founders espoused equal dignity, liberty and justice for all. They laid a foundation for pluralism by accepting religious diversity and by a constitutional design that allowed states with disparate histories and cultures to live together in a federated republic. They challenged earlier views that a republic must be small and homogeneous to succeed. Instead, Americans with a vision for a new society opted for diversity.

Today, similar debates about the small, homogeneous republic vs. the diverse, democratic society are being waged in higher education. The college curriculum, which underwent revolutionary changes at the turn of the century, is changing again to provide students with the skills needed to lead this diverse American democracy in the future. Simultaneously, the curriculum is also changing in order to foster knowledge of global cultures, and of the connections between distant regions and new American communities sprouting up in all parts of the United States.

The question, then, is not whether we should address diversity and multiculturalism in the curriculum, but how to do it in ways that strengthen our democratic commitments. Drawing from myriad traditions, we must keep in mind always the founding commitments to liberty, equality, justice and voice, not only for individuals but for all the communities and cultures that are the nursery of our democracy.

In this spirit, the Association of American Colleges and Universities has released a set of recommendations for addressing diversity in the college curriculum. Economic realities have already answered the question whether students "ought" to learn about global cultures. We have warned that it would be a mistake to view courses on world cultures and United States diversity as interchangeable, or that giving attention to U.S. diversity can be optional. "Education for United States democratic and cultural pluralism," we observed in a recent report titled "American Pluralism and the College Curriculum," "is just as important as global study and deserves its own space and time in the curriculum." This study should include knowledge of diverse cultural traditions and histories, including one's own. The goal is to graduate students who are both prepared and inspired to take responsibility for the future of our diverse democracy.

Column A and another from Column B and then shout: 'Bingo! I'm educated,' " says Robert Zeminsky, director of the Institute for Research on Higher Education. Instead, Zeminsky says, schools need to help students grow other skills as well. "We're focused on the question of whether the student develops a real capacity to learn and to apply his knowledge to the world," he says.

Applying knowledge to the here and now is important, argues Schneider of the Association of American Colleges and Universities: "There is and there should be a determination in the world of higher education to engage learning with important contemporary issues, to make it more relevant to the present." For instance, she says, students should be able to learn about the creation of the American republic more than 200 years ago and, at the same time, compare it with the fight by Nelson Mandela and others to create democratic institutions in South Africa today.

Efforts to make knowledge more relevant are vital, says City College's Moses, because they offer students more opportunities to learn and connect what they've learned to other knowledge. "We must provide multiple points of entry for students to give them what they want," she says. ∎

OUTLOOK

Liberal Arts Revival

Educators may argue about the direction liberal arts education should take, but most involved in the debate agree on one thing: In the future, liberal educations will become more, not less, important than they are today.

Ironically, it is the changing nature of work that is brightening the future for liberal arts education, the experts say. Vocational study, while still valued, does not have the flexibility to effectively prepare many of the people who are entering the new world of shifting careers.

"Most of us will have four or five careers in our lifetime," Moses says. "So training you in one area or field won't get you another job."

But a liberal arts education, with its broad fields of study and emphasis on communication and analytical thinking, will give graduates the ability to move from one job to another. "In a way, liberal arts education prepares you for all careers," Moses says.

The question then becomes: How will liberal arts education change, if at all, in the coming decades? Many conservatives see a rollback of multiculturalism and other educational "fads," like interdisciplinary studies. "You can already see some kids rebelling against this stuff,"

Ricketts says. "They want a more traditional education."

The University of Illinois' Douglas agrees. "In a generation or two, this ideological and politically correct stuff will be overturned. People will become disenchanted and demand a return to more traditional methods."

And yet, Ricketts and others say, the change will not come overnight. "The people who hold such views are outfunded and outgunned right now," he says.

Schmidt goes a step further, arguing that things will get much worse for traditionalists before they get better. "This kind of thing is hard to fight because we have lost our moral foundations, and in the postmodern era truth is relative and a lie is not a lie."

But many say that the proponents of traditionalism are screaming into the wind. "They've lost the war even if they are very strategic in their arguments," says Musil at the Association of American Colleges and Universities. While the conservatives are still arguing "about what you can read," everyone else has gotten on with teaching and learning. "They don't realize how much excitement there is on campus today between students and professors."

Magrath of the Association of State Universities and Land Grant Colleges agrees. "This whole idea that we've gone to hell in a handbasket is nonsense," he says. "We have more educated and more cultured people today than we've ever had before." ■

Notes

[1] Cited in *The Chronicle of Higher Education, 1997-1998 Almanac Issue*, Aug. 29, 1997.

[2] Mark Edmundson, "On the Uses of a Liberal Education: As Lite Entertainment for Bored College Students," *Harper's*, September 1997.

[3] Allan Bloom, *The Closing of the American Mind: How Higher Education Has Failed Democracy and Impoverished the Souls of Today's Students* (1987), pp. 62-67.

[4] See Dinesh D'Souza, *Illiberal Education: The Politics of Race and Sex on Campus* (1991), p. 59. For background, see "Academic Politics," *The CQ Researcher*, Feb. 16, 1996, pp. 145-168.

[5] Martha Nussbaum, *Cultivating Humanity: A Classical Defense of Reform in Liberal Education* (1997), p. 55.

[6] Quoted in Edmundson, *op. cit.*

[7] *Ibid.*

[8] *Ibid.*

[9] *Ibid.*

[10] For background see Richard Hersh, "Intentions and Perceptions: A National Survey of Public Attitudes Toward Liberal Arts Education," *Change*, March/April, 1997.

[11] *Ibid.* For background, see "Getting Into College," *The CQ Researcher*, Feb. 23, 1996, pp. 169-192, and "Paying for College," *The CQ Researcher*, Nov. 20, 1992, pp. 1001-1022.

[12] *Ibid.*

[13] *Ibid.*

[14] Edmundson, *op. cit.*

[15] George Roche, *The Fall of the Ivory Tower* (1994), pp. 28-29.

[16] Daniel J. Boorstin, *The Americans: The Democratic Experience* (1973), p. 486.

[17] *Ibid.* pp. 493-494.

[18] *Ibid*, p. 485.

[19] George M. Marsden, *The Soul of the American University* (1994), p. 376.

[20] Robert Orrill (ed.), *Education and Democracy: Re-imagining Liberal Learning in America* (1997), pp. 141-142.

[21] Denise K. Magner, "Professors and Influential Alumni Join Forces to Protect Brooklyn College's Core Curriculum," *The Chronicle of Higher Education*, Oct. 17, 1997.

[22] Quoted in *Ibid*. For background, see "What Should College Students Be Taught?" *Editorial Research Reports*, Jan. 5, 1990, pp. 1-16.

[23] Quoted in *Ibid*.

[24] The National Academy of Scholars, *The Dissolution of General Education: 1914-1993*, 1996.

[25] *Ibid.*

[26] Jeffrey Hart, "How to Get a College Education," *The National Review*, Sept. 30, 1996.

[27] Victoria Benning, "Va. Colleges Are Goofing Off, Group Says," *The Washington Post*, Feb. 14, 1998.

[28] Quoted in *Ibid.*

Bibliography

Selected Sources Used

Books

Bloom, Allan, *The Closing of the American Mind*, Simon & Schuster, 1987.

The late University of Chicago professor traced what he deemed to be the precipitous decline of higher learning. He concluded in the runaway best-seller that students, even at the nation's best universities, were being fed a diet devoid of intellectual and spiritual nourishment. To revive university educational fare, Bloom recommended, among other things, a return to key texts and ideas of the Western tradition.

D'Souza, Dinesh, *Illiberal Education: The Politics of Race and Sex on Campus*, The Free Press, 1991.

D'Souza, a fellow at the American Enterprise Institute, chronicles what he sees as absurd and damaging trends in the academy, from multiculturalism and Afrocentrism to affirmative action. He concludes that "the current revolution of minority victims threatens to destroy the highest ideals of liberal education, and with them enlightenment and understanding, which hold out the only prospects for racial harmony, social justice and minority advancement."

Marsden, George M., *The Soul of the American University: From Protestant Establishment to Established Nonbelief*, Oxford University Press, 1994.

Marsden chronicles the declining role of religion at colleges and universities and the impact on higher education.

Nussbaum, Martha C., *Cultivating Humanity: A Classical Defense of Reform in Liberal Education*, Harvard University Press, 1997.

Nussbaum, a professor of law and ethics at the University of Chicago, argues that multiculturalism and other educational trends attacked by conservatives are supported by the great writers and thinkers of the classical world. For instance, she notes, Plato encouraged the study of other cultures.

Orrill, Robert (ed.), *Education and Democracy: Reimagining Liberal Learning in America*, The College Board, 1997.

Orrill, executive director of The College Board, has put together a collection essays by various scholars on the future of liberal education and its role in preparing students as citizens.

Schmidt, Alvin, *The Menace of Multiculturalism: Trojan Horse In America*, Praeger, 1997.

Schmidt, a professor of sociology at Illinois College, argues against multiculturalism as an ideology. In the end, he writes, it will lead to a nation fragmented along ethnic lines.

Articles

Edmundson, Mark, "On the Uses of a Liberal Education: As Lite Entertainment for the Bored College Students," *Harpers*, September 1997.

Edmundson, a professor at the University of Virginia, examines the attitudes of the current crop of college students and finds them wanting. Instead of looking to be challenged and changed by courses, undergraduates today want to be entertained, he writes. Edmundson blames their attitude on the prevailing consumer culture — TV and computers in particular — which has created a generation of students that seeks instant gratification, even in education.

Hart, Jeffrey, "How to Get a College Education," *National Review*, Sept. 30, 1996.

Hart, a professor at Dartmouth College, bemoans the lack of basic knowledge that so-called educated people have. At Dartmouth, he writes, freshmen arrive with little or no understanding of their culture, and many leave the same way, since the school has few liberal arts requirements.

Leatherman, Courtney, "10 Years After Bloom's Jeremiad Scholars Weigh Its Significance," *The Chronicle of Higher Education*, Jan. 17, 1997.

Leatherman examines the debate sparked by *The Closing of the American Mind* 10 years after its publication. She finds that the book and the issues it raised are still being debated.

Magner, Denise K., "Professors and Influential Alumni Join Force to Protect Brooklyn College's Core Curriculum," *The Chronicle of Higher Education*, Oct.. 17, 1997.

Magner details the recent battle over the fate of the core curriculum at Brooklyn College and the thus-far unsuccessful attempt to "reorient" it away from the 10 broad survey courses.

Reports

American Association of Colleges and Universities, *The Academy in Transition: Contemporary Understandings of Liberal Education*, 1998.

The report examines the changes that are taking place in American higher education, from new methods of instruction to the role of technology.

National Association of Scholars, The Dissolution of General Education: 1914-1993, 1996.

The association, which favors more liberal arts requirements, traces the decline of mandatory courses at 50 top universities.

6 Encouraging Teen Abstinence

KATHY KOCH

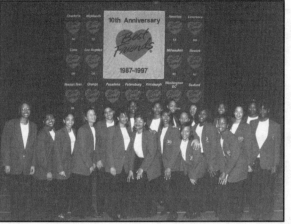

S aying "no" to sex, drugs and alcohol has been easy for 18-year-old Latasha Lewis. The secret of her success: She had Best Friends by her side.

"Best Friends taught me to stand up for what I believe in," says the Ohio Wesleyan University sophomore. "It gave me the extra support I needed to stand up to peer pressure. And it's an extra shoulder to lean on when you're not at home."

Lewis and 800 other students from across the country gathered recently at the group's annual rally in Washington, D.C., to salute the program, whose adult mentors help girls from the fifth to eighth grade avoid premarital sex and finish high school.

In doing so, participants are clearly going against the national grain. Girls of all races are experimenting with sex at younger and younger ages, experts say. The percentage of girls who have had sex before age 15 jumped from 11 percent in 1988 to 19 percent in 1995. The number of boys who had sex before 15, meanwhile, remained stable at 21 percent. [1]

Yet 84 percent of young girls say they want to know "how to say 'no' without hurting the other person's feelings." [2]

Best Friends is one of thousands of groups teaching both girls and boys to say no, and now there is federal money to help. Under a controversial "abstinence-only" block grant program — a dividend of the 1996 welfare reform law — grant recipients must teach teens to remain chaste until marriage. To send teens an unambiguous message, Congress said the money could not be used to teach teens about contraception or how to protect themselves from sexu-

From *The CQ Researcher,*
July 10, 1998.

ally transmitted diseases.

Because of the restrictions, many governors hesitated at applying for the grants. But eventually all 50 governors applied, alarmed that America has the highest teen birth rate in the industrialized world and faces increasing numbers of illegitimate babies, who often end up on welfare.

The grants account for about half of the $837.5 million the welfare reform bill obligated state and federal agencies to spend over five years to discourage childbearing among teens and unmarried adults.

The federal funding gave a big boost to the growing abstinence movement, which seeks to reinsert "values" and personal responsibility into teens' sexual behavior. [3] The conservative-led movement picked up steam in the 1990s, and now thousands of American youths are joining chastity clubs, signing abstinence pledge cards and proudly declaring their virginity.

"Ten years ago, abstinence was almost something you couldn't mention," says Peter Brandt, executive director of the National Coalition for Abstinence Education, an ad hoc group monitoring implementation of the block grants. "Now the culture is embracing it."

National statistics appear to confirm the trend toward abstinence, but only among older teens from the suburbs. From 1990 to 1995, the

percentage of all teens ages 15-19 who had ever had intercourse declined from 55 percent to 50 percent, reversing steady increases since the 1970s. Most of the decrease was among black and white suburban teens. And only 38 percent said they had had sex in the last three months, compared with 42 percent in 1988, suggesting some teens are having sex less frequently. [4]

"Abstinence is unquestionably in vogue," says Rebekah Saul, a policy analyst for the Alan Guttmacher Institute, which conducts research and policy analysis in reproductive health issues.

Abstinence may be gaining in the suburbs, but the number of sexually active, inner-city black teenagers remains about the same as in 1988. Hispanic teenagers, on the other hand, are having sex at significantly higher levels today than in 1988, according to the National Center for Health Statistics.

But while their older siblings may be cooling their jets, younger teens apparently aren't getting the message. "[Teachers] talk about not having sex before marriage, but no one listens," says 13-year-old Shana, from Denver. "I use that class for study hall." [5]

The jury is still out, however, on whether teaching abstinence results in fewer pregnancies, especially when taught without birth-control information.

In 1992, with broad bipartisan support and an extensive media campaign, California launched the largest statewide abstinence-only effort ever initiated. Some 187,000 middle-schoolers in 31 counties attended fairs, rallies and assemblies urging them to postpone sex. They received five hours of instruction on how to resist peer pressure to have sex. Three years and $15 million later, participants were no less likely to avoid sex, pregnancy or sexually transmit-

Teen Sexual Activity Varies Widely

Fewer than 30 percent of U.S. 15-year-olds had had intercourse in 1995. But more than half of the 17-year-olds and three-quarters of the 19-year-olds were not virgins.

Teens 15-19 Who Have Had Sexual Intercourse, 1995

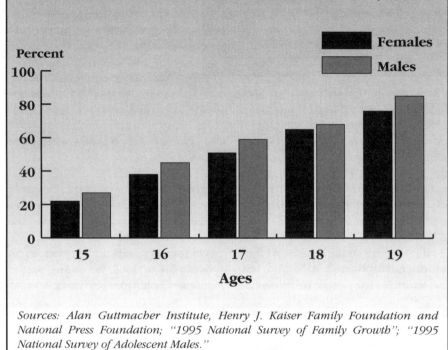

Sources: Alan Guttmacher Institute, Henry J. Kaiser Family Foundation and National Press Foundation; "1995 National Survey of Family Growth"; "1995 National Survey of Adolescent Males."

ted diseases (STDs) than teens in a control group. [6]

In December 1995, Republican Gov. Pete Wilson scrapped the much-heralded program, saying, "We need a much more comprehensive strategy to deal with out-of-wedlock pregnancy."

Yet eight months later, while putting final touches on the welfare reform bill, Congress quietly voted to spend $250 million over five years for abstinence-only programs. Since the states will chip in $187.5 million in matching funds, the total being spent for abstinence education is $437.5 million. Congress also promised an additional $400 million bonus over four years to the five states showing the greatest drop in unwed motherhood without increasing abor-

tion rates.

Americans have been arguing about what to teach kids about sex for decades. As a result, sex education has always been a strictly local affair — a patchwork of curricula based on the widely divergent sensibilities of the nation's different communities. Nonetheless, 93 percent of U.S. high schools today offer some kind of sexuality or HIV-AIDS education.

Congress' new abstinence-only law added a few caveats to the perennial chastity vs. birth control debate. The law not only prohibits teaching about contraception but also requires teenagers to be taught that adults in America are expected to refrain from extramarital sex because it "is likely to have harm-

ful psychological and physical effects."

Reflecting the new wrinkle in the controversy, more than 600 sex-ed battles are now being fought in school districts throughout the country, according to the nonprofit Sexuality Information and Education Council of the U.S. (SIECUS). In 1994, by comparison, only 200 local sex-ed battles were being fought.

Polls show that while most parents want their teenagers to abstain from sex at least until they finish high school, the majority also want schools to teach about contraception. [7]

Refusing to provide contraceptive information leaves teenagers "defenseless," says Henry Foster, an obstetrician who is special adviser to President Clinton on reducing teen pregnancy. "They don't have the facts on how to protect themselves, yet they are bombarded with media messages" telling them to "just do it."

"You're turning your back on those kids who choose not to abstain," Foster says, abandoning them to cope with raging hormones in a sexually saturated culture that "titillates and stimulates kids in dress, song, dance and images."

Abstinence advocates argue just as vehemently that teaching about "safe sex" is fundamentally dishonest because condoms are not 100 percent effective. Moreover, they say, teaching about birth control gives teenagers tacit approval to have sex. Decades of "safe-sex" education and easier teenage access to confidential services offering contraceptives and abortions have produced a generation of teens who treat sex casually and irresponsibly, they say. As evidence, they cite alarming news reports about sexual behavior among children, from fourth-graders found having oral sex in an empty Washington, D.C., classroom to a syphilis outbreak among 22 affluent Atlanta girls who gave public health officials 450 names as potential past sex partners.

By giving teens "non-directive" sex

education, wrote Patricia Funderburk Ware, former director of the Bush administration's adolescent pregnancy program, society has "abdicated its responsibility to instill values in this generation of young people. We've left childrearing to the TV executives and video producers." [8]

A California gang member seemed to echo Funderburk's concerns. Then 17-year-old Eric Richardson, whose gang was accused of raping hundreds of girls, some only 10, told a reporter in 1993: "They pass out condoms, teach sex education and pregnancy-this and pregnancy-that. But they don't teach us any rules." [9]

Birth-control proponents, meanwhile, say that the declines in teen sexual activity, births and abortions prove that their efforts are working. (See graph, p. 96.) Indeed, they say, the rates are down because teens use birth control more than ever before: From 1975-1995, the percentage of teenagers who used condoms the first time they had sex tripled, increasing from 18 percent to 54 percent.

But abstinence groups say birthrates are down because teens are abstaining. "It's due to less sex, not more protected sex," Brandt says.

Family planners warn, however, that switching to abstinence-only education could reverse the positive trends. "We'd be taking the reverse path from the Europeans, who have the lowest rates of STDs, teen pregnancy and abortions" even though their teens are just as sexually active as Americans, says Gloria Feldt, president of the Planned Parenthood Federation of America.

Sex education is universally taught and contraception easily accessible in many European countries, Feldt notes. In addition, sexually active European teens generally use condoms and birth control pills simultaneously, while American teenagers in recent years primarily have used condoms and dramatically re-duced their use of "the pill." (See sidebar, p. 106.)

To move the debate forward, the bipartisan National Campaign to Prevent Teen Pregnancy persuaded the perennially warring camps — both represented on its board — to adopt the goal of reducing adolescent pregnancies by one-third by 2005. Both sides agreed, moreover, that a clear message should be sent: Teenage pregnancy — especially if you're not married — is not OK.

"It's a breakthrough, really," says Kristin A. Moore, president of Child Trends, a Washington-based research firm, and a member of the campaign's Board of Trustees. "It's a very pragmatic approach that basically tries to get the adults to stop arguing and concentrate on solving the problem." The campaign left it up to the opposing sides to "do what they do best" to bring the pregnancy rate down.

But lowering the pregnancy rate faces big obstacles:

• Although teen birthrates have dropped in recent years, a million American teenagers — 76 percent of them unwed — still get pregnant every year, according to the Alan Guttmacher Institute. And U.S. teens have twice as many pregnancies per capita as their counterparts in England, Wales or Canada and nine times more than in the Netherlands or Japan.

• Although U.S. teens are having less sex, younger kids are becoming sexually active earlier and earlier, especially in urban areas.

• STDs are rampant among U.S. teens, with 3 million new cases reported each year. STD rates are 50-100 times higher in the U.S. than in other industrialized countries, according to the Centers for Disease Control and Prevention (CDC).

• The percentage of American girls ages 15-17 who were unmarried when they gave birth has more than tripled, from 23 percent in 1950 to 84 percent in 1996. [10]

As educators and health officials grapple with the nation's high teen birthrate, these are some of the questions they are asking:

Is abstinence-only education good for teenagers?

Today's teenagers face a much more dangerous sexual landscape than their baby boom parents did during the sexual revolution. In the 1960s, syphilis and gonorrhea — both easily treatable with penicillin — were the most common STDs. Today, there is HIV-AIDS as well as more than 20 other newly discovered sexually transmitted diseases. And one in five Americans are infected with a penicillin-resistant viral STD. [11]

But the new abstinence-only grants stipulate that grant recipients can only teach students to abstain from sex. They are not permitted to discuss birth control.

"Sex is a serious business, and it's for adults only," says Elayne Bennett, founder of Best Friends and wife of former Education Secretary William J. Bennett. "When one spends a lot of time instructing teens on all the various paraphernalia for protecting themselves, the message is that it's perfectly safe to do this as long as you protect yourself. But we know that [using protection] does not protect against many STDs."

"The public debate on this whole issue has centered around condoms," Brandt says. "That was a mistake. The reality of the situation is that sexual abstinence is the only way for kids to avoid out-of-wedlock pregnancies and STDs."

Obstetrician Joe S. McIlhaney Jr. of Austin, Texas, agrees so strongly with the abstinence approach that he quit his medical practice and founded the Medical Institute for Sexual Health to counteract what he calls the government's "dishonest" message that condoms can make sex "safe."

What You Should Know About Teen Sex

■ Although teen birthrates have dropped in recent years, a million American teenagers ages 15-19 still get pregnant every year — 76 percent of them unwed. [1]

■ Although teens overall are having less sex, younger kids are becoming sexually active earlier, especially in urban areas. For example, in 1995, 17 percent of 15-year-old girls were sexually active, compared with 3 percent in the 1950s. More black youths (24 percent) initiate intercourse before age 13 than Hispanic (8.8 percent) or white students (5.7 percent). [2]

■ Sexually transmitted diseases (STDs) are rampant among U.S. teens, with 3 million new cases reported each year. STD rates are 50-100 times higher in the United States than in other industrialized countries. [3]

■ Only 70 percent of adolescent mothers finish high school. Teen mothers and their children have more health problems than adult mothers and their children. The federal government spends $39 billion a year to support families begun by teen mothers. [4]

■ Children of teenagers have more social and behavioral problems than other children, and they are more likely to become teen parents later.

■ Children raised by unwed mothers are more likely to end up in prison. Some 70 percent of long-term prison inmates grew up without fathers, as did 60 percent of rapists and 75 percent of teens charged with murder. [5]

■ Fatherless children are 40 times more likely to experience child abuse and three times more likely to fail at school and commit suicide. [6]

[1] Fact Sheet, Alan Guttmacher Institute, 1996.
[2] "Sex and America's Teenagers," Alan Guttmacher Institute, 1994, and "Youth Risk Behavior Surveillance, 1995," Centers for Disease Control and Prevention.
[3] "Facts in Brief," Alan Guttmacher Institute, 1993.
[4] Advocates for Youth.
[5] The Hudson Institute.
[6] Ibid.

McIlhaney says condoms fail to prevent pregnancy up to 13 percent of the time and don't protect against AIDS 31 percent of the time. Such failure rates are "unacceptable when compounded over five to 10 years" of premarital sexual activity, he says, since most teens don't use condoms consistently and correctly, especially when alcohol or drugs are involved.

But the CDC says the 31 percent AIDS failure rate cited by McIlhaney is from an outdated and "flawed" 1993 study by researcher Susan C. Weller. [12] In fact, two newer, larger studies show that condoms are "highly effective" against AIDS, according to the CDC. The new studies show condoms fail less than 2 percent of the time, when used correctly and consistently. [13]

McIlhaney also points out that condoms don't protect against the human papilloma virus (HPV), an STD raging among today's teens. The virus causes venereal warts and is suspected as a major cause of cervical cancers and precancerous cervical changes, both increasing among young women in recent years, he says.

Condoms do not protect against chlamydia, the nation's most rampant STD, which can cause sterility if left untreated, he argues. The CDC says there is little research as to whether condoms protect against chlamydia. McIlhaney also says that condoms are not very effective against genital herpes, which is increasing among teenagers faster than among the general population.

McIlhaney points out that sexually active younger teens are up to 10 times more susceptible to pelvic inflammatory disease (PID) than adult women because teen reproductive systems are undeveloped. "PID is the most rapidly increasing cause of infertility in the U.S. and is a primary reason for the 600 percent increase in ectopic pregnancies since 1970," McIlhaney writes. [14]

Given all this evidence, promoting condom use among teenagers is dangerous, McIlhaney says. "The best that 'safer-sex' approaches can offer is some risk reduction. Abstinence, on the other hand, offers risk elimination," he writes.

Critics say McIlhaney's anti-condom approach is dangerous, especially for the 50 percent of teens already sexually active. "Young people may get the impression that condoms are not effective" and stop using them, warns SIECUS President Debra Haffner.

Presidential adviser Foster agrees that a strong abstinence message is wise for younger teens, but he says it's dangerous to let teens enter high school uninformed about how to protect themselves. "We should tell kids to abstain, but they also need to know how to protect themselves from diseases," Foster says. "They aren't going to stay middle school kids forever."

Because teens often do the opposite of what adults advise, keeping them ignorant about protecting themselves is irresponsible, he says, especially in the AIDS era.

Telling kids to "just say no" leads to what public health experts call the "swept away" syndrome, in which teens know they are supposed to abstain so they don't carry condoms. Then they end up having sex in the heat of the moment, without protection.

Even though polls show most Americans want contraception taught in schools, abstinence advocates say parents should be the ones to tell kids about birth control.

"It's nice to say that the parents should be the ones to educate their kids about sex," Foster says, "But what if the parents never learned all the facts themselves?"

"When you've got a 12-year-old girl whose mother is a drug addict and her daddy's in prison, who teaches her?" asked Gilbert Burnett, a retired judge who runs a pregnancy-prevention program in North Carolina. "What do we do? Forget about her?" [15]

Sex educators also object strenuously to Congress' requirement that educators teach that marriage is the standard for human sexual activity in the United States, and that extramarital sex is psychologically and physically harmful. It's "unrealistic, irresponsible and hypocritical" to tell kids that "when more than 90 percent of the marriages in this country are not virginal," says Barbara Huberman, director of training for Advocates for Youth, which seeks to reduce teenage pregnancy and AIDS. A 1994 study found that fewer than 7 percent of men and 20 percent of women ages 18-59 were virgins when they married, and 77 percent of America's 74 million single adults had had sex within the last year. [16]

"The concept of chastity until marriage may have made more sense 100 years ago when teenagers reached puberty in their middle teens and marriage closely followed," Haffner says. Today, the average American girl hits puberty at 12 $\frac{1}{2}$ and marries at 25.

"They're asking young people to deny powerful hormonal urges for more than 12 years," Huberman says. "We set kids up for failure by telling them to remain chaste all that time."

But expecting a young person to practice birth control 100 percent effectively and remain disease-free for 12 years is also unrealistic in today's world, says Family Research Council analyst Gracie Hsu. "Isn't that setting them up for failure?" she asks.

Do abstinence-only programs work?

Several eighth-graders used to be pregnant each year at Nathan Hale Middle School in suburban Chicago. But after three years of the abstinence-only program Project Taking Charge, the school graduated three pregnancy-free classes in a row.

Among Best Friends participants in Washington, D.C., only 5 percent of the 15-year-olds in the program had had sex, compared with 63 percent of the youths throughout the city, according to an independent researcher. By the time they graduated, only 14 percent of participants had engaged in sexual intercourse, compared with 73 percent citywide. [17]

Abstinence advocates have dozens of similar success stories. The problem, social scientists say, is that none of the abstinence studies have been conducted scientifically. Even though the federal government has funded abstinence-only programs since 1981 through the Adolescent and Family Life Act (AFLA) program, proponents have not published "a single peer-reviewed study showing that they work," Haffner points out (see p. 101).

The abstinence coalition points to findings from the National Longitudinal Study on Adolescent Health, published last September in the *Journal of the American Medical Association* (*JAMA*). Known as the "Add Health" study, it found that teens who had taken abstinence pledges were "sig-

nificantly" less likely to engage in early sexual activity than teens who had not.

"The Add Health study now places scientific research soundly on the side of the abstinence message," said a coalition letter last December to state officials who administer abstinence-only grants. The study "raises serious questions" about sex-education programs that teach both abstinence and contraception, the letter said.

When authors of the Add Health survey heard about the coalition's letter, however, they sent out a clarification of the coalition's "erroneous" interpretation of their findings.

"They have . . . imputed causality where there is no causality," says Robert W. Blum, one of the authors. "You cannot look at the data and say that an abstinence pledge leads to virginity. This is not a random population of kids in America who make abstinence pledges. There's a religious and ethnic skew to it. The abstinence pledge is just one piece of a constellation of factors we see in kids who are less likely to have intercourse."

To determine which sex-education programs work best, the Campaign to Prevent Teen Pregnancy last year published an extensive evaluation of 33 sex-ed studies. After examining six abstinence-only studies, the evaluation found that the abstinence-only programs do not delay sexual activity. But the evidence is inconclusive, the evaluation said, because all of the studies were methodologically flawed except one — the one showing that California's much-touted program didn't work. [18]

"The jury is still out," says Douglas Kirby, author of the campaign's evaluation.

Abstinence opponents also cite a study published in *JAMA* in May — the first-ever comparing the chastity-vs.-condoms approaches. It found that over several years, abstinence-only was not as effective as a safer-

Most Teenage Mothers Are Unmarried

The percentage of teenage mothers ages 15-19 who were unmarried in 1996 was nearly six times the percentage in 1950. The increase reflects sharply rising birthrates among unmarried teenagers and a decline in teenage marriages since the mid-1970s.

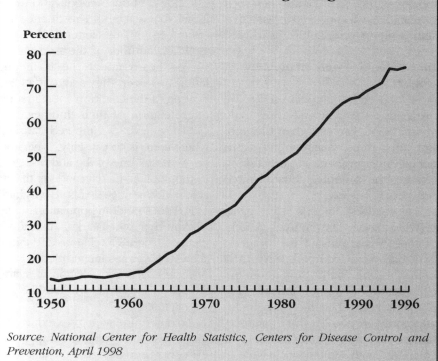

Births to Unmarried U.S. Teenagers Ages 15-19

Source: National Center for Health Statistics, Centers for Disease Control and Prevention, April 1998

sex program at preventing inner-city African-American teens from having sex. The safer-sex program had stressed abstinence as the safest way to avoid STDs and pregnancy but also taught about condoms. [19]

Given the lack of "clear and compelling data" showing significant and consistent benefits from abstinence-only programs, said a *JAMA* editorial, "it is difficult to understand the logic behind the decision to earmark funds specifically for abstinence programs. "Unfortunately," it continued, debate over the issue appears "ideologically motivated rather than empirically driven."

But the Family Research Council's Hsu says the results of the *JAMA* study

cannot be generalized, because it was conducted among African-American youths living in a "sex-saturated" community. You cannot expect a message that is so "counter-cultural" to have an impact after only two four-hour Saturday morning sessions, she says.

Do contraception-education programs encourage teen sex?

Abstinence advocates argue that youths receive a mixed message when adult authority figures explain how to obtain and use contraceptives, even if they tell them chastity is best. "It's talking out of both sides of your mouth," and it undermines parental directives to abstain from

sex, Brandt says.

"Giving kids contraception information gives them permission to have sex," Hsu says.

"By now," Moore counters, "there are at least 16 studies showing that sex-ed does not increase sexual activity among kids. But it remains a very widely held belief."

"That's like saying that driver's ed increases traffic accidents," says Gloria Feldt, president of the Planned Parenthood Federation of America. "It's silly."

Yet abstinence proponents turn the driver's education analogy on its head, especially when describing programs like those in more than 400 U.S. high schools, which provide students with free condoms. "Just because you give a kid driver's education doesn't mean you give him a car," Brandt says.

Giving teens condoms, they argue, takes away one of their excuses for avoiding sex, leaving them with one less weapon in their anti-peer-pressure arsenal.

The Family Research Council cites two studies that it says show that either pregnancy or sexual activity increased at San Francisco and Dallas schools after they began distributing condoms. [20]

Yet Kirby, who authored both studies, says that the council selectively chose anomalies in each study, though they both concluded that there was no overall impact from making condoms available. "For instance, out of 36 measures of sexual activity, 33 showed that there was no impact, two showed that the program actually delayed sexual activity and one showed that it hastened the onset of intercourse," he says. "They highlighted the one statistic that showed sexual activity increased. I looked at all 36 factors and concluded that there was no impact on sexual activity."

In addition, he said, numerous

studies since then show "absolutely overwhelming" evidence that sex-education programs that teach contraception do not increase sexual activity. The most comprehensive was Kirby's own massive evaluation of studies of 33 sex education and HIV-prevention programs, *No Easy Answers,* for the National Campaign to Prevent Teen Pregnancy.

"Sexuality- and HIV-education curricula do not increase sexual intercourse, either by hastening the onset of intercourse, increasing the frequency of intercourse or increasing the number of sexual partners," Kirby says. "We have more data supporting that than anything else." Some of the programs, however, did the opposite: They either delayed sexual activity, reduced the frequency or reduced the number of sexual partners, he notes.

In 1993, the World Health Organization published an extensive review of 35 studies of sex-education programs, some dating back to the 1970s. "The overwhelming majority of studies over time, despite various methodologies and countries of study, found no evidence that sex-education encourages sexual experimentation or increases activity," said a CDC fact sheet. One study did vary from the trend — an abstinence-only program that actually increased the level of sexual activity in young people, according to the CDC.

On the other hand, the recent *JAMA* study comparing safe-sex programs with abstinence-only programs among inner-city youths (*see above*) found that teens in the safe-sex program were having sex less than either the abstinence-only or the control group participants when interviewed six and 12 months later. Similarly, a recent study of condom availability in school-based health centers in Philadelphia showed a marked decline in the number of students engaging in sexual activity — from 75 percent to 66 percent — and increased condom

use among sexually active teens who used the health centers. [21]

Most experts now agree overwhelmingly that the best sex-education programs teach both abstinence and how to reduce the risk of pregnancy and STDs.

Apparently, most Americans agree. While 95 percent of Americans believe that teens should receive strong messages to abstain from sex — at least until they are out of high school — 60 percent want kids to have access to contraceptives if they are sexually active. Less than 25 percent believe teenagers should never be able to obtain contraceptives. [22]

"The concern is how do you present the risk-reduction message without unduly encouraging sexual activity?" says former Bush official Ware.

Kirby's evaluation found that the most effective programs focused on clear, directive messages aimed at encouraging specific behaviors, like delaying intercourse or using contraception. "These programs gave a clear message by continually reinforcing a clear stance on these behaviors," he says. "They did not simply lay out the pros and cons of different sexual choices and implicitly let the students decide which was right for them. Rather, most of the facts, activities, values and skills were directed toward convincing the students that abstaining from sex, using condoms or using other forms of contraception was the right choice."

Kirby's comments would appear to bolster the conservatives' claim that the "non-directive," values-free method of teaching sex education is not effective.

Ware sees the abstinence-only movement as a backlash to the values vacuum that resulted from the moral relativism of earlier eras: "It was the idea that nothing was wrong unless you personally decided it was wrong," she says. "In the last few years, we've seen the consequences of that.

"Our young people are killing each

other, doing drugs, having babies out-of-wedlock and generally exhibiting behavior that is frightening adults. The adults are now saying, 'Wait a minute. Maybe it's asking too much for young people to make decisions about things that we as adults even have trouble making.' " ∎

BACKGROUND

'Chastity Act' Passed

Congress has actually been funding community-based abstinence-only education programs since 1981, when it passed the Adolescent Family Life Act (AFLA), commonly known as the "chastity act."

Conceived during the first year of the Reagan administration as the conservative "alternative" to family planning, AFLA was the result of a quiet political deal — conservatives agreed not to block federal funds for family planning clinics if liberals supported AFLA. [23]

Sponsored by Republican Sens. Jeremiah Denton, R-Ala., (1981-87), and Orrin G. Hatch, R-Utah — who believed family planning programs encourage teen sexual activity and abortion — the bill was inserted into a budget bill without hearings or floor votes in either house.

Partly to win liberals' support, the original bill stipulated that two-thirds of AFLA funds would be used to support already-pregnant teens and one-third to promote abstinence. That ratio was reversed in 1997 and '98.

Like the current abstinence-only program, AFLA sprang from social conservatives' deep conviction that too much emphasis and money have been given to "comprehensive" sex-education and contraception-based pregnancy-prevention efforts. Both programs were "consciously constructed to steer funds toward conservative 'pro-family' groups and away from family planning and sexuality education providers," wrote Saul of the Guttmacher Institute. [24]

Conservatives say the Clinton administration has weakened the program, turning it into "AFLA lite" through liberal interpretations of agency rules. For instance, they note, in 1997 a Planned Parenthood affiliate in northern Michigan received AFLA money to teach seventh-graders to resist sex. Conservatives have pinned their hopes on the "purer" version of abstinence education, as defined in the welfare reform law.

Critics of the statute said its eight-point definition of abstinence was a bold attempt to legislate morality — particularly its call for all adults to abstain from sex unless married. In a statement clarifying congressional intent, the authors admitted, "This standard was intended to put Congress on the side of social tradition — never mind that some observers now think the tradition outdated. That both the practices and standards in many communities across the country clash with the standard required by the law is precisely the point." [25]

Although the federal government has disbursed $186 million in AFLA grants over the past 16 years — including about $50 million for abstinence programs — no long-term scientifically rigorous evaluations of the programs were conducted.

Initially, the 1996 welfare reform law did not earmark funds to evaluate the $250 million in abstinence-education grants it was mandating either. After a barrage of criticism, however, Congress set aside $6 million for evaluations.

Welfare Reform Debate

I n the mid-1990s, teenagers and their babies were swept up into the highly politicized debate over

how to overhaul the welfare system. The debate quickly centered on reasons for the decline of the American family, as evidenced, in part, by skyrocketing rates of illegitimacy among both teens and adults. Conservatives blamed a welfare system that rewarded illegitimacy and penalized marriage among poor parents.

"Preventing teen pregnancy and out-of-wedlock births is a critical part of welfare reform," said President Clinton in sending his welfare-overhaul proposal to Congress in June 1994. "To prevent welfare dependency, teenagers must get the message that staying in school, postponing pregnancy and preparing to work are the right things to do."

His proposal put less emphasis on the Reagan-Bush era's abstinence-only approach and more reliance on sex education, contraception and abortion. The president's proposal was ignored in 1995 by the new Republican-led Congress as it debated welfare reform.

In his 1995 State of the Union address, Clinton challenged the nation to fight "our most serious social problem, the epidemic of teen pregnancies" and out-of-wedlock births.

The "epidemic" of out-of-wedlock births became a major rallying point for conservatives seeking to overhaul welfare in 1995 and '96, partly because of an influential 1993 *Wall Street Journal* column by the late Charles Murray. Titled "The Coming White Underclass," it predicted that the problems generally attributed to the demise of the black inner-city family — violence, crime and poverty — would rapidly spread to white neighborhoods because of rising illegitimacy rates among white teenagers.

The number of illegitimate babies born to white teenagers more than tripled from 1970 to 1995, from 10.9 per 1,000 to 35.5 per 1,000. Meanwhile, the percent of black babies

born out of wedlock — while three times as high as the rate among whites — actually declined modestly, from 96.9 per 1,000 to 92.8 per 1,000. [26]

When viewed from a historical perspective, fewer teenagers are giving birth today than in 1957, at the height of the baby boom. But the baby boomers' teenagers are not getting married first, like their moms did. (*See chart, p. 100.*)

Today, for a variety of reasons, women are postponing marriage until much later, and skyrocketing illegitimacy is common throughout the industrialized world. More out-of-wedlock births occur in Great Britain and France than in the U.S. And most involve adult women, not teenagers.

Douglas Besharov, a resident scholar at the American Enterprise Institute, sees the drop in marriage rates as a function of women's political and social emancipation. "In the post-industrial age, when the earning power of men and women becomes quite equal, that creates a very different relationship between men and women and makes it easier for women to leave unhappy relationships." [27]

But declining marriage rates alarm other conservatives. They see premarital and extramarital sex, as well as the increasing acceptance of out-of-wedlock childbirth by both teens and adults, as major threats to the institution of marriage. Hence, a primary goal in the welfare reform bill was not just preventing teen pregnancy but stamping out premarital and extramarital sex among all teens and adults.

In the end, Congress imposed a five-year lifetime limit on eligibility for welfare. It also required parenting teens under 18 to live at home and finish high school to receive benefits.

Conservatives argued that the abstinence grants merely "level the playing field" between the amount of federal funds spent on family planning and the amount spent promoting abstinence. "This amount simply brings federal financing for absti-

Chronology

1950s *Teen birthrates hit an all-time high, but most baby boom mothers are married when they give birth.*

1957
The teen birthrate peaks at 96 births per 1,000, then begins a steady decline.

———— • ————

1960s *Out-of-wedlock births rise as women begin marrying later.*

1965
Sen. Daniel P. Moynihan, D-N.Y., warns that out-of-wedlock childbearing is threatening the black family and causing social disruption in the black community.

———— • ————

1970s *As the baby boom generation enters adolescence, teen births surge, and out-of-wedlock births among teens continue to rise.*

1970
President Richard M. Nixon creates a comprehensive family-planning program for poor women at federally subsidized clinics, through Title X of the Public Health Service Act.

1972
The Social Security Act is amended to require that states provide family planning services to "minors who are sexually active." Changes to Title IX of the 1972 Education Amendments prohibit public schools from barring pregnant and parenting students from class.

1973
The Supreme Court's *Roe v. Wade* decision legalizes abortion, which spurs publication of statistics that make it possible to calculate reliable teen pregnancy rates.

1976
The Alan Guttmacher Institute declares adolescent pregnancy an "epidemic" in the U.S.

———— • ————

1980s *Out-of-wedlock births become the norm for teen childbearing; battles over sex education ensue between advocates of abstinence and birth control.*

1981
Congress passes the so-called "chastity bill" — the Adolescent Family Life Act — providing grants for community-based, abstinence-only education programs. The programs not only encourage teens to delay sexual activity but also to consider adoption (instead of abortion) if they are already pregnant.

1985
The Guttmacher Institute notes that the United States has the highest teen pregnancy, abortion and birthrates in the industrialized world.

1987
After two decades of decline and then a 10-year leveling-off period, the teen birthrate begins a four-year climb.

1989
In *Webster v. Reproductive Health Services,* the Supreme Court makes it more difficult for teens to obtain abortions.

1990s *Teen birthrates decline as contraception use increases and community-based abstinence programs gain in popularity. Chastity-vs.-condoms battles proliferate as some parents oppose "comprehensive" sex-education curricula taught in some schools.*

1993
New York City schools chief Joseph Fernandez is fired amid criticism of his program to give away condoms in schools.

1994
President Clinton declares that preventing teen pregnancy and out-of-wedlock births is a critical part of his welfare reform plan.

1995
In his State of the Union address, Clinton challenges "parents and leaders all across this country to ... make a difference" against "our most serious social problem, the epidemic of teen pregnancies" and out-of-wedlock births.

1996
The privately funded, bipartisan National Campaign to Prevent Teen Pregnancy is created in February with the goal of reducing teen pregnancy by one-third by 2005. In August a welfare-reform bill is signed into law providing $250 million over five years for abstinence-only education.

1997
All 50 states apply for abstinence-education grants, which must be matched with 75 percent state funding. An estimated 600 local battles are being fought over sex education.

Asking Hollywood Writers . . .

One childlike face after another flashed onto the television screen. The pubescent, pimply complexions, sometimes with braces flashing, belied the adult pain in their eyes. One by one, with wrenching simplicity, the teenagers spoke of dashed dreams.

They were just a few of the 1 million teenagers who get pregnant every year in America.

When the four-minute video ended and the lights came on, several of the 40 veteran television writers and executives in the room "were dabbing at their eyes," says Marisa Nightingale, media programs manager for the National Campaign to Prevent Teen Pregnancy.

Nightingale uses the powerful video, which was donated by Ogilvy and Mather public relations, to brief magazine and television writers and executives. As part of the campaign's goal to reduce teen pregnancy by one-third by 2005, she's asking Hollywood to help get the message across to teens that adolescence and pregnancy don't mix.

"We cannot hope to reduce the high rates of teen pregnancy in this country without engaging the vast power of the media," says campaign Director Sarah Brown. "The media can be just as persuasive in convincing young people that parenting is not child's play as they are in informing them that the ZIP Code for Beverly Hills is 90210."

Contrary to popular belief, Nightingale says, Hollywood executives are not deaf to public opinion. "They're all enthusiastic to help," she says. "Every time I go to L.A., I'm overwhelmed by how positive the response is. They're tired of getting beat up" by the public and politicians.

"The media [are] speeding the moral breakdown of our society," said Sen. Joseph I. Lieberman, D-Conn., in a speech last September at the University of Notre Dame. He and former Education Secretary William J. Bennett, a Republican, have been leading what they call the "Revolt of the Revolted," giving voice to the "disgust millions of Americans feel toward the growing culture of violence, perversity and promiscuity" in the media.

Congress responded to complaints about TV sex and violence in 1996 by passing legislation requiring a "V-chip" to be installed in all new American-made TV sets beginning this fall. The technology will allow parents to screen out shows carrying certain ratings. [1]

Nightingale's friendly reception in Hollywood may reflect her efforts to build bridges and form a partnership with film and TV executives, rather than attack them. Realizing that screen and magazine writers "are allergic to being told what to write," she is careful not to sound directive in her approach. "They are hungry for ideas. But the minute you act like you know what a good story line is, you're out of there."

Instead, she offers 10 messages about teen pregnancy, any one of which writers can use "at their own pace and in their own way" to develop their own story lines, she says. One message says that, contrary to what parents think, teens want to know what adults think about sex, love and relationships.

"Our surveys show that kids are looking for guidance from their parents," she says. That message particularly resonated with a group of daytime soap opera writers Nightingale briefed recently, since their audiences are adult women, most of whom are parents.

The Henry J. Kaiser Family Foundation, in Palo Alto, Calif., has worked for years to get Hollywood to stop portraying teenage sex as not having consequences.

"Now, when a couple hops into bed, there are no consequences. We'd like to change that," says Vicky Rideout, director of Kaiser's entertainment, media and public health programs. "Our purpose isn't to get sex off

---

nence up to parity with annual Title X financing to promote teenage use of contraceptives," Richard A. Panzer, author of a book on teenage sex education, wrote in a letter to *The New York Times*. [28]

Title X of the Public Health Service Act, signed into law in 1970 by President Richard M. Nixon, created a comprehensive family planning program for poor women through federally subsidized clinics. For the past two decades, conservatives have attacked the program, primarily because many of the clinics provide abortions. About 13 percent of the Title X clinics are affiliates of the Planned Parenthood Federation of America.

But conservatives also argue that by allowing teenagers to obtain birth control pills — and sometimes abortions — without parental notification or consent, the clinics encourage teen sexual activity and undermine parental authority. The Title X program has been a dismal failure, they say, because sexual activity, STDs and out-of-wedlock birthrates have skyrocketed among teens over the 30-year life of the program, notwithstanding the recent drop in teen sexual activity.

Family planning proponents bristle at any effort to equate funds spent on family planning clinics with the amounts now being spent on abstinence education.

"It's absolutely ludicrous to say that this levels the playing field," Feldt says. Title X clinics provide health care like Pap smears, medical exams and testing for STDs for adult women, she points out, and fewer than 10 percent of the clients are under 18. "That's totally different from providing sex education in the schools.

"Furthermore," she adds, "any birth control counseling done in the

... To Cut Down on Irresponsible Sex

TV, but to get the entertainment community to think more about the impact of what they are doing."

But she also sees a potential "sex educator" role for television. "TV can be a very important source of information for kids about sex," she says. The Media Project, a partnership between Kaiser and Advocates for Youth, periodically briefs television writers to inform them about teen pregnancy, sexually transmitted diseases (STDs) and other health issues and operates a hotline writers can call if they have a question about rates of STDs or pregnancies.

In February, the Media Project briefed television writers and producers in Los Angeles about the results of a Kaiser survey showing where teens learn about sex. About 54 percent said they learned about sex and birth control from television. A third said some teens have sex because television and movies make it seem "normal" for teens to be sexually active.

"We've also measured the impact when information is included in a show," Rideout says. "We survey people before and after the show, and we find that it's an incredibly effective way to get a message across. When we explain this to the writers, they are surprised and a little frightened. It's not a responsibility that they asked for."

Yet, Rideout says, she agrees with Nightingale that "a lot of writers care about what they do." She points to several examples of responsible TV programming that have resulted from the groups' efforts:

• MTV did a series of humorous, attention-grabbing public service ads offering 25 different ways to say "Put on a condom."

• The NBC drama "ER" has done several segments focusing on teen pregnancy, including one dealing with the "emergency" contraception pill, which can be taken within the first 72 hours of unprotected sex.

• Two ABC soap operas are weaving a message about teen pregnancy prevention into their story lines over the next two years.

Kaiser has found that parental concern about sex on TV has escalated in the past two years. In a 1996 Kaiser survey about "family hour" shows, 43 percent of parents said they were concerned about sexual content (compared with only 40 percent who were worried about violence). Last April, a new Kaiser survey found that 67 percent of parents were "greatly concerned" about sex, compared with 62 percent who were worried about violence.

"There's been a lot of brouhaha about violence on TV," Rideout says, "but almost no studies of the impact of sexual content on kids."

The WB network's titillating, new teen soap opera, "Dawson's Creek," may be the last straw. The controversial and highly popular show featured a 15-year-old having an affair with his 30-something English teacher.

"It raised a lot of hackles for parents," Nightingale says.

"That show alone could counteract our entire program," says Peter Brandt, executive director of the National Coalition for Abstinence Education, which has lobbied for years to get $50 million a year in federal grants for community-based programs that teach kids to abstain from sex. "We should have used the $50 million to buy out 'Dawson's Creek' and pay them not to produce."

But Nightingale isn't giving up. This summer she will try to get WB network shows, including "Dawson's Creek," to put in a word for responsible sex.

---

[1] For background, see "Children's Television," *The CQ Researcher,* Aug. 15, 1997, pp. 721-744.

---

clinics includes encouraging abstinence and encouraging young people to talk to their parents."

Furthermore, Haffner points out, "The federal government does not spend a penny for comprehensive sex education in the schools, and it never has."

"The welfare reform law created a dedicated funding stream for abstinence education," Feldt says, noting that the abstinence funds are "entitlements" and do not have to get annual appropriations. "There is no federal funding stream dedicated specifically to providing responsible, balanced sex education. There ought to be, but there isn't." ■

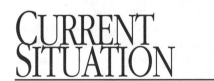

CURRENT SITUATION

Sex-Ed Battles

Although Clinton signed the welfare reform law, he does not see it as an effort to force states to replace existing sex education programs with abstinence-only programs.

"The policy of the administration is that we should encourage abstinence among our young people," Clinton said. "The question of contraception is one that should be resolved at the local level involving all sectors of the local community. There is no national policy on that, and there will not be." [29]

Meanwhile, sex education and illegitimacy issues continue to clog legal and legislative agendas at the local, state and federal levels.

Now that all states have received block grants for abstinence-only programs, some legislatures and school boards are overhauling their existing

Heartland Honor Societies Face a Dilemma . . .

In America's heartland, communities are facing a problem that inner cities have long wrestled with — skyrocketing rates of unwed teen parenthood. To send a clear message that it is not OK, some communities have drawn a line in the sand at the National Honor Society's front door.

This spring, two small towns in Ohio and Kentucky blocked three academically qualified high school girls from membership in the prestigious society. All were either unwed teen mothers or pregnant at the time.

Elsewhere, however, pregnant teens are quietly inducted. Last year in Tipton, Ind., for instance, the high school salutatorian was an unwed mother as well as an honor society member. "We don't believe in shaming kids," says Tipton school Superintendent Tom Fletcher.

But in Xenia, Ohio, and Williamstown, Ky., the faculty selection committees said that the three pregnant or parenting girls in their communities did not qualify for society membership because they did not meet its "character" criterion. The girls failed the character standard not because they were unwed mothers — federal law prohibits schools from discriminating against pregnant or parenting teens — but because they had obviously engaged in premarital sex, school officials said.

Xenia school Superintendent James Smith said that his school's standard has been on the books since 1952, and that it has been equally applied to exclude boys who were known to be unwed fathers. But Amanda Lemon, the 18-year-old teen mother who was excluded in Xenia, asked, "What about the people who have had sex, and then had abortions? I was told by one of the people [at school] that

they do know people on the National Honor Society that had had abortions, but that I have visual evidence."

"What do you think that makes people think?" she continued. "You can have sex and use protection and you can be in the National Honor Society. You can have sex and have an abortion, and you can be in the National Honor Society. But if you have sex and make the choice to keep your baby and do the morally right thing, then you cannot be in the National Honor Society."[1]

The exclusions set off a firestorm of controversy that erupted onto editorial pages and on television and radio talk shows across the country, opening up what some say is a much-needed national debate about what is acceptable sexual behavior for teenagers.

Given the reactions to the honor society moms — opinions were split about 50-50 on whether they should be inducted — clearly America hasn't reached a consensus on the issue.

The controversy raised numerous thorny questions that honor society selection committees have been grappling with in recent years: Should only virgins be allowed to join the honor society? If so, how will the society prove their chastity? Is it legal (or fair) to exclude sexually active girls, whose "mistakes" cannot easily be hidden, but not the boys? Should students be asked to swear they have never had sex before they can join?

How many honor society male members have secretly fathered a child? If a local council hears a rumor that a boy has fathered a child, should they demand a paternity test? How many of the society's female members have had an abortion? Do they have more "character" than someone

sex education curricula to qualify for the abstinence-only grants.

Florida, for instance, now requires public school health education to teach "an awareness of the benefits of sexual abstinence as the expected standard." In Arizona, the Legislature funded an abstinence-only program despite a recent public opinion poll showing 80 percent opposition to the program.

"We are gravely concerned that these abstinence-only-until-marriage guidelines are changing the landscape of sexuality education in America," Haffner says. "Good programs that are effective are being replaced by fear-based education programs."

In South Carolina, where a recent

poll found that 84 percent of citizens want sex education instruction time increased, a bill has been introduced in the state Senate limiting class time spent on sex education and refocusing instruction on abstinence.[30]

Despite Haffner's fears, only a handful of states have mandated that schools revise their sex-education courses to fall in line with Congress' abstinence curriculum. Most are using the money for programs that supplement — rather than replace — existing sex-education curricula. Most are targeting younger youths, 9-14 years of age, for the abstinence message. There is widespread agreement that abstinence is especially appropriate for younger teens, although

some conservatives want the message sent to all teens.

According to the Maternal and Child Health Bureau, which administers the grants, only 29 out of the 155 groups receiving grants this year are school-based, and only half will teach classes during school hours. The rest of the abstinence courses are being offered by city or county health departments, community groups, church-affiliated groups and universities.

The National Coalition for Abstinence Education says it is quite pleased with the "excellent and very creative" abstinence programs that most states have developed. Initially, however, about 30 proposals did not abide by the legislative intent of the law, Brandt says.

... Over Admission of Unwed Teen Mothers

who chooses to keep her child?

"I respect what [Amanda] has done," in keeping her baby and staying in school, Smith says. "But is she a good role model for teen mothers, or is she a good role model for the National Honor Society? Therein lies the debate."

The messages teens are receiving from Washington are equally confusing. On the one hand, the government urges pregnant teens to finish high school and forbids schools from kicking them out. Yet, those who "do the right thing" by finishing school and excelling at the same time are told they are not exhibiting character worthy of the National Honor Society.

The National Campaign to Prevent Teen Pregnancy trumpets what it calls a "clear message" to America's teens: that teen pregnancy is not OK. But the group is silent on whether that means kids should remain chaste or just be very prudent in choosing and using birth control.

Congress voted in 1996 to send its own "clear message" to teens: Do not have sex until you get married. It pledged $437.5 million in state and federal funds over the next five years to send that message, as well as $400 million to discourage unwed motherhood. In the same legislation, Congress said that all Americans are expected to refrain from sex unless married. But in a country where 77 percent of the single adults had had sex within the last year and a president accused of multiple sexual indiscretions receives consistently high approval ratings, some editorialists question which "clear message" teenagers are getting about non-marital sex?

The National Association of Secondary School Principals, which administers the National Honor Society, says the society is not just an academic organization. To qualify for membership a student must exhibit four qualities: scholarship, community service, leadership and character.

"Membership is an honor," says Pat Scanlan, spokeswoman for the association. "It is not a right." The association allows each local faculty selection council to decide, based on local sensibilities, how they define the four criteria. "It's impossible for us to decide on individual cases. That's up to the local chapters."

When cases have arisen in the past, the association has advised local chapters that pregnancy, whether within or out of wedlock, "cannot be the basis for automatic rejection." It could be construed as discriminating against someone based on gender, since boys don't get pregnant, she says.

William Galston, a University of Maryland professor and chairman of the campaign's task force on religion and values, says the current debate is a perfect chance for local communities to clarify their values and the messages they want to send kids about sex among teens.

"If I were in a position of authority at one of these schools, I would convene a school or town meeting and say, 'Here are the four general criteria for induction into the honor society. I intend to interpret the character criterion in such-and-such a way as the definition of honorable behavior in handling one's sexuality. If you disagree with me, let's have that discussion right now.'"

"You can't have a person in authority suddenly jumping up and saying, 'Surprise!'"

---

[1] Quoted on CNN "Talkback Live," April 28, 1998.

"Overall, we think it's going quite well," Brandt says. "We're seeing a much broader approach to the problem. States are addressing the kids almost holistically." Many of the programs take a communitywide approach, involving the medical profession, service organizations, the business community, peer groups and after-school as well as in-school programs, he says.

Meanwhile, states are also scrambling to compete for the $20 million "illegitimacy bonuses" the federal government will award to the five states that achieve the greatest reduction in out-of-wedlock births. Some states, like Georgia, Mississippi and Oklahoma, are incorporating the federal abstinence-only criteria into their welfare programs in hope they will help bring down illegitimacy rates. Other states are looking for ways to expand family planning services for low-income women.

Federal Initiatives

At the federal level, congressional conservatives are seeking restrictions on birth control and abortion services for teenagers. They have introduced bills requiring parents of teenagers to be notified before their children can obtain contraceptive services from a federally funded Title X clinic. Since Republicans took majority control in Congress, there have been three efforts to require parental consent for teen birth-control counseling at such clinics. The last attempt, in September, failed by only 19 votes, so proponents have vowed to try again this year. Illinois Republican Rep. Donald Manzullo has also introduced a similar bill, which has been referred to the House Commerce Committee.

Congressional action is also expected this session on highly controversial legislation making it illegal for an adult to take a minor across state lines to evade laws requiring parental notification before an abortion can be performed. Emotional hearings were held in May on measures pending in both houses, foreshadowing what is likely to be an intense debate when the bills come to the House and Senate floors. Sen. Hatch has vowed to send Clinton such a bill before Congress adjourns.

Targeting Unwed Dads

Alarmed at both skyrocketing STD rates and out-of-wedlock births, legislators, prosecutors, social workers and public health providers are increasingly focusing the spotlight on unwed fathers.

"Changing the reproductive behavior of males is a crucial element of strategies to prevent the transmission of STDs," said a 1997 Urban Institute study. Most STDs can be prevented through consistent condom use, the study said. [31]

But it's the increasing fatherlessness of America's children that most worries policy-makers.

"All of the problems tearing apart the fabric of our society have deep roots in this exploding epidemic of out-of-wedlock births," said California Gov. Wilson in 1996 in his sixth State of the State address.

The lack of a father in the home can have a devastating impact not only on the child but also on the community, said a 1997 Hudson Institute study. For instance, 70 percent of long-term prison inmates grew up without fathers, as did 60 percent of rapists and 75 percent of teenagers charged with murder. Compared with children raised in two-parent homes, fatherless children are 40 times more likely to experience child abuse and three times more likely to fail at school, require psychiatric treatment and commit suicide, the study said. [32]

Forty states have enacted strategies to encourage male reproductive responsibility. They range from beefing up statutory rape laws to in-creased efforts to establish paternity. Some states are vigorously enforcing child-support laws and excluding school-age unwed fathers from extracurricular activities.

As welfare reform goes into effect and states begin moving millions of single welfare mothers into the work force, attention is also being focused on how to get unwed fathers involved in their children's lives.

"Providing jobs to single mothers is not enough," said the Hudson Institute. "Welfare stands at the center of a larger social crisis: the demise of marriage and the increasing disappearance of fathers from families."

The study recommended a number of measures state welfare officials can take to entice the fathers to either marry the mother of their child or become more involved in their children's lives. For instance, welfare offices can give preferential treatment to married parents in distributing discretionary benefits, like Head Start and public housing slots. States could require mothers to cooperate with visitation orders as a condition for receiving welfare benefits, or let fathers satisfy the work requirement for families on aid.

Growing concern about the impact of children growing up in fatherless households has led to the fatherhood movement, exemplified by the recent Million Man and Promise Keepers marches on Washington.

In addition, pioneering fatherhood programs have been established across the country, ranging from education/outreach programs at health clinics to school- or church-based peer-mentor programs.

Even at Operation Fatherhood in Trenton, N.J., where an evaluation of the program has been less than glowing, officials say participants have gotten more involved in their children's lives. "We may not have made the biggest strides," says Director Dolores Bryant, "but we are definitely working small miracles one at a time." [33]

■

OUTLOOK

Parents' Influence

As the last of the baby boomers' teenagers reach puberty, the total U.S. teen population is expected to surge by 13 percent, or 2.5 million additional youths ages 15-19, by 2008. In addition, as Hispanic immigration continues climbing, the absolute number of teen births will jump, demographers say, even if the birthrate doesn't. [34]

Eyeing that coming increase, most experts now agree that prevention is not just about chastity or condoms. It requires a holistic approach addressing the psychological, behavioral, moral, social and cultural variables that predispose teenagers to get pregnant.

Many veterans of the sex-education wars say that youth-development programs have been the most successful at preventing teen pregnancy. "A lot of people think youth development is the way to go," says Brian L. Wilcox, director of the Center on Children, Families and the Law at the University of Nebraska and a board member of the Campaign to Prevent Teen Pregnancy.

"This is an area that shows great promise that everybody can agree on," says William Albert, a spokesman for the campaign. Youth-development programs are comprehensive approaches, offering everything from dropout prevention to supervised after-school recreational activities. They usually offer adult mentoring and encourage kids to establish career goals and help them develop skills to achieve them. Most also involve teens in community service work, he says.

At Issue:

Are "abstinence-only" sex-education programs good for teenagers?

JOE S. MCILHANEY JR.

President, Medical Institute for Sexual Health, Austin, Texas

FROM INSIGHT MAGAZINE, *SEPT. 29, 1997*

*W*e have had at least 20 years of an educational message that says, basically, "If you can't say no, act responsibly." Yet these safe/safer/protected sex curricula have been tried and found wanting in terms of preventing the skyrocketing damage to our teens and their long-term physical, emotional, social, spiritual and economic health. It is time for an honest and open-minded look at a new sexual revolution: abstinence until . . . marriage. . . .

Non-marital teen pregnancy all too often has a devastating impact on teen parents and their children. Indeed, teen pregnancy has received much analysis because of the long-term effects not only to the mother and child but to the father, to extended families and ultimately to society. . . . [O]nly 30 percent of girls who become pregnant before age 18 will earn a high-school diploma by the age of 30, compared with 76 percent of women who delay child bearing until after age 20. And 80 percent of those young, single mothers will live below the poverty line, receive welfare and raise children who are at risk for many difficulties as they grow to adulthood. . . .

In addition to pregnancy, adolescents and young adults are in the age group at highest risk for contracting STDs [sexually transmitted diseases]. . . .

The statistics for disease and pregnancy are not in dispute. The concern is in what we should do about preventing these problems from occurring and devastating young lives. This is where the controversy starts.

The prevailing opinion for the last two or three decades has been that kids will do it anyway, so we have to give them condoms and contraceptives so they can be protected. Education programs have given a nod to abstinence as the only 100 percent safe choice outside of marriage but then have gone on to spend much time and emphasis on the "how to's" of safer sex. . . .

The bottom line is that although studies show that "safer sex" approaches do not increase sexual activity among students, none of these programs has dramatically lowered the number of teens who choose to be sexually active, who have to deal with pregnancy or who acquire STDs. Nor have they dramatically increased contraceptive use among those who are sexually active.

Why should abstinence be emphasized in schools? The best that "safer sex" approaches can offer is some risk reduction. Abstinence, on the other hand, offers risk elimination. When the risks of pregnancy and disease are so great, even with contraception, how can we advocate anything less?

DEBRA HAFFNER

President, The Sexuality Information and Education Council of the United States (SIECUS)

FROM INSIGHT MAGAZINE, *SEPT. 29, 1997*

*W*e believe young people should receive comprehensive sexuality education that will serve as a foundation for a lifetime of sexual health. This education is designed to assist people to develop a positive view of sexuality, provide them with information about taking care of their sexual health and help them acquire the skills to make decisions. . . . Abstinence education is an important part of this program. A goal of comprehensive sexuality education is to help young people exercise responsibility and resist pressure to become prematurely involved in sexual relationships. SIECUS believes, however, that it also is important to teach young people about a full range of issues related to sexual health and behavior. . . .

By contrast, there is no evidence that abstinence-only programs work. No published evaluations are available to show that these programs truly help young people postpone sexual relationships. And, in fact, an analysis of a recent $5 million abstinence-only program in California found that it not only did not increase the number of young people who abstained but, in one school, actually resulted in more students engaging in sexual intercourse after participating in the course. . . .

Unfortunately, proponents of these abstinence-only programs scored a huge victory last year. They convinced Congress to create a new federal entitlement program for abstinence-only education as part of welfare reform. It provides nearly $88 million [a year] in federal and state funding for programs that must have as their "exclusive purpose teach social, psychological and health gains to be realized by abstaining from sexual activity." . . .

The program requires adults to teach young people that "abstinence from sexual activity is the only certain way to avoid out-of-wedlock pregnancy, sexually transmitted diseases and other associated health problems." This may give them the dangerous impression that contraception and condoms aren't worth using. Many fear-based, abstinence-only programs discuss contraception only in negative terms. This message threatens to reverse significant strides American youth have made during the last two decades to delay sexual activity or else protect themselves. . . .

There is no question that young people want help saying no. Too many young people still are having sexual intercourse too early. Too many of them report that they regret their experiences. Too many are pressured by their friends, the media and older partners. We must teach teens the skills to handle the challenges of dating, intimacy and sexual limit-setting.

Why Did Black Teens' Birthrate Decline?

Social scientists have theories, but no firm answers, as to why the birthrate for black teenagers is declining faster than for any other ethnic group.

Some say it's probably due to more effective birth control. Others say it represents a dramatic shift in sexual mores. Still others contend it heralds the beginning of a rebirth of conservative values among black teenagers.

From 1991 to 1996, birthrates declined 5-12 percent for all teenagers. But among African-Americans the rate dropped a dramatic 21 percent, to 91.7 births per 1,000 — the lowest rate ever recorded. For younger black teenagers 15-17, the drop was even more dramatic, 23 percent, while the rate for blacks 18-19 fell by 16 percent. [1]

Hispanic teenagers now have the highest birthrate in the country, at 101.6 births per 1,000. Their birthrate declined only 5 percent.

In explaining the drops, statisticians point to the growing popularity of the contraceptives Depo-Provera, which is injected once every three months, and Norplant, an implant that lasts up to five years. By contrast, birth control pills, which are becoming less popular among American teens, must be taken daily.

"Two principle changes in contraceptive use among black teenagers occurred between 1988 and 1995," says statistician William D. Mosher of the National Center for Health Statistics (NCHS). "There were big decreases in the use of the [birth control] pill (down from 75 percent to 38 percent), and sizable increases (24 percent) in the use of implants and injectibles."

Overall, 8.4 percent of all black teenagers use implants or injectibles, compared with 2.6 percent of all white teenagers, he says.

Henry Foster, the teen pregnancy adviser to President Clinton, sees a different reason for the decline of teen births among blacks. Foster, an obstetrician, says that the growing black middle class has taken an aggressive stance against teen pregnancy. Affluent black women and their influential sororities have begun mentoring young black girls and accessing private and government funds to fight teen pregnancy, sexually transmitted diseases and substance abuse, he adds.

Patricia Funderburk Ware, former Bush administration director of the Office of Adolescent Programs, sees the decline as the first wave of a much bigger cultural revolution in the black community. But she says it's coming primarily from the inner cities, not the suburbs.

"We see what happens when these kids don't have a father," Ware says. "They're in the streets killing each other. We aren't telling our kids anymore that [casual sex] is OK.

"I don't think the white community is telling their kids that yet. They haven't suffered as much. Their daughters haven't had so many abortions that they can't have another one. They haven't become infertile from the sexually transmitted diseases or haven't been traumatized enough by going from one broken sexual relationship to another."

Ware notes that a majority of youths 14-18 rated declines in the family as the No. 1 problem facing the nation, according to a recent poll. [2] Moreover, she says, NCHS statistics show that 44 percent of teen girls who identified themselves as virgins said it was against their religious or moral values to have premarital sex.

Led by inner-city teenagers, she says, "We are beginning to see a real possibility for a swing in the proverbial pendulum toward a more drastic and long-lasting decrease in sexual activity rates among teens."

But if inner-city teens are in the vanguard of change, it has not yet shown up in national statistics. According to preliminary findings by the NCHS, even though the number of teens 15-19 who are sexually active dropped 42 percent from 1988 to 1995, most of the decline occurred among black and white teens in the suburbs.

"Suburban youth were much more likely than central city or rural youth to have lower levels of sexual activity in 1995 compared with 1988," according to Joyce Abma, an NCHS statistician. And, she notes, among black and white inner-city youths, there was no difference in levels of current sexual activity between 1988 and 1995. [3]

[1] "Teenage Births in the United States; National and State Trends, 1990-96." National Center for Health Statistics, April 1998.

[2] "The State of the Nation's Youth," Horatio Alger Association of Distinguished Americans Inc., 1996.

[3] Joyce Abma and Freya L. Sonenstein, "Teenage Sexual Behavior and Contraceptive Use: An Update," National Center for Health Statistics, April 28, 1998.

"I'm optimistic about these sorts of programs, especially if combined with family life education," Wilcox says. But, he warns, "They take enormous investment. I'm worried that we'll try to replicate some of the more successful programs on the cheap, and then they won't work."

And as most who work on the problem agree, it can't be solved by Washington alone but through the commitment of the entire society.

"The federal government can only provide guidance and information," says Clinton adviser Foster. "It's too big and too divisive for a one-size-fits-all solution."

As a Phoenix grandmother and guardian of two teenagers told a Campaign to Prevent Teen Pregnancy focus group last year: "Let's face it.

The media, entertainment, news, sports, the society in general, politicians, everybody needs to get more responsible. How can we expect teenagers to be responsible for themselves when we're showing grownups on TV not being responsible and getting away with it?"

Studies increasingly show that, contrary to popular belief, parents have more influence over whether their teens will get pregnant than any other factors. Not only is communication needed but also a strong sense of connectedness between parent and child, says Blum, the "Add Health" study co-author.

"Our data shows screamingly loudly that far more overriding than whether there is parental sex education is the sense of connection between parent and child," he said.

Perhaps more surprisingly, teenagers want to know what their parents have to say about whether or not they should engage in sex. "Our most recent survey shows that teenagers really want to hear from their parents about sex and sexuality," says campaign spokesman Albert. "Not just one talk about the birds and the bees. It needs to be an ongoing conversation over a lifetime."

The campaign recommends that parents first clarify in their own minds how they feel about teenage sexuality in today's world, and then clearly relay those values and attitudes to their children. That might be difficult for baby boomer parents who might be conflicted about their own teenage sexual histories or fearful that their kids will ask them about their own sexual past.

"Somehow, over time, we have lost a cultural consensus on what is acceptable teen sexual behavior," Brandt says. Perhaps a benefit of the abstinence legislation is that it has opened up a national debate and is getting society to focus on the issue, he says.

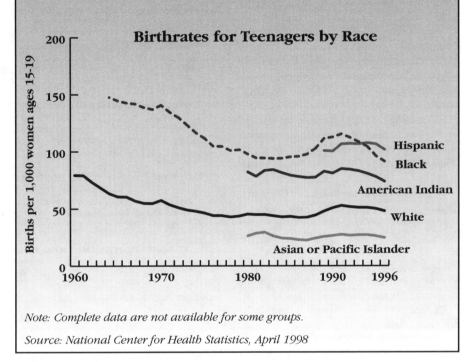

Birthrate for Black Teens at Record Low

The birthrate for black teenagers ages 15-19 fell 21 percent from 1991 to 1996 to the lowest rate ever: 91.7 births per 1,000. Birthrates for other teens dropped from 5-12 percent during the same period. Despite the sharp decline for blacks, their birthrates and those for Hispanic teens are higher than for other groups.

Birthrates for Teenagers by Race

Hispanic
Black
American Indian
White
Asian or Pacific Islander

Note: Complete data are not available for some groups.

Source: National Center for Health Statistics, April 1998

The Family Research Council would like to focus that debate less on teen sexual activity and more on all non-marital sex. "We believe the real problem is out-of-wedlock sexual behavior," Hsu says.

"We're uneasy as a society about the social and cultural balance that we've struck in the last generation," says William Galston, a University of Maryland professor and chairman of the campaign's task force on religion and values. "We're searching for adjustments that are tolerable. I doubt very much that we will return to the sexual mores of the 1950s. I do think we are fumbling our way toward a new balance, and not just a simple repetition of the distant past." ■

Notes

[1] Preliminary figures in a National Center for Health Statistics study due in August.
[2] Marion Howard and Judith Blamey McCabe, "Helping Teenagers Postpone Sexual Involvement," *Family Planning Perspectives*, January/February 1990.
[3] For background, see "Teaching Values," *The CQ Researcher*, June 21, 1996, pp. 534-557.
[4] "National Survey of Family Growth," August 1997.
[5] Quoted in Ron Stodghill II, "Where'd You Learn That?" *Time*, June 15, 1998.
[6] Douglas Kirby et. al., "The Impact of the Postponing Sexual Involvement Curriculum Among Youths in California," *Family Planning Perspectives*, May/June 1997.
[7] For background, see "Parental Rights," *The CQ Researcher*, Oct. 25, 1996, pp. 946-969.
[8] Patricia Funderburk, "None, Not Safer, Is

the Real Answer," *Insight,* May 9, 1994. For background, see "Children's Television," *The CQ Researcher,* Aug. 15, 1997, pp. 721-744 and "Sex, Violence and the Media," *The CQ Researcher,* Nov. 17, 1995, pp. 1017-1040.

[9] Jane Gross, "Where Boys Will be Boys and Adults Are Befuddled," *The New York Times,* March 29, 1993.

[10] National Center for Health Statistics, April 1998.

[11] "Facts in Brief," Alan Guttmacher Institute, 1993.

[12] See Susan Weller, "A Meta-Analysis of Condom Effectiveness in Reducing Sexually Transmitted HIV," *Social Science and Medicine,* June 1993.

[13] I. DeVincenzi et al, "A Longitudinal Study of Human Immunodeficiency Virus Transmission by Heterosexual Partners," *The New England Journal of Medicine,* No. 6, 1994, pp. 341-346 and A. Saracco et al, "Man to Woman Sexual Transmission of HIV: Longitudinal Study of 343 Steady Partners of Infected Men," *Journal of Acquired Immune Deficiency Syndromes,* Vol. 6, 1993, pp. 497-502.

[14] "The Sexually Transmitted Disease Epidemic," published by the Medical Institute of Sexual Health.

[15] Quoted in Christina Nifong, "Paying Cash for Good Behavior," *The Christian Science Monitor,* March 25, 1998.

[16] E. Laumann et al, *The Social Organization of Sexuality* (1994).

[17] Study data were provided by Best Friends.

[18] Douglas Kirby, *No Easy Answers: Research Findings on Programs to Reduce Teen Pregnancy,* National Campaign to Prevent Teen Pregnancy (1997).

[19] John B. Jemmott III, et al., "Abstinence and Safer Sex HIV Risk-Reduction Interventions for African American Adolescents," *Journal of the American Medical Association,* May 1998.

[20] Douglas Kirby, et al, "An Assessment of Six School-Based Clinics," Center for Population Options, 1989, and "Six School-Based Clinics: Their Reproductive Health Services and Impact on Sexual Behavior," *Family Planning Perspectives,* January/February 1991.

[21] F. Furstenberg et al, "Does Condom Availability Make a Difference?" *Family Planning Perspectives,* May/June 1997.

[22] "A Summary of the Findings from National Omnibus Survey Questions About Teen Pregnancy," National Campaign to Prevent Teen Pregnancy, May 1997.

[23] See "Preventing Teen Pregnancy," *The CQ Researcher,* May 14, 1993, pp. 409-432.

[24] Rebekah Saul, "Whatever Happened to the Adolescent Family Life Act?" *The Guttmacher Report,* April 1998.

[25] Ron Haskins and Carol Statuto Bevan, "Abstinence Education Under Welfare Reform," University of Maryland, 1998.

[26] National Center for Health Statistics, *op. cit.*

[27] Quoted in Tamar Lewin, "Family Decay Global, Study Says," *The New York Times,* May 30, 1995.

[28] Letter to *The New York Times,* May 16, 1997.

[29] Remarks upon nominating Henry Foster as surgeon general, Feb. 2, 1995.

[30] The South Carolina Council on Adolescent Pregnancy Prevention conducted the poll.

[31] "Involving Males in Preventing Teen Pregnancy," Urban Institute, 1997.

[32] Wade Horn and Andrew Bush, "Fathers, Marriage and Welfare Reform," Hudson Institute, 1997.

[33] Quoted in *The Washington Post,* June 8, 1998, p. A1.

[34] Hispanics, at 38 percent of all immigrants, account for the largest share of U.S immigration. Most Hispanic immigrants are Mexican-Americans, who traditionally have more babies in their teen years than whites, blacks or even other Latinos.

FOR MORE INFORMATION

Alan Guttmacher Institute, 120 Wall St., New York, N.Y. 10005; (212) 248-1111; www.agi-usa.org. The institute promotes the prevention of unintended pregnancies as well as a woman's freedom to terminate unwanted pregnancies.

Henry J. Kaiser Family Foundation, 2400 Sand Hill Road, Menlo Park, Calif. 94025; (650) 854-9400; www.kff.org. Devoted exclusively to health, the foundation focuses on U.S. health policy, reproductive health, HIV and health and development in South Africa.

Medical Institute for Sexual Health, P.O. Box 4919, Austin, Texas, 78765-4919; (512) 451-7599; www.mish.org. MISH is a non-profit medical education organization that espouses abstinence as the only safe way to avoid disease and pregnancy before marriage.

National Campaign to Prevent Teen Pregnancy, 1776 Massachusetts Ave., N.W., Suite 200, Washington, D.C. 20036; (202) 478-8500; www. teenpregnancy.org. This bipartisan, nonprofit organization aims to reduce teen pregnancy by one-third by 2005. It doesn't take a position on abstinence or sex education.

National Coalition for Abstinence Education, P.O. Box 536, Colorado Springs, Colo. 80901-0536; (719) 531-3388. This group of community-based abstinence-only education programs monitors implementation of the $50 million per year in abstinence grants under the Welfare Reform Act of 1996.

Sexuality Information and Education Council of the United States, 130 West 42nd St., Suite 350, New York, N.Y. 10036-7802; (212) 819-9770; www.siecus.org. SIECUS promotes comprehensive education about sexuality and advocates the right of individuals to make responsible sexual choices.

Bibliography

Selected Sources Used

Books

Lichter, S. Robert, Linda S. Lichter and Stanley Rothman, *Prime Time: How TV Portrays American Culture*, Regnery Publishing, 1994.
This comprehensive study focuses on how prime-time entertainment has portrayed American society from the 1950s to the '90s. In a lengthy chapter on TV, it notes, for instance, that during the 1976-77 season there were seven references to casual extramarital sex for every one time marital sex was mentioned.

Lind, Michael, *Up From Conservatism*, The Free Press, 1996.
Lind, a conservative-turned-moderate, argues that conservative intellectualism is dead as a result of the rise of the radical right of Pat Robertson, Patrick Buchanan and anti-government militias. He contends that the epidemic of illegitimacy is a myth, knowingly perpetrated on the public by conservatives manipulating statistics in order to dismantle the welfare system.

Luker, Kristin, *Dubious Conceptions: The Politics of Teenage Pregnancy*, Harvard University Press, 1996.
Luker argues that both liberals and conservatives have "constructed" an epidemic of teenage pregnancy. She traces the way popular attitudes came to demonize young mothers and examines the social and economic changes that have influenced debate on the issue.

***Teenage Pregnancy: Opposing Viewpoints*, Greenhaven Press, 1997.**
This collection of essays offers opposing viewpoints on the most controversial issues surrounding teenage pregnancy, including whether it really is a problem.

Articles

Funderburk, Patricia, "None, Not Safer, Is the Real Answer," *Insight, The Washington Times*, May 9, 1994.
The former Bush administration official argues that teaching youngsters to abstain from sex is better than teaching them how to protect themselves from pregnancy and sexually transmitted disease. She says that by not giving teenagers clear messages in sex-education classes, adults have failed to give today's teenagers any values.

McIlhaney, Joe S., "Are abstinence-only sex-education programs good for teenagers?" *Insight, The Washington Times*, Sept. 29, 1997.
An obstetrician-turned-activist writes that given the enormous health risks from rampant sexually transmitted diseases, it is irresponsible to teach teenagers that "safe" sex is possible.

Reports and Studies

Horn, Wade, and Andrew Bush, "Fathers, Marriage and Welfare Reform," Hudson Institute, 1997.
The authors argue that welfare helped cause the demise of marriage and the increasing disappearance of fathers from families and outline ways states can promote marriage-friendly welfare policies.

"Into a New World," Alan Guttmacher Institute, 1998.
This comprehensive study looks at sexual relationships, marriage and childbearing among the world's adolescents and young women. Numerous charts and graphs compare data on education levels, ages of first sexual experiences, age of first marriage and childbearing in 46 developing and developed countries.

Jemmott, John B. III, et al., "Abstinence and Safer Sex HIV Risk-Reduction Interventions for African American Adolescents," *Journal of the American Medical Association*, May 20, 1998.
This first-ever study comparing chastity vs. condoms found that abstinence-only was not as effective as a safer-sex program at preventing inner-city teens from having sex. The safer-sex program had stressed abstinence as the safest way to avoid STDs and pregnancy but also taught about using condoms.

Kirby, Douglas, "No Easy Answers: Research Findings on Programs to Reduce Teen Pregnancy," National Campaign to Prevent Teen Pregnancy, March 1997.
Kirby, a respected teenage sexuality researcher, evaluated 33 sex-ed studies and found that abstinence-only programs do not delay sexual activity.

Kirby, Douglas, et al, "The Impact of the Postponing Sexual Involvement Curriculum Among Youths in California," *Family Planning Perspectives*, May/June 1997.
This massive study of the Education Now and Babies Later (ENABL) program in California, the largest statewide abstinence-only effort ever initiated, found that participants were no less likely to avoid sex, pregnancy or STDs than teens in a control group.

Sonenstein, Freya L., et al, *Involving Males in Preventing Teen Pregnancy*, Urban Institute, 1997.
Researchers examine the crucial role that males play in teen pregnancy and STD prevention, and evaluate 23 programs around the country that focus on male behavior as a means of preventing pregnancy.

7 Drug Testing

KATHY KOCH

For Julie Izard, just married and looking for part-time work, organizing social activities at her apartment complex in Alexandria, Va., sounded perfect. Since the pay was minimal and the job only involved a few evenings a week, she viewed it almost as a volunteer position.

So she was surprised when she was sent to a nearby laboratory for a drug test. "I thought it was kind of funny," Izard says, since it wasn't a high-security job and she wouldn't be in charge of people's safety.

Drug testing has become a prime weapon in the nation's war on drugs, and more and more typical citizens like Izard — not just drivers, pilots, train operators and high-security government employees — are being asked to provide urine samples.

Nearly three-quarters of America's biggest companies hand job applicants a plastic cup as part of the recruiting process. A decade ago, only 21 percent of U.S. companies drug-tested recruits.

Most companies only test job applicants. Others screen both applicants and "safety-sensitive" employees — such as those who operate machinery. Still others test any employees who appear to be using drugs.

Increasingly, however, employers are requiring random testing of all employees — raising the hackles of some employees, unions and civil libertarians.

Momentum for the exponential growth in drug testing has come from several sources:

• The federal government — Transportation and Defense Department rules require drug testing for certain safety-sensitive jobs in both the public and private sectors; and the 1988 Drug-Free Workplace Act requires federal contractors or grant recipients to maintain drug-free workplaces.

• Courts — A series of decisions recognizes private employers' right

From *The CQ Researcher,* November 20, 1998.

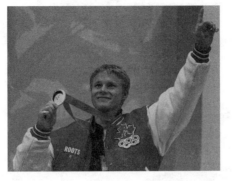

to test employees and applicants.

• Insurance companies — Insurers favor testing as a means of reducing accident liability and controlling health-care costs.

• Testing laboratories — Laboratories aggressively market their testing services to companies, schools and government agencies.

But clearly, much of the momentum for drug testing has come from Congress. "Over the past 15 years, Congress has passed laws requiring workplace drug testing of more than a tenth of the work force, or about 12 million individuals," says J. Michael Walsh, who designed the federal employee drug-testing regime.

Yet the same Congress has refused to undergo drug testing itself. Judges and political candidates are also exempt from mandatory drug testing, the courts have said (*see p. 128*).

Meanwhile, federal, state and local governments are widening their drug-testing net to cover even more citizens. Besides government employees, drug tests are now given to welfare mothers, prisoners, college-loan recipients and, sometimes, students wanting to join school clubs. And at the urging of President Clinton, Congress and some states are considering requiring all teenagers applying for a driver's license to be tested.

Some experts predict that eventually anyone receiving public money of any sort will have to be tested. Louisiana already requires random drug testing of anyone who receives anything of economic value from the

state — and those who balk can lose their job, license, loan, scholarship, contract or public assistance.

Local school boards also are expanding drug testing. For years, middle- and high-school athletes have undergone testing. [1] Now some school districts are requiring anyone participating in extracurricular activities to be tested. A few districts test any student who parks a car on school property. A handful of private schools have tested their entire student bodies, something public schools so far have been prohibited by the Constitution from doing, although at least two Texas school districts are toying with the idea.

Perhaps nowhere are the "bladder cops" — as some critics call drug testers — more prevalent than in the scandal-plagued sports world. (*See story, p. 124.*)

Civil libertarians and privacy advocates complain that the ever-widening drug-testing net dangerously erodes Americans' constitutional rights. While polls show most people agree that testing workers in safety-sensitive positions is appropriate, the trend toward testing new groups is "an evisceration of the Fourth Amendment in the name of the drug war," says Ethan Nadelmann, director of the Lindesmith Center, a drug-policy think tank.

Other critics call drug testing "chemical McCarthyism" because an improperly administered test could yield a false-positive result from the use of legitimate prescription drugs or even eating a poppy-seed bagel. Innocent job seekers or employees can lose their jobs. Sixty percent of companies fire an employee who tests positive for drugs; only 23 percent retain them, referring them for drug treatment.

If fired for a positive drug test, an employee usually cannot collect unemployment insurance. And employees who are injured on the job and test positive after the accident will probably be fired and become

Marijuana Was Most Frequently Detected

More than half of the employees who tested positive for drugs in 1997 had used marijuana.

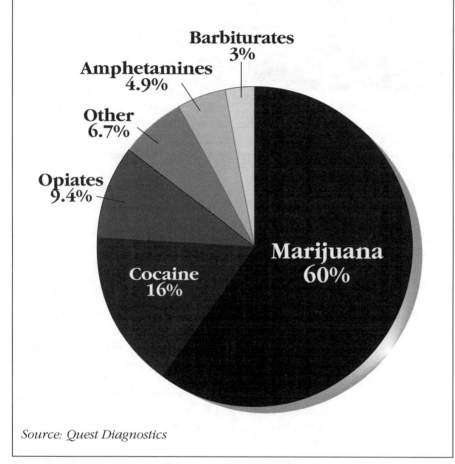

Barbiturates 3%

Amphetamines 4.9%

Other 6.7%

Opiates 9.4%

Cocaine 16%

Marijuana 60%

Source: Quest Diagnostics

ineligible for health benefits, workers' compensation or unemployment insurance.

Critics complain workplace drug testing gives employers unprecedented police power over what employees do during off-duty hours and unfairly targets those who use marijuana, which can remain in the system weeks longer than other "hard" drugs.

Proponents, however, say the magnitude of the nation's drug-abuse problem, and the cost of drug abuse to society — in lost productivity, workplace accidents, tardiness, absenteeism, workplace theft and in-

creased health-care costs — justifies testing, even if it infringes on individual privacy rights. [2]

"This problem is bleeding America," says Mark de Bernardo, executive director of the Institute for a Drug-Free Workplace, a coalition of businesses, business organizations and individuals. "The United States is the world's leader in substance abuse. We have 6 percent of the world's population, but we engage in 60 percent of the world's illicit drug use."

Last year, 13.9 million Americans — 6.4 percent of the population — used illicit drugs on a regular basis, a 10 percent increase from the 1992

record low of 5.8 percent. But the current rate is about half the 25 million who used illicit drugs in 1979, when drug use in America reached its peak and began declining, a decade before drug testing came into vogue.

Drug-testing advocates argue that because 74 percent of illicit drug users are employed, the workplace is an excellent place to catch them. "Employers have the most effective weapon in the war on drugs," de Bernardo says. "If your job is contingent on your being drug-free, it creates a powerful incentive for you to get off and stay off drugs.

Moreover, de Bernardo says, "Once an employer has a drug-testing policy, fewer drug abusers apply, and some [abusing] employees voluntarily leave."

Many abusers then seek work in small companies, he says, because only 3 percent of small firms — which employ half the nation's work force — have drug-testing programs. But twice as many employees in small firms use illegal drugs as in large firms.

To close the small-business "escape hatch," Congress last month appropriated $10 million for the Drug-Free Workplace Act of 1998 to encourage small companies to establish testing programs.

Polls show employees generally accept drug testing as a necessary evil, although there are still those who chafe at what they see as an unwarranted invasion of their privacy. Employees have filed dozens of court suits in the last 15 years, along with a handful of students, even though most students and parents favor drug testing because it gives students an excuse to resist peer pressure to use drugs. (*See story, p. 118.*)

These are some of the questions being asked by those debating this issue:

Does drug testing deter drug use?

"There are lots of books and research to show that drug testing deters drug use," de Bernardo says. "Individual companies have seen dramatic decreases in positive drug-test rates."

He is quick to add that drug testing alone isn't a deterrent. It must be accompanied by a comprehensive substance-abuse prevention program that includes four other components: a written anti-drug policy, an anti-drug education program, rigorous enforcement and a treatment program for addicted employees.

Drug-testing proponents often cite a 1988 U.S. Navy study showing that drug use among enlisted men went down from 48 percent in 1980 to 5 percent in 1988 after a comprehensive substance-abuse prevention program with random drug testing was instituted. [3]

Indeed, a 1987 Navy personnel survey showed 83 percent considered random testing the Navy's strongest deterrent to drug abuse. "Significantly, 27 percent also said that they would resume their use of illicit drugs if the Navy discontinued its drug-testing program," according to the Institute for a Drug-Free Workplace. [4]

Another study showed a 50 percent drop in positive drug tests — from 22.9 percent to 11.6 percent — at the Southern Pacific Railroad after a year of "reasonable-suspicion" drug testing. [5]

Walsh says drug testing "keeps mainstream working folks from casual recreational use."

Workplace drug testing will deter drug use among those recreation users, most of whom are employed suburbanites, said Rep. Gerald B.H. Solomon, R-N.Y., as he argued for the bill to encourage small businesses to start drug testing. "If we were to solve that problem," he said, it would eliminate U.S. demand for drugs, "and in Colombia they would be making bathtubs instead of [exporting] drugs into this country."

Proponents also point to American Management Association (AMA) statistics showing the percentage of

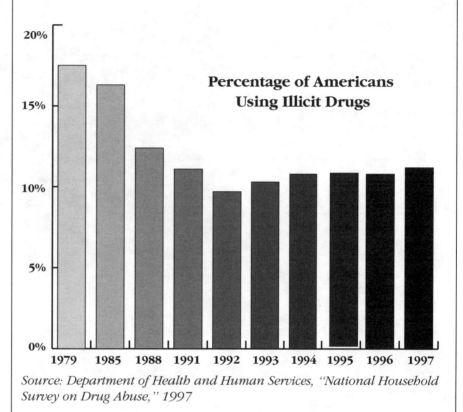

Americans' Drug Use Is Rising

Americans' drug use has been rising since 1992, but it was still 35 percent less in 1997 than it was in 1979, when U.S. drug use reached an all-time high.

Percentage of Americans Using Illicit Drugs

Source: Department of Health and Human Services, "National Household Survey on Drug Abuse," 1997

employees testing positive for drugs declined from 8.1 percent in 1989 to 1.9 percent in 1995. [6]

But Eric Greenberg, AMA's director of management studies, says the declining figures do not prove drug use is actually declining. That's because employers have been expanding the total pool of persons tested to include all employees, not just those suspected of drug use. If you test more employees who show no obvious signs of drug use, "Naturally, the test-positive ratios will go down," he says.

"When companies didn't expand the pool of employees covered, the percentages stayed the same," he says. "This is why I say those statis-

tics do not show that drug testing is a deterrent."

Lewis Maltby, director of the Office of Workplace Rights at the American Civil Liberties Union (ACLU), which opposes random drug testing, agrees. "When you go from suspicion-based testing to random testing, the number of hits are going to go down," he says.

Maltby argues that anti-drug education programs may be more of a deterrent. Companies that combine drug testing with education programs consistently have lower test-positive ratios than firms that rely solely on testing.

But some companies are cutting both their drug-education and supervisor-training programs, which teach

They Decided to Fight the System...

Hollister Gardner is hardly a rebellious teenager. He maintained an "A" average while serving as president of the National Honor Society, drum major in the band and treasurer of Future Farmers of America (FFA) at his West Texas high school.

But Gardner rebelled last year when he was told that he would have to pass a drug test to keep participating in such extracurricular activities.

Having never been involved in drugs, he chafed at the implication that he was guilty unless proven innocent. He believes the Fourth Amendment of the Bill of Rights protects U.S. citizens from such warrantless searches without "reasonable suspicion" that someone is guilty.

So he never signed the consent form. His 12-year-old sister, Sarah, and his 13-year-old cousin Molly also refused to sign theirs.

When the school notified Hollister that he could no longer attend after-school activities, he sued the Tulia Independent School District board, whose members include his father, Gary, the only board member who opposed drug testing when it was instituted. Representing himself in federal court, Hollister argued the board's drug-testing policy is unconstitutional.

"The school district can't test just because they feel like testing," he said. "People fought and died for these rights, and they are not to be given up to the Tulia School Board just because they think they can take them from you."[1]

The elder Gardner agreed with his son's decision. "To my eyes, it's almost a duty," he says. "It was something he just had to do." No trial date has been set in the case, which is pending in Amarillo's federal court.

The school district contends its policy is legal because in 1995 the U.S. Supreme Court upheld the Veronia, Ore., school district's policy of randomly testing all high school athletes. In that case, the court said random, suspicionless drug tests were justified because the drug crisis in the Veronia district had reached "epidemic proportions."

Gardner, now a sophomore at Angelo State University, says the drug problem in rural Tulia was not severe enough to justify warrantless searches. "I don't use drugs," he told

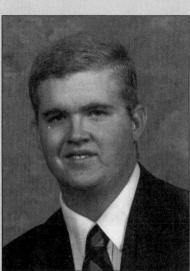

Hollister Gardner

a newspaper reporter at the time, "and no one I know in my organizations uses them."[2]

Tulia School Superintendent Mike Vinyard says the school board instituted drug testing after a 1994 survey showed 27 percent of students in grades 7-12 had used drugs at least once, and 10 percent said they had used marijuana prior to the survey. Six percent of junior high kids said they had smoked marijuana before class.

Although the survey showed Tulia's drug use was below the state average, Vinyard says, "We think any drug use is serious." He said "about a dozen students" have tested positive since the program began in January 1997.

Most parents like the policy, he says, because fear of random testing gives students an excuse to resist peer pressure to use drugs. "The Gardner family is really the only critic of the program," Vinyard says. "Most parents would like to randomly test all students rather than only those in extracurricular activities."

At least two other Texas school districts apparently feel the same way. The Texas Association of School Boards has reviewed at least two proposals from school districts wanting to require all students to be randomly drug tested. Shellie Hoffman, the association's director of legal services, would not reveal the names of the districts.

If adopted, they would become the first public school districts in the country to test all students. The policy would undoubtedly be challenged legally, says Jim Harrington, director of the nonprofit Texas Civil Rights Project. "The Supreme Court has made it very clear that drug testing can only be applied in certain cases, such as where there is a pervasive drug culture, violence or physical danger for athletes, or where students are considered role models," he says.

Hollister says that while parents may favor drug testing, many students supported him. "I had quite a few people come up to me and thank me for sticking up for their rights," he says.

But standing up for one's rights is costly, he says. Not unexpectedly, he and his family have paid emotionally,

managers to spot drug abuse — a policy that could prove "penny-wise but pound-foolish," Maltby says. Only 6 percent of surveyed companies rely only on drug testing, says

the AMA report.

Drug-testing opponents say there are no peer-reviewed, scientific studies to show that drug testing deters drug use. "The decline in drug use in

this country began in 1979," says Maltby. "Nobody was doing drug testing in 1979."

"The era of drug testing began in 1985-1986, yet since 1991, drug use

... When Ordered to Take Drug Tests

academically and financially for their stand. "I warned him if he refused to sign, he would get more flak than he ever thought about, and that they might not even let him graduate," remembers Hollister's father.

Hollister was not allowed to show his pig at the agricultural fair with other members of his FFA group, and his sister Sarah was told she could not play in the band. The school later allowed protesting students to stay in after-school activities until the case is settled.

The family also paid about $6,000 for transportation, court fees and administrative costs, says Gary Gardner, who calls himself "just a small dirt farmer." The costs were especially burdensome because of the huge losses Texas farmers suffered due to bad weather this year. "Any other year it wouldn't have been so bad," he says.

Hollister has even greater respect for the Constitution now. "Our family has always understood what the Constitution meant," he says. "Now I've really developed a love for it."

A lifelong love for the Constitution also led Georgia history teacher Sherry Hearn to stand up against drug testing. And she, too, has paid a high price.

Three years away from retirement, the award-winning Savannah, Ga., high school teacher lost her job — and nearly lost her pension — when she refused to take a drug test on demand.

For 27 years Hearn, who was her county's Teacher of the Year in 1994, had taught her American history students that the Fourth Amendment protects citizens against unreasonable searches and seizures by police. Not surprisingly, she had been an outspoken critic of her district's policy of allowing "lockdowns," or periodic, unannounced, schoolwide searches — using drug-sniffing dogs — to ferret out illegal guns or drugs. Many school districts, including 400 in Texas alone, use drug-sniffing dogs to search school grounds.

During the two-hour lockdowns in Savannah, students and teachers must stand in the hallways, while dogs search each room, bookbag and purse, and students are scanned with metal detectors.

Hearn maintains such searches without specific information that someone may possess drugs or weapons are an invasion of constitutional rights and a dreadful message to be sending students. She had opposed the tactics at faculty meetings, to her principal, the school board and to police officers who conducted the lockdowns.

Then during a lockdown on April 4, 1996, police say they found a partially smoked marijuana cigarette in Hearn's car. But police refused to show her the evidence, claiming it had been accidentally destroyed. Hearn refused to submit to a drug test without first seeing her lawyer, especially since the officers had searched her car without her permission, in clear violation of the school's written policy.

School board officials claim Hearn was fired for insubordination. She claims she was targeted by police because she had objected to the lockdowns.

No action was taken against the officers who searched her car without permission. And the school board never investigated a tip police received giving them the initials of a student who had bragged to classmates that he had "planted" the marijuana in Hearn's car.

"The board feels very strongly about its drug-free workplace policy, and we feel equally strongly that we can't pick and choose who gets to follow the rules," Chatham County School Board President Karen Matthews told The Associated Press. [3] Hearn's case is pending before the U.S. District Court in Atlanta.

Since she was fired, Hearn has been unable to find a full-time job at any Georgia public school. She believes she was blackballed for standing up for her rights. "How else would you explain someone with my qualifications not being able to find a job, when we have a teacher shortage in Georgia?" she asks.

She finally was hired at a juvenile detention center, and is enrolled again in the state's pension program.

Knowing how much standing up for her rights has cost her, if she had to do it over again would she take the test? She hopes not. "It would endanger my credibility with my students, which I spent 27 years building up."

More important, she says, "I would be voluntarily surrendering my rights. Anytime you accept any sort of violation — no matter how minor — of your basic liberties there are those who will take increasing liberties. Eventually, you won't have any left."

---

[1] Allan Turner, "Defending his rights; Student risking all to oppose drug testing," *The Houston Chronicle,* Feb. 2, 1997.

[2] *Ibid.*

[3] John Cheves, "Fired Chatham teacher sues," *Florida Times-Union,* April 17, 1997.

---

among teenagers has been going up," points out Allen St. Pierre, executive director of the NORML Foundation, which wants to legalize marijuana.

Critics like St. Pierre claim the statistics used to "prove" that testing deters drug abuse are "twisted and manipulated" by proponents, many of whom are connected to the testing industry.

"It's really hard to prove that drug testing is a deterrent in itself," says William Sonnenstuhl, professor of industrial labor relations at Cornell University. "If you look at the railroad industry, the first industry in which drug testing was implemented, they were not successful until the unions started educating their members to stop drinking and covering up for members who used alcohol or drugs on the job."

"I don't think drug testing deters anyone, except for the novices," Sonnenstuhl continues. "Skillful drug users know how to beat the tests. It just becomes a game they have to play."

In 1994, the National Academy of Sciences (NAS) reviewed all of the literature on drug testing and found "no conclusive scientific evidence from properly controlled studies that employment drug-testing programs widely discourage drug use or encourage rehabilitation." [7]

Drug-testing opponents say that rather than testing teenagers for drug abuse, it is cheaper to teach them how to say no to drugs.

"There are lots of peer-pressure resistance classes available to schools," says Jim Harrington, director of the Texas Civil Rights Project. "And they are much cheaper than drug testing."

Proponents say the "tough love" zero-tolerance approach encourages abusers to get treatment.

But skeptics point out that when an applicant fails a drug test, 98 percent of large employers reject his application, and 63 percent fire existing employees who test positive, rather than referring them to a company-supported drug rehab program. [8] Those fired workers are then usually ineligible for unemployment or health benefits, as well as workers' compensation if they were injured on the job before testing positive. Thus, say critics, most can't afford to join a drug-treatment program.

The "dumping" of drug abusers back into the community, unemployed and without benefits, "encourages their entry into illegal economies," says Paul M. Roman, research professor of sociology and director

of the Center for Research on Deviance and Behavioral Health at the University of Georgia.

Workplace testing also misses those most seriously addicted to drugs who are usually unemployed, say critics. Other argue that some drug abusers merely substitute alcohol or harder drugs, such as heroin or cocaine, that are more difficult to detect through urinalysis because they only stay in the body for a few hours.

Nadelmann says, "If you want to get bombed on Saturday night now, and you need to be 'clean' on Monday morning, instead of smoking a joint, which will stay in your system longer, you'll switch to cocaine or heroin."

Does drug testing protect worker and public safety?

Proponents say companies with drug-testing policies have safer workplaces, better overall job performance, reduced liability for accidents and injuries and reduced medical and insurance costs.

"Without question, substance abusers account for higher rates of accidents in the workplace," says de Bernardo. "Lots and lots of studies link illicit drug use to impairment, and impairment to safety and health concerns."

"No one doubts that employers with effective substance-abuse policies have fewer workplace accidents," said Thomas J. Donohue, president of the U.S. Chamber of Commerce. As a result they have fewer workers'-compensation claims. Several states, he said, now offer employers who have such programs discounted rates on insurance premiums. [9]

In addition, "Employers consistently report reduced rates of employee violence and crime" after implementing a comprehensive substance-abuse policy, Donohue added.

Dan Wurzburg, corporate safety director for Sordoni Skanska construction-management firm in Parsippany,

N.J., said, "In the construction industry, having a drug-free workplace program means that the company can absolutely be assured that it will have a better safety record, and fewer accidents mean lower costs and lower insurance premiums."

According to data in the recent bill to encourage small businesses to set up workplace drug-testing programs, accidents involving drug users are 300-400 percent higher than among non-users.

In the Southern Pacific Railroad study, personal injuries and accidents dropped dramatically after drug testing was implemented. Personal injuries, for instance, dropped from 2,234 in 1983 to 322 in the first six months of 1988. Train accidents caused by human error decreased from 911 to 54 during the same period. [10]

But opponents question the statistics used by advocates to show that drug abusers cause more workplace accidents. For instance, the claim that 47 percent of workplace accidents are caused by drug abusers — used by Congress in October to justify spending $10 million to encourage workplace drug testing in small companies — "is absurd on the face of it," Sonnenstuhl says. "Such statistics are based on a series of assumptions "inferring causation where what has been shown is only correlation."

Workplace accident reports show that most accidents result from "a series of management or supervisory decisions that create or tolerate unsafe work environments, equipment and practices," Sonnenstuhl says.

"To blame drug users is to shift focus and remedial efforts from a strategy that has been proven successful [ie., reducing hazards and educating workers about workplace safety] to one of dubious assumptions, merits and promise," sociologist William Staudenmeier says.

Sonnenstuhl says drug testing is being sold to employers and employees as a question of job safety. But

Experts Question Hair Testing

New drug-testing techniques being introduced are considered less invasive than urinalysis and almost impossible to "beat." Hair testing, for instance, can detect drug use as far back as three months. By comparison, urinalysis only detects heroin and cocaine within hours or days of use, and marijuana for up to 70 days.

Not surprisingly, some of the new techniques raise thorny questions about accuracy, privacy and the purpose of drug testing.

Ethan Nadelmann, director of the Lindesmith Center, a drug-policy think tank, argues that testing hair, sweat and saliva is more — not less — invasive because it delves more deeply into one's past history. And because hair and saliva contain DNA, they reveal information about medical conditions and genetic makeup that some employees may not want to reveal to their bosses.

"Hair testing opens the door to genetic testing by employers," says Lewis Maltby, director of the Office of Workplace Rights at the American Civil Liberties Union (ACLU), noting that companies could refuse to hire someone based on inherited medical conditions, which the applicant may not even know about. Although hair testers claim they wouldn't look at DNA, the procedure stirs controversy on several other fronts.

In hair testing, a snippet of hair from the back of the neck (or the armpit of a bald person) is tested for drug residues. The developer of the technique, Boston-based Psychemedics Corp., says it detects four times more drug users than urinalysis.

Florida entrepreneur H. Wayne Huizenga, founder of Blockbuster Entertainment and Waste Management Inc. and owner of the Miami Dolphins, is a major stockholder in Psychemedics and helped raise the company out of debt in 1989. With Blockbuster and Waste Management as major clients, the firm has grown to more than 1,400 clients today, including General Motors and The Sports Authority.

"Hair testing will continue to grow dramatically," says company General Counsel William Thistle. "It's inevitable once companies see the advantages."

Sales have more than doubled in the last five years, as more firms adopted the process. Several police departments have signed on as well, including New York City and Chicago. At least 40 private schools have begun testing students' hair, among them De la Salle High School in New Orleans, which randomly tests its entire 860-member student body.

(Public schools are generally thought to be prohibited by the Fourth Amendment from testing entire student bodies.)

Psychemedics has lobbied Congress to require the Health and Human Services Department (HHS) to adopt hair testing for all federal employees, but so far the agency has resisted.

"We in the federal government are not confident of it at this time," says Donna Bush, chief of drug testing for the Substance Abuse and Mental Health Services Administration (SAMHSA).

The National Institute on Drug Abuse, the Food and Drug Administration, the College of American Pathologists and the Society of Forensic Toxicologists are all concerned that hair testing may be unfairly biased against persons with coarse black hair, such as African-Americans, Asians or Hispanics. Some tests have shown that coarse hair shows much higher concentrations of drugs than lighter hair after ingestion of the same amount of drugs.

"There is no study, any time, any place, anywhere, that shows that Psychemedics' testing procedures have a racial bias," Thistle says. "I've been involved in hair testing since 1989, and at no time has there been a racial-discrimination lawsuit on the grounds that hair testing is racially biased."

Other scientists claim hair testing doesn't differentiate between drugs absorbed into the hair from environmental contamination, such as being at a concert where marijuana is smoked.

For these reasons, the ACLU strongly opposes hair testing. "Every reputable scientific organization in America rejects the use of hair testing for employment purposes," Maltby says.

Thistle says the ACLU should favor hair testing because it is not biased against marijuana users like urine testing. "With a urine test, the chances of finding a marijuana user are greater than finding a cocaine or heroin user," he says. "With hair testing, all drug users are uniformly caught."

Further, he says, the company's special decontamination procedure, which includes washing hair samples in various solutions for nearly two hours before conducting the tests, eliminates contamination due to passive absorption.

While Psychemedics' decontamination procedures may be carefully performed, critics say no one knows whether other hair testing labs are being as careful, because hair testing is unregulated. There are no national standards for hair analysis as there are for urinalysis.

John Baenziger, special commissioner of toxicology at the College of American Pathologists, says his group does not support hair testing yet because it is "not being done uniformly" and the procedures being used in labs "are not being looked at in a critical fashion."

more and more, all employees are being tested, including clerks and receptionists. As a result, "drug testing becomes just a moral cover for 'You shouldn't be using drugs.' "

Critics argue vociferously that drug testing does not test one's current fitness for duty, especially in the case of marijuana, which can show up in the urine for up to 70 days after consumption, long after the effects of the drug have worn off. Meanwhile, other drugs and alcohol are washed out of the system within a few hours, they point out. And cocaine doesn't show up immediately after being ingested.

Because of these discrepancies, "Most people who fail tests are totally sober, and most who are stoned pass," Maltby says.

"We've got reams and reams from the government itself that show urinalysis doesn't test impairment," St. Pierre says. "All the testimony before Congress has said that having marijuana metabolites in your urine does not prove impairment."

"So drug testing is not done to protect the public health, it is mainly done for the symbolism," he says. "Logic has totally been thrown out the door, as it has for most of this war on drugs."

If companies really wanted to protect workplace safety, they would go after alcohol use, say critics. "The biggest problem regarding workplace safety, bar none, is alcohol," St. Pierre says. Most urinalysis does not check for alcohol levels.

"Alcohol is an enormous problem," de Bernardo acknowledges. "Any employer who addresses drug abuse and not alcohol is foolish."

Critics of drug testing often favor impairment testing as the best way to protect public safety. "There are better ways to protect the public safety than to invade somebody's privacy," Maltby says. "It is absolutely clear that impairment testing protects the public safety better than urine testing."

Impairment testing, also called performance testing, involves using computerized video programs to test eye-hand coordination by requiring the employee to use a "joy stick" to keep a cursor in the middle of a screen. An employee takes several practice tests to establish his "baseline" capability, and then is tested randomly — or daily for those with safety-sensitive positions — to see whether he is impaired.

Yet, Donna Bush, chief of drug testing for SAMHSA, says, "At this time we've not seen evidence in the peer-reviewed scientific literature that impairment testing works." "Performance testing is easily manipulated," says de Bernardo.

Walsh agrees. "There's not much data to show that it really works. And there's no data at all to show that it would detect drug use. If I'm an illicit drug user, I would have every incentive not to do well on the baseline."

Walsh and de Bernardo say such tests do not detect illegal drug use because they do not differentiate as to whether someone is impaired because he has been using drugs or he is merely fatigued because he was up all night with a sick child.

"Performance testing doesn't determine whether someone is engaged in illegal behavior," says de Bernardo. "It protects people's jobs who don't deserve that protection."

For that reason, urinalysis advocates also do not favor another method being used by police officers in some states to test driver impairment. They use new devices shaped like binoculars, which test the reactions of the pupils to flashes of light. "It shows if you are under the influence of something," says Maltby, but it doesn't determine whether it's alcohol or illegal drugs. ∎

BACKGROUND

War on Drugs

In 1971, President Richard M. Nixon declared the nation's first "war on drugs." But drug use continued, especially among youths, until it peaked in 1979.

By then, drugs like marijuana and cocaine had become socially acceptable in many quarters. For instance, in 1979, 19 percent of Americans 18-25 had used cocaine in the preceding 12 months, according to the National Institute on Drug Abuse. [11] As marijuana became regarded as a "soft drug" like alcohol and tobacco, 11 states decriminalized possession of small amounts, one legalized it and 29 others made possession of small amounts a misdemeanor, writes Beverly Potter, co-author of *Drug Testing at Work*. In 1977, President Jimmy Carter even called for decriminalization of marijuana possession.

In 1978-79, as drug use was reaching its peak in America, an anti-drug backlash developed, led by the "parents movement," which later became the Atlanta-based anti-drug group National Families in Action. In 1980-81, the military vowed to clean up its ranks and began random, suspicionless drug testing.

By 1982, President Ronald Reagan had declared a second "war on drugs," and drug testing outside the military came into vogue. In 1986, the president and his senior advisers submitted urine samples to be screened for the presence of illegal drugs. The symbolic gesture was designed to encourage private employers to test their workers, and to reduce employee opposition to testing.

Sociologist Staudenmeier calls Reagan's push for private employers to do drug testing "privatized social control." The Fourth Amendment prohibits the government from requiring the general population to provide urine samples, he points out. "We find the president of the United States appealing to employers to use their power to accomplish what the state cannot: widespread urine testing of American citizens," he wrote. [12]

But there was scant public outcry as companies increasingly began asking

Chronology

1960s *Marijuana, hallucinogens and other drugs become widespread among middle-class youth during the counterculture revolution. Drug use becomes rampant among Vietnam soldiers.*

1968
Mandatory drug testing in the military begins as addicted Vietnam vets begin returning home.

———— • ————

1970s *Marijuana and cocaine become socially acceptable in many quarters, even as the country launches its first "war on drugs."*

1971
President Richard M. Nixon declares the first "war on drugs."

Aug. 3, 1977
President Jimmy Carter calls for decriminalization of marijuana possession.

1979
Drug use peaks. Eleven states decriminalize possession of small amounts of "pot," one legalizes it and 29 others make possession a misdemeanor. Anti-drug backlash develops, led by the "parents movement."

———— • ————

1980s *Cocaine becomes the drug of choice among urban professionals. Crack cocaine, a highly addictive form of cocaine, causes skyrocketing crime rates. Only 5 percent of high-*

school seniors smoke marijuana daily, compared with 10 percent in 1978.

1982
President Ronald Reagan declares a second "war on drugs."

July 1985
Arkansas court rules that "the excessive intrusive nature" of drug testing student athletes without reasonable suspicion is not justified by its need.

1986
In a symbolic gesture, Reagan and his senior advisers submit urine samples to be screened for the presence of illegal drugs. In September Reagan issues Executive Order 12564, calling for a "drug-free workplace" in all federal agencies.

November 1988
Congress passes Drug-Free Workplace Act, requiring federal contractors or grant recipients to maintain drug-free workplaces. Many employers set up voluntary testing programs. Employees begin suing, claiming drug testing is a violation of individual privacy rights. Courts allow suspicionless drug testing.

1989
President George Bush unveils his National Drug Control Strategy, encouraging comprehensive drug-free workplace policies in the private sector and in state and local government. In *National Treasury Employees Union v. Von Raab* decision, Supreme Court upholds random drug testing when a "special need" outweighs individual privacy rights.

1990s *President Bush expands the federal drug-testing program to include all White House personnel. Clinton expands the Reagan-Bush drug-testing policies. Drug use increases.*

1991
Congress passes the Omnibus Transportation and Employment Testing Act, extending drug and alcohol testing to 8 million private-sector pilots, drivers and equipment operators.

1992
Drug use begins increasing. Clinton is elected president.

1995
In *Vernonia School District v. Acton*, the Supreme Court rules that random urinalysis of high school athletes is justified because the drug crisis in the school district has reached "epidemic proportions."

1996
Marijuana arrests are up 80 percent, mostly for possession. Teenage drug use becomes a hot campaign issue. Just before the election, Clinton proposes mandatory drug tests for all teens seeking driver's licenses.

1998
In June Congress rescinds federal student loans to any student convicted of a drug charge. In August Congress refuses to order tests for members of Congress and their staffs. In October the Supreme Court lets stand a rural Indiana high school's policy of testing all students in extracurricular activities and passes the Drug-Free Workplace Act of 1998.

Athletes vs. Drug Testers

Athletes have long been subjected to drug testing for performance-enhancing drugs, which are often dangerous to an athlete's long-term health and give users an unfair advantage over athletes that don't use them. [1]

But the use of banned performance-enhancing drugs appears to be on the rise, despite stepped-up testing. Athletic drug testing has become a constant cat-and-mouse game, as athletes continually try to outsmart the drug testers, and the laboratories keep improving their detection technology.

This year several drug-testing scandals have rocked the sports world, including:

• In July the top team in the prestigious Tour de France bicycle race was disqualified amid news that some cyclists were using the banned synthetic hormone EPO. The hormone, which increases the red blood cell count, gives athletes greater endurance by putting extra oxygen into the blood. But it is extremely dangerous and has been blamed for dozens of athletes' deaths.

• Irish swimmer Michelle de Bruin was banned for four years from swimming competitions after manipulating a test sample.

• Chinese swimmer Yuan Yuan was arrested at Sydney airport on her way to the World Swimming Championships in Perth. She was carrying 13 vials of human growth hormone, which her coach later said were his. He was suspended for 15 years.

• In February Canadian snowboarder Ross Rebagliati's Olympic gold medal was taken away after he tested positive for marijuana; it was returned after he appealed, claiming it was due to secondhand smoke.

Closer to home, controversy swirled around Mark McGwire, the record-breaking St. Louis Cardinals slugger who broke Roger Maris' single-season home-run record on Sept. 27. McGwire was using the controversial performance enhancer androstenedione, a testosterone-boosting precursor to anabolic steroids developed by East Germany's state-sponsored athletic drug program in the 1970s.

"Andro" rapidly elevates testosterone levels, producing a temporary energy surge described by East German swimmer Raik Hannermann as a "volcanic eruption." [2] It is sold in U.S. health food stores as a nutritional supplement.

Because andro is allowed in Major League Baseball (MLB), McGwire was cheered on to victory while taking the drug. But Olympic shotputter Randy Barnes was banned for life by the International Amateur Athletic Federation (IAAF) in July after he tested positive for the same substance, which some scientists say is extremely dangerous.

Because experts disagree over whether androstenedione should be considered an anabolic steroid and thus be banned because it is available only by prescription, sports organizations treat it differently. The IAAF, the International Olympic Committee (IOC), the National Football League and the National Collegiate Athletic Association have all banned it.

But MLB and the National Basketball Association have not, and the National Hockey League prohibits only illegal drugs. [3]

Such dramatic inconsistencies in athletic drug testing have led many to call for reform of international drug-testing laws so they are clear, consistent and enforceable.

Complicating the situation was the U.S. government's loosening of laws governing food supplements in 1994, which allowed products like androstenedione to be marketed in the U.S. as a food. Such products were not available over-the-counter under old Food and Drug Administration rules. Now, foreign athletes come to the United States shopping for banned performance-enhancers.

Other supplements, like the muscle-building amino acid creatine, are now widely used by high school and professional athletes alike. Creatine hit the headlines last summer, when both McGwire and his closest home run competitor, Sammy Sosa of the Chicago Cubs, admitted using it. Creatine is considered safe, but the long-term effects are unknown.

With new "natural" performance drugs and masking agents constantly being developed, drug testers have difficulty figuring out how to detect the new substances, and deciding whether they should be legal.

"In today's world, athletes who are determined to cheat know that natural substances are the way to go," said Don Catlin, a professor of medicine and pharmacology at the University of California at Los Angeles and a member of the IOC medical commission. The new substances, including androstenedione, are popular with athletes because they are currently undetectable through testing, and so new that many leagues have not formed policies about their use, he said. [4]

The IOC has called for establishment of an independent international agency to coordinate drug testing for Olympic athletes. The proposal will be discussed at a sports drug summit in February in Lausanne, Switzerland.

The Association of Professional Team Physicians recently called on MLB to ban androstenedione. Even if it does, there will probably be other questionable supplements on the market soon.

"There's a whole cornucopia of other things right behind it," said Catlin. "That's where things are going." [5]

---

[1] See Richard L. Worsnop, "Athletes and Drugs," *The CQ Researcher*, July 26, 1991, pp. 513-536.

[2] Quoted in Scott M. Reid, "Special Report: Slugger's drug widely banned," *The Denver Post*, Aug. 25, 1998

[3] Under federal law, anabolic steroids are a controlled substance, available only by prescription.

[4] Kirk Johnson, "Mac's use of drug raises issues beyond sports," *The (Charleston, S.C.) Post and Courier*, Sept. 1, 1998.

[5] *Ibid.*

employees for urine samples. Following a barrage of press articles in 1986 about crack cocaine and crack babies, public attitudes about drugs took a sharp right turn. A *Time*/CBS survey found that 72 percent of full-time workers said they would voluntarily submit to drug testing, and 25 percent of full-time factory workers said they had a colleague who used drugs. [13]

Several high-profile accidents in the 1980s involving drugged or drunken drivers and pilots added fuel to the national anti-drug sentiment. In 1981, a Navy pilot, apparently high on marijuana, crashed into the deck of the U.S.S. *Nimitz*, destroying several planes and causing more than $100 million in damages. Marijuana was also implicated in the 1987 Conrail-Amtrak train collision in Maryland, which killed 16 people. And alcohol was blamed for the 1989 *Exxon Valdez* accident in Alaska, which caused one of the worst oil spills in U.S. history. [14]

The public began to demand that those responsible for the safety of others — such as pilots, surgeons and police officers — be drug-free. In addition, the highly publicized deaths of University of Maryland basketball star Len Bias and Cleveland Browns' footfall player Don Rogers led to a public outcry about drug use among sports stars. Drug testing was touted as part of the solution to both problems.

Meanwhile, with increased availability bringing lower costs, cocaine had became the drug of choice among successful young urban professionals. Crack cocaine had also entered the picture, a highly addictive form of free-base cocaine, blamed for skyrocketing urban crime rates.

In the late 1980s, then-Attorney General Richard L. Thornburgh called drug testing by employers the moral thing to do. "That's really what started this whole process and has been driving it all along," Sonnenstuhl says. "The responsibility has to be put at the foot of the federal government for inciting all of this stuff."

Despite all the hysteria about skyrocketing drug use in the 1980s and Reagan's push for drug testing, total drug use nationwide had begun a steady decline in 1979 that continued until 1992. Cocaine and crack use continued to flourish in the 1980s among a small percentage of the population, but marijuana use, particularly among students, declined. By the late 1980s, for instance, only 5 percent of high-school seniors smoked marijuana every day, compared with 10 percent in 1978. [15]

Workplace Testing

Nonetheless, in September 1986 President Reagan issued Executive Order 12564, calling for a "drug-free workplace" in all federal agencies and ordering that employees in "sensitive positions" be tested for illegal drug use. The rule allowed anyone who tested positive to be fired after a single offense, but mandated that second offenders must be fired. President George Bush later expanded the program to include testing for all White House personnel. Today, 1.7 million employees in 111 federal agencies are tested, with those in safety-sensitive positions usually tested on a random basis.

Congress expanded the drug testing net with the Drug-Free Workplace Act of 1988, which required federal contractors or grant recipients to maintain drug-free workplaces. Although drug testing wasn't mandated, many employers set up testing programs.

In 1989, President Bush unveiled his National Drug Control Strategy. It said the federal government "has a responsibility to do all that it can to promote comprehensive drug-free workplace policies."

Two years later, Congress passed the Omnibus Transportation and Employment Testing Act of 1991, which extended mandatory drug and alcohol testing to 8 million private-sector pilots, drivers and equipment operators.

President Clinton has expanded the Reagan-Bush drug-testing policies to prisons, where those "who commit a lion's share of the crimes in this country are in a controlled environment," said White House senior adviser Rahm Emanuel. "We have to slam shut the revolving door between drugs and crime. Through mandatory testing, you will force a change in their behavior that will break the link." [16]

Arguing that most drug offenders get arrested sooner or later, the administration pushed through Congress a law requiring states to test and treat prisoners and parolees for drugs before they can receive federal prison-construction funds. It also increased the number of residential treatment centers in federal prisons and more than tripled the number of inmates being treated for substance abuse. [17]

Critics say the administration's anti-drug policies are nothing more than a war on casual marijuana users, because they are the ones most often "caught" with current drug-testing methods.

"Despite criticism that this administration is soft on drugs, FBI data clearly demonstrate that Clinton's war on marijuana smokers is the toughest ever waged in our nation's history," says St. Pierre of the NORML Foundation. Marijuana arrests have risen 80 percent since 1990, according to the FBI. Nearly 642,000 people were arrested for marijuana offenses in 1996, St. Pierre says, 85 percent for possession.

Legal Challenges

As soon as drug tests began appearing in schools and workplaces, individuals, unions and the American Civil Liberties Union (ACLU) began challenging the practice in court. Plaintiffs typically claimed drug testing violated individual privacy rights or Fourth Amendment protections against unreasonable search and seizure by government agents.

Until the mid-1980s, the lower courts had consistently ruled that — except in the military — it was unconstitutional to randomly drug test without "reasonable suspicion" that someone was using drugs.

But in the mid-1980s, as the "war on drugs" gained momentum and public attitudes toward drugs shifted, courts began allowing suspicionless drug testing when the state was seen to have an administrative interest that overrode an individual's right to privacy. This "administrative exception" was applied to jockeys, prison guards, nuclear plant employees, public school teachers and Customs Service employees.

In a precedent-setting 1989 case involving customs inspectors — *National Treasury Employees Union v. Von Raab* — the Supreme Court for the first time allowed random, suspicionless drug testing when there is a "special need" that outweighs the individual's privacy rights. The courts spent the next decade defining "special need."

Civil rights scholars viewed the *Von Raab* ruling as a major departure for the court because it was holding individual privacy rights as less important than the state's interest in winning the war on drugs. [18]

The decision is tantamount to jettisoning the need to establish probable cause before searching private homes because the state has a strong interest in eliminating crime, argued law scholar Jeannette C. James. [19]

But perhaps no case shocked civil libertarians more than *Vernonia School District v. Acton*, in which the Supreme Court ruled in 1995 that

suspicionless, random urinalysis of high-school athletes was justified because the drug crisis in the school district had reached "epidemic proportions." Yet the Vernonia district had found only 12 positive drug tests in four and a half years. Just 10 years earlier the court had struck down as unreasonable a New Jersey school's athlete drug-testing program in a school district where 28 students tested positive for drugs in a single year.

Justice Antonin Scalia — who had written a scathing dissent in *Von Raab* — wrote the majority opinion in the *Vernonia* case.

Scalia argued that student athletes have even less privacy rights than the general student body because they are role models and because they dress and shower in close proximity to one another. He also said that school drug testing was a response to drug usage by athletes.

"Obviously his view of the evils of drugs had changed between 1989 and 1995," says Paul Armentano, publication director of NORML. ∎

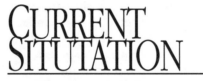

CURRENT SITUTATION

Teen Drug Use Rises

After the *Vernonia* ruling, more school districts instituted random drug testing of athletes, driven in part by new national surveys showing that declining teen drug use had suddenly reversed itself in 1992 and was rising steadily.

Indeed, drug use among teenagers became a hot campaign issue in 1996, after the annual "National Household Survey on Drug Abuse" showed that teen drug use had more than doubled during Clinton's first term. [20] Repub-

lican presidential candidate Bob Dole blamed Clinton for the upswing, pointing out that he had slashed funding for the White House drug-policy office (which Clinton later restored) and had hired employees who had used drugs in the past.

Clinton pointed out that the increase in teen drug use was a multiyear trend that started before he was even sworn into office. Administration officials also noted that from 1992-1995 Congress consistently cut anti-drug education funds administered under the Safe and Drug-Free Schools program. Critics have called the program ineffective because there are few restrictions on how the money is spent, and it is allocated on a per-capita basis, rather than targeted at districts with severe drug problems.

Officials in the White House Office of National Drug Control Policy also pointed to opinion polls showing student attitudes about the dangers of marijuana had begun to change in 1990. Clinton's drug czar, Barry R. McCaffrey, said that from 1990-1993, the percentage of high-school seniors viewing marijuana use as risky fell. [21]

Joseph A. Califano, Jr., president of the National Center on Addiction and Substance Abuse at Columbia University, blamed the increased teen drug use on baby boomer parents' complacency about drugs. Califano released a survey showing that two-thirds of babyboomer parents who used drugs in their youth expected their children to do the same, and 40 percent felt they had little influence over their teenagers' decisions about drugs.

"What is infuriating about the attitudes revealed in this survey is the resignation of so many parents to the present mess," Califano said. [22]

Shortly before the election, Clinton proposed encouraging states to impose mandatory drug tests for all teens seeking driver's licenses. "Our message should be simple: no drugs, or no driver's license," Clinton said in his weekly radio address. Republicans called the proposal an election-year gimmick.

Since the 1996 election, teen drug use has continued rising, even as more schools have implemented or expanded testing programs. The percentage of youths ages 12-17 using illicit drugs increased from 9 percent to 11.4 percent from 1996-1997, still far below 1979's record high of 16.3 percent. Teen drug use had dropped to an all-time low of 5.3 percent in 1992.

Perhaps even more worrisome for parents and officials are the latest statistics showing that drug use among 12- and 13-year-olds increased from 2.2 percent to 3.8 percent from 1996-97. [23]

Some schools have responded to rising teen drug use by requiring testing not only for athletes but also for all students participating in extracurricular activities, such as band, drama and student council. Other schools test students who drive to school.

Privacy Issues Raised

Parents generally like testing programs, and some even want all students tested.

"The majority of kids support drug testing because it gives them an excuse to say 'no' to drugs," says Robert Weiner, spokesman for the White House Office of National Drug Control Policy. "The administration has been strongly supportive of giving schools that tool," he says.

But some parents and teenagers have sued their local school boards, claiming testing is an unconstitutional invasion of privacy.

However, on Oct. 5 the Supreme court let stand a rural Indiana high school's policy of requiring mandatory drug testing for all students in extracurricular activities. After a con-

cerned parent sued the Rush County School Board, an Indiana appellate court had ruled that the policy does not violate students' privacy rights, even though the school district is not experiencing a serious drug problem. [24]

"We're getting closer to that line where you can expect to be tested just because you show up at school," said Kenneth J. Falk, an attorney for the Indiana Civil Liberties Union, which represented the plaintiffs. [25]

On the other hand, "Kids now can say, 'I can't experiment because my number may come up,' " said Rush County School Board lawyer Rodney V. Taylor. [26]

Although the court's inaction is not a precedent-setting decision, the ruling it left in place remains binding in Indiana, Illinois and Wisconsin. Critics say it opens the door for similar policies in other states. Several school districts had been waiting for the court to decide the case before they expanded their testing programs.

Civil libertarians and some editorial writers were stunned by the court's inaction.

"Drug abuse among teenagers is alarming, but so is the ease with which the Rehnquist court has disregarded fundamental constitutional protections guaranteed to citizens under the Fourth Amendment," said a *St. Petersburg Times* editorial. "Historically, suspicionless searches have been deemed to violate personal privacy and the protection against unreasonable searches and seizures. There may be compelling reasons to allow such searches, such as when public safety mandates it. But that's certainly not the case here." [27]

Critics point out that besides infringing on the Constitution, such programs target the wrong kids. High achievers who spend their free time playing in the band are not likely to be using drugs, they argue.

Politicians Not Tested

In other recent Supreme Court action on drug testing, the court last March 2 denied an appeal by two government economists who balked at taking random drug tests because they have access to the Old Executive Office Building next-door to the White House.

But the court has rejected drug testing for judges and politicians. The justices struck down a Georgia law requiring candidates for state office to take drug tests. Because urinalysis intrudes on a person's right to privacy, it should be used only when the risk to public safety "is substantial and real," the high court said. [28]

Meanwhile, lawmakers in the last two years introduced more than 60 bills requiring drug testing in one form or another; most were never acted upon.

The law providing $10 million to help small businesses establish drug-free workplaces was the only major drug-testing legislation approved. It also ordered the Small Business Administration to study the extent and costs of drug use in the workplace.

While Congress pushed for more small businesses to do drug testing, it refused to submit to drug testing for congressmen and their staffs, claiming it was too undignified and possibly unconstitutional.

"It's not fair to require more and more Americans to undergo drug testing, when the same Congress that passed the laws expanding the practice over the last 15 years won't submit to the same level of scrutiny themselves," St. Pierre says.

On the opening day of the 105th Congress, the House had passed a rules package requiring all representatives and their staffs to undergo random drug testing. But the rule was never implemented, due to opposition from both Republican and Democratic leaders, some of whom feared that the results of positive drug tests might be used against them by a political opponent.

"Of course, the information would be used against them," St. Pierre says. "That's exactly the way drug testing is being used across the country. We deny welfare mothers custody of their children, we deny students access to student loans, we deny employees access to workers' compensation or health benefits. Everybody is being punished for positive drug tests except the people who forced these laws on the country. It's rank hypocrisy."

"We have a few well-placed people who don't want this," said Rep. Joe L. Barton, R-Texas, who co-sponsored the bill with House Rules Committee Chairman Solomon. [29] ■

OUTLOOK

Questions of Fairness

Under the Drug-Free Workplace Act of 1998, more small companies are expected to begin asking their employees for urine samples. Some fear that cash-strapped firms may cut corners by only performing the one-step screening test, which is more likely to turn up false-positives. Congress recommended that the more comprehensive two-step testing be done, but many employers already reject job applicants based solely on the single-screening tests.

In large companies, drug testing is here to stay, predicts de Bernardo of the Institute for a Drug-Free Workplace. "There will be no retreat on drug testing," he says. "The numbers of companies testing increases every year." He predicts more large companies will expand their "for-cause"

testing programs to include universal random testing.

"It's by far the fairest type of testing you can do," he says. "It is inherently objective and has a greater deterrent impact." Testing only for "reasonable suspicion" is inherently subjective and open to abuse by an employer with a grudge, he adds.

But as employers expand their testing, they may run into a new obstacle: hemp seed oil. Sold in health food stores, hemp oil reportedly lowers cholesterol, fights viruses, increases calcium absorption and reduces inflammation. Because it comes from the same family as the marijuana plant, hemp oil can cause a user to test positive for marijuana.

Observers predict that marijuana smokers will start using the supplement to mask their marijuana use.

Others worry that as drug testing becomes more widespread, the confidentiality of the results may be compromised. "This information will become part of student records, insurance records and other databases, regardless of the reason that someone tested positive and how long ago it happened," says Alexander Robinson, public policy director of the Drug Policy Foundation.

Questions about fairness are already being raised about new tests using hair, sweat and saliva. The new techniques are considered less intrusive than urinalysis, and thus less subject to legal challenge. They are also expected to detect more drug users, because they are almost impossible to "beat."

Some say the expanding use of hair and urine testing is leading the country closer to a police state.

"You have a police-state mentality," Robinson says. "Incentives have been established in schools rewarding students who turn in other students. State and local ordinances reward kids who turn in their parents."

At the White House, Weiner ac-

knowledges that a "vocal few" see drug testing as moving toward a police state.

"People are making a huge deal out of this *horrendous* violation of individual rights," he says, "but it's also a violation of civil liberties to go through an X-ray machine at an airport, or to wear a seat belt. Their concerns about Americans' civil liberties are important, but the law has to support the general good. There's nothing wrong with drug testing when you have a national consensus."

Some opponents hope for a public backlash. "The hope is that proponents will go so far there will be some backlash," Nadelmann says. If not, drug testing could lead a desensitized public down "a slippery slope to greater and greater loss of freedom. Bit by bit, we are slowly getting used to greater and greater intrusion."

Some observers are concerned that so many students nationwide have acquiesced to drug testing without thinking much about its long-term impact on their privacy rights.

"As these students, now inoculated with an intolerant attitude, take power, invasions of privacy will become more widely implemented because they will be seen as prime American values," wrote Arnold Trebach and Scott Ehlers of the Drug Policy Foundation. [30]

Cornell's Sonnenstuhl argues that rather than curtailing constitutional rights, invading privacy and turning employers into policemen, "The best way to prevent alcohol and drug abuse in the workplace is for supervisors to do the job they were hired to do — monitor job performance and use discipline to encourage abusers to get treatment," he says. "Most large corporations are not training their supervisors to do their jobs."

But at a steel foundry in Portland, Ore., Pat Bishop has no doubts about testing.

At Issue:

Is workplace drug-testing effective?

Michael Walsh
President, the Walsh Group, P.A., a Bethesda, Md., research and consulting firm, and former executive director of the President's Drug Advisory Council.

FROM HR NEWS, APRIL 1996.

i n 1994, the National Academy of Sciences (NAS) issued a report, "Under the Influence: Drugs and the American Workforce," in which the principal finding was that there is little or no data in the scientific literature to demonstrate the effectiveness of drug-free workplace programs in reducing substance abuse.

My colleagues at the American Civil Liberties Union have taken this to mean that these programs don't work. The fact is that the NAS found no evidence that the programs don't work either; there simply wasn't conclusive evidence one way or the other.

But from a national perspective, there are positive signs of success. Since the widespread implementation of drug-free workplace programs in the mid-1980's, we have seen a significant decline in the use of drugs by employed individuals. Data from the "National Household Survey on Drug Abuse" (conducted by the National Institute on Drug Abuse and, more recently, by the Substance Abuse and Mental Health Services Administration) indicate that the number of full-time workers that are current users of illegal drugs has dropped by more than 6 million over the last 10 years.

Over the last 15 years "employee drug testing" has become a standard business practice in the American workplace. A recent survey conducted by the American Management Association (AMA) indicates that nearly 80 percent of surveyed firms test employees for drugs.

Since 1987, company drug testing in the United States has increased by more than 300 percent. With the increased prevalence of illegal drug use, most executives believe that the absence of pre-employment testing would be an open invitation to drug users. The approximately 80 "Forensic Urine Drug Testing" laboratories certified by the U.S. Department of Health and Human Services are currently processing about 60,000 specimens a day, and many employers who conduct employee testing programs use labs certified by other organizations or use on-site test procedures.

This phenomenon of workplace drug testing evolved slowly over more than a decade. During that time policies, procedures, and technology have changed considerably. In general, most organizations don't have "drug-testing programs." Rather, "testing" has become the foundation for a comprehensive programmatic approach to substance abuse. Prevention and deterrence are the key concepts of most workplace programs, not detection, but when a worker develops a problem the standard practice is to get the substance-abusing employee into treatment, and back to work.

Lewis L. Maltby
Director, American Civil Liberties Union National Task Force on Civil Liberties in the Workplace.

FROM HR NEWS, APRIL 1996

m ounting evidence suggests that drug testing does not work, or at least that the claims of those who make their living selling testing are greatly exaggerated.

The most important evidence comes from the National Academy of Sciences. The academy's Institute of Medicine recently released a report which examines all the major studies regarding drugs and the workplace and summarizes the state of our knowledge. This report casts doubt on the effectiveness of drug testing. The critical assumption on which all drug-testing programs are based is that those who use illegal drugs are less productive than other employees.

The academy, after reviewing all the evidence, found no consistent relationship between drug use and the quality of an employee's work. No relationship was found between drug use and productivity, or between drug use and the rate of workplace accidents. In some areas, drug use did make a difference. Drug users had slightly higher rates of absenteeism.

The ultimate question for an employer is whether urine testing is cost-justified. Here, too, the academy found little support of the industry's claims. Some studies found that drug testing was not cost-effective. Others reached the opposite conclusion, but were described by the academy as "deeply flawed." Overall, the academy concluded that, "decisions by organizations to adopt such programs have often been made without a well-grounded consideration of the likely benefits."

One reason the expenses of drug testing are so hard to justify is that few drug users are ever identified. According to the National Institute on Drug Abuse, only 3 percent of all random drug tests are positive. When one considers the cost of programs required to identify these few people, serious questions emerge. The federal government recently found that the average cost of a confirmed positive test result is $77,000. Is it really worth this much money to learn that a file clerk is smoking marijuana on a Saturday night?

Non-testing employers do not ignore the problem of drug abuse. They simply choose to deal with it differently. Many companies rely on careful employee selection and thorough performance evaluation and quality-control systems to create a high-quality workforce, avoiding those with any performance-impairing problems, including drug abuse.

The truth is that there are many strategies for dealing with employee drug abuse. Urine testing is one strategy, but is not the only one. There are other approaches, and mounting evidence from impartial sources indicates that urine testing may not be the best way.

The Marijuana Debate Goes on

Discussions about drug testing invariably turn to marijuana and the age-old questions: Is it harmful? Addictive? Does it act as a "gateway" to harder drugs? Marijuana residues stay in the body longer than other drugs, thus causing more marijuana users to get "caught" by urinalysis than users of other drugs.

"Drug testing is all about marijuana," says John P. Morgan, professor of pharmacology at City University of New York Medical School, who supports legalization of marijuana. "It's a critical weapon in the government's war on recreational marijuana users," he adds, noting that more people have been arrested for possession of marijuana during the Clinton administration than any other.

Critics like Morgan say drug testing should focus on more dangerous and addictive drugs like cocaine and heroin, or alcohol and tobacco, rather than "pot."

But testing proponents contend that marijuana is dangerous, addictive and a gateway to harder drugs and that cracking down on marijuana will indirectly stem the demand for heroin and cocaine.

"It's easy for people to underestimate the impact that marijuana has,"says Mark de Bernardo, executive director of the Institute for a Drug-Free Workplace, which promotes workplace testing. "There are a lot more casual users of alcohol, who don't get addicted, than there are users of illicit drugs" who don't get addicted."

According to a recent report by the National Center on Addiction and Substance Abuse (CASA) at Columbia University, teens 12-17 who use marijuana are 85 times more likely to use cocaine than non-marijuana users. [1]

CASA President Joseph A. Califano contends that the gateway effect means that recent increases in marijuana use among teens will translate into 820,000 more children who will try cocaine in their lifetime, of whom 58,000 will become addicts. Califano wrote that the statistical link between smoking pot and using harder drugs presents "a convincing case for a billion-dollar-a-year investment to move biomedical research on substance abuse and addiction into the big leagues at the National Institutes of Health, along with heart disease, cancer and AIDS." [2]

But Morgan calls the addiction and gateway arguments the "Big Lie" being promulgated by "more and more people, including urine testers and prevention, treatment and education specialists, whose livelihoods depend on the war on marijuana."

"For the large majority of people," Morgan says, "marijuana is a terminus rather than a gateway drug. More than 72 million Americans have tried marijuana at some point in their lives," including the president, the Speaker of the House and the secretary of Health and Human Services, he points out. "Yet in the over-30 population, only 0.8 percent of the population is continuing to use marijuana on a daily or even near-daily basis." [3]

"The lies and exaggerations about marijuana's dangers do little to discourage young people from trying marijuana, and may even have the opposite effect," Morgan writes in his new book, *Marijuana Myths, Marijuana Facts, A Review of the Scientific Evidence*.

Co-authored with Lynn Zimmer, associate professor of sociology at Queens College, the book analyzes the data supporting each of 20 arguments against marijuana used by government agencies and drug testing proponents. "Over and over, we discovered that government officials, journalists and even many 'drug experts' had misinterpreted, misrepresented or distorted the scientific evidence," wrote the authors.

The gateway theory tries to establish a causal relationship when only a statistical association exists, Morgan says. "Most people who ride a motorcycle have ridden a bicycle," he writes. "However, bicycle riding does not cause motorcycle riding."

Regarding marijuana dependence, Morgan cites a study by two pharmacologists who independently ranked the dependence potential of caffeine, nicotine, alcohol, heroin, cocaine and marijuana. Both ranked marijuana and caffeine as the least addictive, and one said marijuana was less addicting than caffeine. [4]

However, treatment specialists report anecdotal evidence of psychological dependence on marijuana, especially by heavy marijuana users. [5] But drug-testing opponents contend that almost all heavy marijuana users are also heavy alcohol users, who probably self-medicate to deaden pre-existing emotional pain.

A study released last March by the National Institute on Drug Abuse (NIDA) apparently supports that finding. It found that teenagers with prior serious anti-social problems are at high risk for marijuana dependence. "This study provides additional important data to better illustrate that marijuana is a dangerous drug that can be addictive," said Alan I. Leshner, director of the institute. [6]

Yet in its "Facts Parents Need to Know" fact sheet on its Web site, NIDA concedes that "Most marijuana users do not go on to use other illegal drugs."

The government also says marijuana is "a hugely significant cause of car crashes," and that marijuana users are "jamming hospital emergency rooms and drug treatment centers," according to White House Office of National Drug Control Policy spokesman Robert Weiner.

"Those are all absolutely false statements," Morgan says. "There's no scientific basis for them." He cites a 1993 Department of Transportation study that said, "Of the many psychoactive drugs, licit and illicit, that are available and used by people who drive, marijuana may well be among the least harmful." [7]

In the largest such study ever undertaken, Australian

researchers at the University of Adelaide found that drivers using marijuana were no more likely to be involved in an accident than those who were drug-free. [8]

Morgan concedes that "inexperienced marijuana users and inexperienced drivers, in particular, may be unable to drive safely even after small doses of marijuana."

Weiner's claim that hospital emergency rooms are "jammed" with marijuana users is based on federal Drug Abuse Warning Network (DAWN) statistics showing recent increases in the number of patients mentioning marijuana in hospital emergency rooms.

Morgan points out that marijuana use is on the increase, and inexperienced users may suffer acute anxiety the first time they use it. But, he says, even though marijuana is the most widely used illicit drug in America, it is mentioned in emergency cases less often than most other illicit drugs, and less than over-the-counter drugs. For instance, in 1993, 47 percent of the drug "mentions" by adolescents were for over-the-counter pain medications, compared with about 8 percent for marijuana.

In addition, he points out, marijuana is rarely mentioned alone. About 80 percent of the marijuana "mentions" also involved alcohol use, he says. "When a patient mentions marijuana, it does not mean marijuana caused the hospital visit," Morgan writes.

Out of more than 500,000 drug-abuse episodes reported by emergency rooms in 1994, only 1.6 percent — or slightly more than 8,000 — involved only marijuana. "And none of the marijuana-only mentions were hospitalized," he says.

Further, he says, evidence of marijuana use was found in only 587 of the 8,426 drug-related deaths in 1993. "In all of those cases, other drugs were found as well," he says. "Marijuana did not cause a single overdose death."

But, argues de Bernardo, "Today's marijuana has 22 times the THC [9] that it had in the 1960s. It's much stronger, more addictive and more dangerous."

After examining statistics from the University of Mississippi's Potency Monitoring Project (PMP), Morgan concludes, "There is no reason to believe that today's marijuana is stronger or more dangerous than the marijuana smoked during the 1960s and '70s." [10]

Independent analyses of marijuana in the 1970s showed an average purity of 2-5 percent. Since 1980, average marijuana potency has fluctuated between 2-3.5 percent, he writes, with no consistent upward or downward trend. But comparing potency data across the 1970s and '80s is misleading, he says, because PMP samples in the '70s were typically from low-potency sources. Improved storage practices and measurement methods in the '80s may have increased the amount of THC detected.

Even if today's marijuana were more potent than in the 1960s, it would not necessarily be more dangerous or produce more intense effects on the body, Morgan says.

"There is no possibility of a fatal overdose from smoking marijuana, regardless of THC content," he writes. In fact,

he says, since the main danger from marijuana is damage to the lungs, higher-potency marijuana may be slightly less harmful than lower-potency marijuana, because users tend to smoke less of it to achieve the same "high."

The NIDA Web site points out that marijuana smoke contains the same cancer-causing ingredients as tobacco, sometimes in higher concentrations. "Studies show that someone who smokes five joints per week may be taking in as many cancer-causing chemicals as someone who smokes a full pack of cigarettes every day," it says.

Morgan concedes that marijuana smokers are at risk because they inhale more deeply and retain smoke in their lungs longer than tobacco smokers, and "joints" are not filtered. But he says there are no epidemiological studies showing higher rates of lung cancer in marijuana smokers than in tobacco smokers, probably because they inhale less smoke overall than cigarette smokers. But, he wrote, heavy smokers of both marijuana and tobacco possibly "have an increased risk of lung cancer." [11]

Drug-testing proponents also point out that about 100,000 people seek treatment for marijuana dependency each year. Morgan argues that many of those were referred to treatment centers by employers or courts, after they tested positive for marijuana. Most do not meet the official definition for "dependency," Morgan says, but either the court or the boss has given them the choice of seeking treatment, being fired or serving time, he says.

"Which would you choose?" he asks.

---

[1] "Cigarettes, Alcohol, Marijuana: Gateways to Illicit Drug Use," Center on Addiction and Substance Abuse, Columbia University, October 1994.

[2] From an editorial written by Califano in September 1997 and distributed to several newspapers.

[3] Morgan's statistics come from the "1994 National Household Survey on Drug Abuse, Population Estimates," Substance Abuse and Mental Health Services Administration, 1995.

[4] P.J. Hilts, "Is Nicotine Addictive? It Depends on Whose Criteria You Use," *The New York Times*, Aug. 2, 1994.

[5] For background, see Sarah Glazer, "Preventing Teen Drug Use," *The CQ Researcher*, July 28, 1995, pp. 666-689.

[6] Thomas Crowley, et. al, "Cannabis Dependence, Withdrawal and Reinforcing Effects Among Adolescents with Conduct Symptoms and Substance Use Disorders," *Drug and Alcohol Dependence*, spring 1998.

[7] H. Robbe and J. O'Hanlon, "Marijuana and Actual Driving Performance," Department of Transportation, 1993, p. 107.

[8] See C.E. Hunter et. al., "The Prevalence and Role of Alcohol, Cannabinoids, Benzodiazepines and Stimulants in Non-fatal Crashes," University of Adelaid, Department of Forensic Science, 1998; Robbe, *op. cit.* (Netherlands study).

[9] THC is the chief psychoactive ingredient in marijuana.

[10] The PMP has been monitoring the potency of marijuana samples submitted by law enforcement agencies since the early 1970s.

[11] Marijuana smokers are only 3 percent more likely than non-smokers to visit doctors for respiratory illnesses like bronchitis, according to researchers at the Kaiser Permanente Medical Care Program, he says.

"We've been randomly testing everyone in the company for the past five years, and during that time the percentage of employees testing positive has gone down from about 5 percent to 1," says Bishop, manager of health services for ESCO Corp.

"We work with molten metal, and our employees support drug testing overwhelmingly. No one wants to work with someone who is drug-impaired." ∎

Notes

[1] For background, see Richard L. Worsnop, "High School Sports," *The CQ Researcher*, Sept. 22, 1995, pp. 825-858.

[2] For background, see Richard L Worsnop, "Privacy in the Workplace," *The CQ Researcher*, Nov. 19, 1993, pp. 1021-1044.

[3] "Winning the War on Drugs — Check the Military," *The Drug-Free Workplace Report*, fall 1990, p. 4.

[4] Marci M. DeLancey, "Does Drug Testing Work?" Institute for a Drug-Free Workplace, 1994.

[5] Robert W. Taggart, "Results of the Drug Testing Program at Southern Pacific Railroad," *Drugs in the Workplace: Research and Evaluation Data*, National Institute on Drug Abuse, 1989.

[6] "Workplace Drug Testing and Drug Abuse Policies: Summary of Key Findings," American Management Association, 1996.

[7] "Under the Influence? Drugs and the American Work Force," National Academy of Sciences, 1994.

[8] American Management Association, *op. cit.*

[9] Chamber of Commerce press release.

[10] Taggart, *op. cit.*

[11] Beverly A. Potter and Sebastian Orfali, *Drug Testing at Work: A Guide for Employers and Employees (1990).*

FOR MORE INFORMATION

Center for Addiction and Substance Abuse, Columbia University, 633 Third Ave., 19th Floor, New York, N.Y. 10019; (212) 841-5200; www/casacolumbia.org. CASA conducts research on drug and alcohol abuse and prevention; it considers marijuana a "gateway" drug.

Drug Policy Foundation, 4455 Connecticut Ave., N.W., Suite B-500, Washington, D.C. 20008-2328; (202) 537-5005; www.dpf.org. This nonprofit research organization studies alternatives to the nation's drug war, including legalization.

Institute for a Drug-Free Workplace, 1225 Eye St., N.W. Suite 1000, Washington, D.C. 20005; (202) 842-7400; www.drugfreeworkplace.org. This business-oriented coalition seeks to improve productivity and safety through detection and treatment of drug and alcohol abuse.

National Clearinghouse for Alcohol and Drug Information, P.O. Box 2345, Rockville, Md. 20847-2345; (800) 729-6686; www.health.org. Provides publications, videotapes and educational materials to help parents talk to their children about drug use.

[12] William J. Staudenmeier Jr., "Urine Testing: The Battle for Privatized Social Control During the 1986 War on Drugs," from I*mages of Issues, Typifying Contemporary Social Problems*, Joel Best, ed. (1989).

[13] Potter, *op. cit.*

[14] *Under the Influence? Drugs and the American Work Force*, National Research Council, 1994.

[15] Potter, *op. cit.*

[16] Quoted in Christopher S. Wren, "Clinton to Require State Efforts to Cut Drug Use in Prisons," The *New York Times*, Jan. 12, 1998.

[17] *Ibid.*

[18] Paul Armentano, "A Look at the Historical Legal Basis for Urine Testing," *NORML Reports*, December 1995.

[19] Jeannette C. James, "The Constitutionality of Federal Employee Drug Testing," The *American University Law Review*, fall 1988.

[20] The survey is published each year by the Substance Abuse and Mental Health Services Administration.

[21] For background, see Sarah Glazer, "Preventing Teen Drug Use," *The CQ Researcher*, July 28, 1995, pp. 674-697.

[22] Quoted in Roberto Suro, "Boomers expect teen drug use, survey finds," *The Washington Post*, Sept. 19, 1996.

[23] Substance Abuse and Mental Health Services Administration.

[24] The case is *Todd v. Rush County Schools.*

[25] Quoted in Frank J. Murray, "High court declines to debate school drug testing," *The Washington Times*, Oct. 6, 1998.

[26] *Ibid.*

[27] "Opening the way to drug tests," *The St. Petersburg Times*, Oct. 13, 1998.

[28] Joan Biskupic, "Court allows drug tests for OEOB pass holders," *The Washington Post*, March 3, 1998.

[29] Quoted in "Different Sauces for Geese and Ganders?" The Associated Press, Aug. 7, 1998.

[30] Arnold Trebach and Scott Ehlers, "The war on our children: destroying the rights of America's youth to save them from drugs," "The Playboy Forum"; *Playboy*, February 1997. Trebach is a professor at American University and editor-in-chief of *The Drug Policy Letter*, published by the Drug Policy Foundation; Ehlers is associate editor.

Bibliography

Selected Sources Used

Books

Holtorf, Kent, *Ur-ine Trouble*, Vandalay Press, 1998.
Holtorf, a physician, has spent years reviewing the scientific data about drug testing. He describes how poorly trained personnel in uncertified laboratories can erroneously cause a job seeker to test positive for drugs and how common foods and medicines can cause false-positive test results.

Jacques Normand, et al., *Under the Influence? Drugs and the American Work Force*, National Academy of Sciences, 1994.
This National Academy of Sciences analysis of all the studies done before 1994 on the effectiveness of workplace drug testing found that "there is as yet no conclusive scientific evidence from properly controlled studies that employment drug-testing programs widely discourage drug use or encourage rehabilitation."

Potter, Beverly A., and Sebastian Orfali, *Drug Testing at Work, A Guide for Employers and Employees*, Ronin Publishing, 1990.
The authors describe how tests work, the civil rights issues involved, how to set up a program and how employees can protect themselves from false-positive results.

Zimmer, Lynn, and John P. Morgan, *Marijuana Myths, Marijuana Facts,* Lindesmith Center, 1997.
The 241-page book, published by billionaire George Sorros' drug-law reform think tank, includes more than 60 pages of bibliography and footnotes listing scores of studies on marijuana and its effects on the human body. Each chapter deals with one of the arguments against marijuana use.

Articles

Armentano, Paul, "A Look at the Historical Legal Basis for Urine Testing," *NORML Reports,* December 1995.
The publications director for the National Organization to Reform Marijuana Laws (NORML) writes about the legal history of drug testing, reviewing major court decisions and how the Supreme Court's position on privacy rights has shifted.

DeLancey, Marci M., "Does Drug Testing Work?" Institute for a Drug-Free Workplace, 1994.
This 116-page report by the institute — a coalition of businesses and individuals that promotes workplace drug testing — provides pages of statistics about the prevalence, cost and effectiveness of alcohol, drug and substance abuse. It also offers testimonials from companies that have established drug-testing programs.

James, Jeannette C., "The Constitutionality of Federal Employee Drug Testing," *The American University Law Review,* fall 1988.
James, a lawyer, focuses on the controversial Supreme Court decision in *National Treasury Employees Union v. Von Raab*. She contends the decision was tantamount to jettisoning the need to establish probable cause before searching private homes because the state has a strong interest in eliminating crime.

Murray, Frank J., "High court declines to debate school drug testing," *The Washington Times*, Oct. 6, 1998.
The author discusses the controversial Oct. 5 decision by the court to let stand a rural Indiana high school's policy of requiring mandatory drug-testing for all students in extracurricular activities, regardless of whether they are suspected of using drugs.

Staudenmeier, William J., Jr., "Urine Testing: The Battle for Privatized Social Control During the 1986 War on Drugs," from *Images of Issues, Typifying Contemporary Social Problems*, edited by Joel Best, 1989.
Sociologist Staudenmeier calls President Ronald Reagan's push for private employers to start drug testing "privatized social control." The Fourth Amendment prohibits the government from requiring the general population to be tested for drugs, he points out.

Trebach, Arnold, and Scott Ehlers, "The war on our children: destroying the rights of America's youth to save them from drugs," *Playboy*, February 1997.
Two Drug Policy Foundation editors argue that current U.S. drug-testing policy is indoctrinating several generations of children with the belief that venerable constitutional privacy guarantees are less important than the need for drug control.

Reports

National Household Survey on Drug Abuse, Substance Abuse and Mental Health Services Administration, 1997.
The annual survey shows that teen drug use has been climbing since 1992.

Taggart, Robert W., *Results of the Drug Testing Program at Southern Pacific Railroad*, Drugs in the Workplace: Research and Evaluation Data, National Institute on Drug Abuse, 1989.
This study showed a 50 percent drop in positive drug tests after a year of "reasonable suspicion" drug testing.

8 Zero Tolerance

KATHY KOCH

On a school bus last fall in rural Mississippi, five high school students passed the time on the long ride home by tossing peanuts at each other.

But the fun ended when the driver got hit. She pulled over, called the police and had the boys arrested for assault, punishable by five years in prison. The criminal charges were soon dropped, but the teenagers were suspended and lost their bus privileges. Unable to make the 30-mile trip to school, all five dropped out.

The recent shooting death of a 6-year-old Michigan girl by another 6-year-old underscores the fear of violence that has invaded America's schools. But the strict, one-strike-and-you're-out policies being imposed to nip school violence and misbehavior in the bud sometimes go too far, critics say. Other examples from the public school crime blotter:

• A 6-year-old boy in York, Pa., was suspended for carrying a pair of nail clippers to school.

• A second-grader in Columbus, Ohio, was suspended for drawing a paper gun, cutting it out and pointing it at classmates.

• A 9-year-old Ohio boy was suspended after writing, "You will die an honorable death" as a fortune-cookie prediction for a class assignment.

• A 12-year-old Florida boy was handcuffed and jailed after he stomped in a puddle, splashing classmates.

• A 13-year-old boy in Manassas, Va., who accepted a Certs breath mint from a classmate was suspended and required to attend drug-awareness classes.

• Jewish youths in several schools were suspended for wearing the Star of David, sometimes used as a sym-

From *The CQ Researcher*, March 10, 2000.

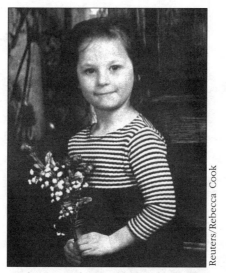

A classmate shot and killed 6-year-old Kayla Rolland last month at school in Mount Morris Township, Mich.

bol of gang membership.

Zero-tolerance policies punish all offenses severely, no matter how minor. School systems began adopting the tough codes after Congress passed the 1994 Gun-Free Schools Act, which required one-year expulsions for any child bringing a firearm or bomb to school.

But zero-tolerance rules in many states also cover fighting, drug or alcohol use and gang activity, as well as relatively minor offenses like possessing over-the-counter medications, disrespect of authority, sexual harassment, threats and vandalism. More than 90 percent of U.S. public schools had zero-tolerance policies for firearms or other weapons in 1997, and more than 85 percent had the policies for drugs and alcohol.

After the massacre last April at Columbine High School in Littleton, Colo., nervous legislators and school boards further tightened their zero-tolerance policies, creating what some critics call a national intolerance for childish behavior. In some jurisdictions, carrying cough drops, wearing black lipstick or dying your hair blue are expellable offenses.

Even writing a paper about murder or suicide can land a student in trouble.

"Things got a lot worse post-Columbine," says John Whitehead, president of the conservative Rutherford Institute, a Charlottesville, Va., group dedicated to protecting civil liberties.

In the current atmosphere, merely displaying the image of a weapon is unacceptable, as Samantha Jones, of Nevis, Minn., learned. The 17-year-old Army recruit was forbidden from using her favorite photo of herself — sitting atop a howitzer at the local VFW post — for her yearbook picture.

"A real vortex has been created that sucks in otherwise good kids who make a single mistake," Whitehead says.

"Some call it zero-zero tolerance," says Paul Kingery, director of the Hamilton Fish Institute on School and Community Violence at The George Washington University.

He discovered that while the number of students expelled for firearms has decreased since 1994, expulsions and suspensions for non-gun offenses have skyrocketed.[1] In Chicago, for instance, expulsions jumped eightfold after zero-tolerance policies were adopted in 1995 for weapons, alcohol and drugs.

Meanwhile, because minor infractions are punished so severely, administrators are ratcheting up punishments for more serious offenses. Two-year and permanent expulsions are on the rise. In Pennsylvania, long-term expulsions jumped nearly 960 percent from 1996 to 1997, Kingery writes.[2]

To accommodate all the expulsions, the number of alternative schools in the United States jumped from 2,604 in 1994, when most zero-tolerance rules were enacted, to 3,380 in 1997, according to the U.S. Education Department.

Only nine states require expelled students to attend an alternative

Most Schools Adopt Zero Tolerance

School systems began adopting zero-tolerance policies after Congress passed the 1994 Gun-Free Schools Act, which required one-year expulsions for bringing a firearm or bomb to school. More than 90 percent of U.S. public schools had zero tolerance for firearms or other weapons in 1997.

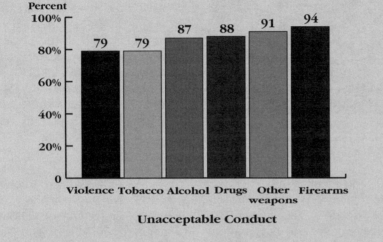

U.S. public schools with zero-tolerance policies, 1996-97

Source: U.S. Department of Education, "Principal-School Disciplinarian Survey on School Violence," 1997.

school. Research shows that expelled students who don't attend alternative classes are less likely to re-enter school and more likely to get mixed up in gang activity and drugs and otherwise run afoul of the law.

Critics say the biggest problem with zero-tolerance policies is their lack of flexibility, which prohibits officials from taking a child's age or past history into account.

"The absolute punishment applies whether you're carrying a nail clipper or a bazooka, Tylenol or illegal drugs," says Nadine Strossen, president of the American Civil Liberties Union (ACLU).

Strossen says school zero-tolerance policies grew out of drug-war laws that abolished discretion and curtailed civil liberties, such as mandatory minimum sentences, three-strikes-and-you're-out laws, civil-asset forfeiture and stop-and-frisk tactics.

"Judges were seen as too lenient," says Eugene Volokh, a professor of law at the University of California at Los Angeles, "and many people perceived that some school administrations tolerated things that shouldn't have been tolerated."

But critics say the zero-tolerance laws that resulted are either too vague or all-encompassing. One such law, an Alabama judge said recently, was unreasonable because it meant that "a sharpened pencil, chemistry supplies and a tennis racket could all be used as weapons." [3]

School administrators defend strict policies, arguing that they're needed because it's difficult to distinguish what is and isn't a weapon or gang-related paraphernalia. They say that students have been caught carrying hairbrushes with blades in the handles, or necklaces with large metal crosses made of knife blades. And

gang symbols can range from a Star of David to a rolled up pants leg.

William Modzeleski, director of the Education Department's Safe and Drug-Free Schools Program, says local zero-tolerance policies go far beyond the federal gun-free schools legislation. "The federal law is very narrowly defined," he says. "It says a child should be expelled for bringing a firearm or bomb to school. Not drug-abusing behavior, not nail clippers, not nail files, not water pistols, not pellet guns."

The federal law also allows local administrators to waive or reduce the one-year expulsion if there are extenuating circumstances. In fact, about one-third of the students expelled for firearms serve less than a year's suspension, he says.

Modzeleski says some schools also may be misinterpreting an Education Department publication on recognizing troubled kids. It recommended that children exhibiting certain behaviors, like writing about death, be referred to a professional counselor. Yet some schools suspend such students.

"We have to send a message that we're serious about no guns and drugs," says Michael Resnick, associate executive director for advocacy and issues management at the National School Boards Association (NSBA). "We can't be fuzzy around the edges about that message."

Educators say they cannot relax their guard because life-threatening incidents continue to plague U.S. schools. Last fall, authorities shut down a Cleveland high school after uncovering a bomb plot. On Dec. 6, a 13-year-old honor student in Oklahoma took a semiautomatic handgun from his backpack and fired 15 rounds at classmates, injuring five. And on Feb. 29, there was the shooting in Michigan of first-grader Kayla Rolland.

While a handful of silly cases make headlines, most zero-tolerance cases involve real weapons, says Vincent Ferrandino, executive director of the National Association of Elementary School Principals (NAESP).

He rejects suggestions that the policies reflect administrators' fear of liability suits if violence should erupt in their schools. "These policies are meant to protect the kids," he says.

But Peter Blauvelt, president of the National Alliance for Safe Schools (NASS), says, "There are a lot of administrators who are comfortable having no discretion, especially when they have to discipline the mayor's child. It's much easier to say they must treat all kids the same because of zero-tolerance laws."

Allowing "flexibility" also allows more racial and ethnic discrimination, Ferrandino contends. But students' advocates say that zero tolerance disproportionately targets minorities, the poor and the disabled.

That was the charge made last fall by the Rev. Jesse Jackson, who led marches in Decatur, Ill., to protest the expulsions of six African-American teenagers for starting a brawl at a football game. White boys, Jackson said, never would have been expelled for two years for a fight that involved no weapons and no injuries.

Similarly, says Judith A. Browne, senior attorney for the Advancement Project, a civil rights group in Washington, D.C., the five Mississippi peanut throwers were treated harshly because they were black and the bus driver white.

Critics say zero-tolerance policies teach children to be intolerant and don't prepare them for making difficult judgments later in life. "School boards somehow expect children to value differences in each other when adults seem unable to differentiate between the behavior of 6-year-olds and 16-year-olds, between an aspirin

Expulsions Hit Black Students Hardest

In some large school districts, black students are three to five times more likely to be expelled than white students, according to a recent survey. Moreover, the percentage of blacks expelled far exceeds blacks' enrollment.

Public school expulsions, by race, 1998-99

SCHOOL LOCATION	PERCENTAGE BLACK	PERCENTAGE WHITE
Austin, Texas		
Enrollment	18%	37%
Expulsion Rate	36%	18%
Boston		
Enrollment	55%	13%
Expulsion Rate	70%	9%
Columbia, S.C.		
Enrollment	78%	20%
Expulsion Rate	90%	9%
Los Angeles		
Enrollment	14%	11%
Expulsion Rate	30%	8%
Miami-Dade County, Fla.		
Enrollment	33%	12%
Expulsion Rate	48%	8%
Providence, R.I.		
Enrollment	23%	21%
Expulsion Rate	39%	13%
San Francisco		
Enrollment	18%	14%
Expulsion Rate	56%	11%

Source: The Applied Research Center, 1999

and cocaine, and between a friendly, first-grade hug and a sexual attack," writes Bethany Baxter, an educational consultant. [4]

As parents, educators and policy-makers debate the pros and cons of zero-tolerance policies, here are some of the questions they are asking:

Are zero-tolerance policies effective?

Proponents credit zero-tolerance policies with recent declines in crime and school weapons cases, even though they acknowledge there is little data to support that claim.

"All we have is anecdotal experience and the broad acceptance among administrators that zero-tolerance policies have been very helpful," says Ronald Stephens, executive director of the National School Safety Center, in Westlake, Calif.

"There is no good, quantitative research to show whether zero-tolerance policies are effective or ineffective," Modzeleski says. "But many educators and law enforcement officials will tell you that because of zero tolerance, we have less violence in schools than we had five years ago."

Federal statistics confirm that the number of crimes in schools per 1,000 students decreased from 155 in 1993 to 102 in 1997. There also were declines in the number of students carrying weapons to school and the number of student fights.

In Baltimore, school officials credit the aggressive zero-tolerance law adopted last spring with a 67 percent drop in arrests and a 31 percent decline in school crime in the first two months of the 1999-2000 school year. [5] And after Texas adopted zero tolerance for drugs and weapons, the percentage of teachers reporting that assaults on students was a "significant problem" dropped from 53 percent in 1993 to 31 percent in 1998. [6]

Moreover, says Stephens, the dramatic increase in the number of alternative schools around the country reflects the fact that zero-tolerance policies have "taken the troublemakers out of the schools and allowed the teachers to get back to the mission of teaching."

But critics argue that if zero tolerance were responsible for either falling street crime or the decline in school weapons-possession, proponents would have statistics showing that crime or weapons possession dropped faster in schools and communities with zero-tolerance policies than in those without them.

"They don't have those statistics," says Jason Zeidenberg, a policy analyst at the Justice Policy Institute.

"It may just be that violent crime and drug use are down everywhere, so they are down in the schools as well," NASS' Blauvelt says.

Despite the lack of compelling statistics, 85 percent of principals, 79 percent of teachers and 82 percent of students credit zero-tolerance policies with keeping drugs out of schools, according to a 1998 Columbia University survey. [7]

However, a 1998 federal government survey of more than 1,000 school principals indicated that there were only minor improvements in

School officials in Kansas suspended senior honors student Sarah Boman, 17, for displaying artwork at school that included a poem written from a madman's perspective. School officials considered it a threat and said Boman can return to school only if she had psychological testing.

KRT Photo/Jaime Oppenheimer

school discipline and drug problems from 1990 to 1996. [8] The percentage of principals reporting "serious problems" with fighting, alcohol use and weapons possession dropped somewhat. But an increase was posted among principals who said tobacco and drug use, drug sales and verbal and physical abuse of teachers were "moderate or serious" problems.

"The bottom line is that the rate of school violence has remained fairly level since the early 1990s," wrote researchers Russell Skiba and Reece Peterson. [9]

The policies are highly effective at sending an unequivocal message to kids, says Gerald Tirozzi, executive director of the National Association of Secondary School Principals. "I can't prove that zero-tolerance policies alone were responsible [for the declines in violence], but with the violence going down, I'd like to think that message is sinking in."

But Skiba, an associate professor of counseling and educational psychology at Indiana University, says the right message may not be getting through, or may be reaching the wrong people. Several studies show that 35 to 45 percent of suspensions are for repeat offenders, he points out. "So we end up punishing honor students to send a message to bad kids. But the data indicate that the bad kids aren't getting the message."

While no studies show conclusively that get-tough tactics work, Skiba says there is good data showing the effectiveness of comprehensive violence-prevention programs focusing on conflict resolution, peer mediation, mentoring and bullying prevention.

Yet zero-tolerance policies are the quickest and cheapest way to put a program in place, Skiba says, "and it makes good rhetoric. We certainly need to set boundaries and limits. But let's not kid ourselves by thinking that we are going to solve school safety problems simply by drawing a line in the sand. Zero-tolerance policies by themselves will not ensure that our schools are safe."

But even proponents agree that the toughest policies won't totally eradicate violence, says John Mitchell, deputy director of education issues at the American Federation of Teachers (AFT). "If a kid is so driven that killing becomes the major thing in their lives, schools can't protect against that just with a zero-tolerance policy," he says. "Other things have to be put into place."

Modzeleski points out that zero-tolerance policies are only effective if they are developed with input from the parents and students and are relevant to the culture of the community and the age of the students. "What you do in Des Moines might be different from what you do in Dubuque," he says. "What is appropriate for a 17-year-old is not necessarily appropriate for a 7-year-old."

Effective programs also include early intervention, violence and gang prevention and programs to promote racial and ethnic tolerance. Efforts to get kids connected to their schools and communities through after-school opportunities, smaller schools, smaller classes and better-prepared teachers are also helpful, he says.

"If the policies are carefully worded, extremely narrowly focused and used in conjunction with a comprehensive violence-prevention program, they can be effective," says Gerald Newberry, executive director of the Health Information Network at the National Education Association (NEA). "And they must be communicated in a way that encourages cooperation, rather than rebellion."

But zero-tolerance measures that turn schools into military or penal institutions "foster anxiety, fear and insecurity — precisely the opposite of their intended effect," the ACLU's Strossen says.

Critics are particularly concerned about zero-tolerance programs run by 14 states that expel students without providing alternative educational opportunities.

"If a child is already ostracized and alienated, the most irrational response is suspension or expulsion," Strossen says. "You want to bring them back into the fold."

Are zero-tolerance policies constitutional?

Strossen maintains that students' rights to privacy, free speech and due process are being abridged by zero-tolerance rules. "Kids have been thrown out of school for completely innocuous things like wearing certain T-shirts, creating works of art or wearing the Star of David," she says.

The Supreme Court has ruled that children have a property interest in public education, and thus the government cannot deprive them of their education without due process, she says. The court ruled in the landmark *Tinker v. Des Moines* case in 1969 that neither students nor teachers shed their constitutional rights at the schoolhouse door, she adds.

"Yet, consistently, we see a whole host of actions being taken that violate civil liberties," Strossen says, "including everything from prosecuting parents when their children are truant, to throwing kids out of school for minor infractions, to censorial discipline for innocuous statements made on students' own Web sites."

Many lawsuits challenging zero-tolerance rules charge that students' rights to free speech were violated. In the wake of schoolyard murders by boys who first wrote about death or made verbal threats or dressed a certain way, teachers are quick to report — and schools prone to expel — a student for what he or she wore, drew or said.

Other challenges to zero-tolerance rules allege that schools failed to follow due-process procedures, Strossen says. Students must be given notice of the charge against them, she says, and allowed to respond to the charge before being penalized.

"But a lot of zero-tolerance policies are being automatically implemented without even giving the student an opportunity to respond," she says. Often the student doesn't even have the right to have a parent or lawyer present.

The Rutherford Institute's Whitehead says the constitutionality of a zero-tolerance code depends on the case and how the code is written. "Some of the policies I've looked at are vague and a bit overbroad, which I think goes to their constitutionality," he says.

Nonetheless, zero-tolerance policies have generally received favorable treatment from the current Supreme Court, which "almost always rules in favor of state laws, police actions and school actions," Whitehead says. "Starting with President [Ronald] Reagan's appointments, the court has shifted to the right," he says. "That has had a big impact on these cases."

For instance, in *Vernonia School District v. Acton*, the court said in 1995 that student athletes have a reduced expectation of privacy and thus could be randomly tested for drugs without probable cause. "In another time, with a different court, you may get a different interpretation," Whitehead says. [10]

Charles B. Vergon, an attorney and professor of educational leadership at Youngstown State University, in Ohio, analyzed about 60 lawsuits brought on behalf of students expelled or suspended for weapons or firearms possession since 1990. In three-quarters of the cases, the schools' right to ensure safety on their premises was upheld, even though in some cases "a reasonable person could have taken a very different posture," Vergon says.

"School districts continue to enjoy substantial deference from the courts in governing the conduct of students at school and coming and going from school, particularly if it enhances the safety of students," he says.

NSBA staff attorney Julie Lewis

Expulsions in Chicago Rose Sharply

The number of students expelled in Chicago more than doubled in 1996-97, a year after the school board passed a strict zero-tolerance policy. Expulsions tripled in 1997-98 and are projected to keep rising.

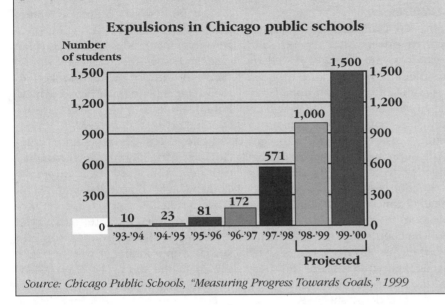

Expulsions in Chicago public schools

Year	Number of students
'93-'94	10
'94-'95	23
'95-'96	81
'96-'97	172
'97-'98	571
'98-'99 (Projected)	1,000
'99-'00 (Projected)	1,500

Source: Chicago Public Schools, "Measuring Progress Towards Goals," 1999

says zero-tolerance policies are usually upheld as constitutional unless they are too vague or overbroad, or the school district violates due-process rules, infringes upon students' free-speech rights or enforces the policies inconsistently.

"Most courts have been flexible in enforcing due process if they see that there was some procedure followed or notice provided," Lewis says. If a principal discusses the accusation with the student, many courts say the student received due process.

Ironically, Lewis says, some school districts are "broadening and broadening and broadening" their zero-tolerance policies, hoping to discourage civil-rights and equal-protection lawsuits. But instead, they now face more due-process and First Amendment suits, she says.

The University of California's Volokh says if zero-tolerance laws are properly written, and the school does not conduct an illegal search or otherwise violate the Constitution,

they're perfectly constitutional. Even expulsions for artwork or writings dealing with death may not violate a student's right to free speech, he says.

In *Tinker v. Des Moines School District*, the Supreme Court held that schools can act if they have "reasonable anticipation" that a student's behavior will cause "material disruption" of school discipline, Volokh explains. For instance, if a student jokes about blowing up the school, the government could argue that it reasonably anticipated that such a joke would interfere with discipline because students would be frightened, rumors would get started or other kids might mimic the threat, he says.

"In the current atmosphere of heightened sensitivity, a school might punish something that in a particular context is disruptive, even though in another context it would be protected," Volokh says. For instance, a university recently removed a bulletin board photo of a military-history professor dressed in a mock Roman

costume holding a sword. "The school said it creates a climate of violence," he says.

Schools' efforts to ban all images of guns are probably constitutional, he says. But they strike him as "a weird kind of fanatical, militant pacifism — an attempt to deny the fact that weapons exist and that sometimes they are useful, and that we pay people to operate them," he says. "Some schools are behaving in ways that are just plain silly," he says. "But silliness is not unconstitutional."

Are zero-tolerance policies fairly and consistently applied?

One of the rationales for zero-tolerance policies both in schools and law enforcement was to remove discretion from authorities and ensure that everyone would be treated equally.

"If you have a policy that clearly articulates what won't be tolerated, what the penalties are and it is consistently applied, that should minimize the extent to which you have discriminatory practices," says Tirozzi of the principals' association.

A discretionary policy allows authorities to consciously or subconsciously treat people from one group differently from those of another, Volokh says. "Zero-tolerance policies theoretically would diminish police discretion and the chance of racist enforcement," he says.

But critics argue that when zero-tolerance policies are actually applied in the real world, blacks, minorities, poor people and disabled students are expelled and suspended at higher rates than whites. Similarly, the critics say, racial stereotyping by police causes a disproportionate number of blacks and minorities to be stopped, frisked or arrested. For example, Strossen says, African-Americans make up 13 percent of the population and 13 percent of drug users. But blacks make up 74 percent of those incarcerated for drug use, she says.

The Decatur case brought this long-simmering controversy to the forefront. Lawyers for the six suspended youths produced statistics showing that 82 percent of Decatur students expelled in the past three years were African-American, although only 48 percent of the student population is black.

In addition, a recent survey of 12 large school districts showed that in some districts black students are three to five times more likely to be expelled than white students are. For instance, in Phoenix, blacks made up only 4 percent of the high school population but received 21 percent of the expulsions or suspensions. By comparison, only 18 percent of the whites — representing 74 percent of the enrollment — were suspended. Similarly, in San Francisco blacks account for 16 percent of the enrollment but 52 percent of the exclusions. [11]

Even the Department of Edu-cation's own figures show that in 1997 black students represented 17 percent of public school enrollment nationwide but 32 percent of those suspended — a disparity that has remained consistent since 1975.

"The recent school shootings were done primarily by white kids," Zeidenberg points out. "But African-American kids are the ones being disproportionately expelled and suspended. Is it really fair for them to bear the brunt of America's panic about school violence?"

However, "A numerical disparity does not by itself prove discrimina-

tion," Norma Cantu, assistant secretary of Education for civil rights, told the U.S. Commission on Civil Rights on Feb. 18. "It does not tell us the cause of the disparity."

The judge in the Decatur case agreed that disparate statistics alone don't prove discrimination. Judge Michael McCuskey upheld the students' suspensions on Jan. 11 after finding that the school district had not violated their civil rights. "Because the students failed to show that any similarly situated Caucasian students were

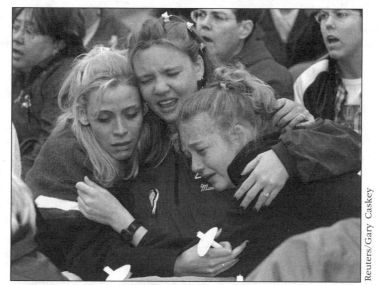

Students attend a prayer vigil in Denver last April following a shooting spree by two Columbine High School students that left 15 people dead. The killings prompted many schools to strengthen their zero-tolerance policies.

Reuters/Gary Caskey

treated less harshly," he wrote in his ruling, "they failed to establish that race played any role in the School Board's expulsion decision."

Volokh agrees that raw, disparate numbers don't prove discrimination. "There may be a disproportionate amount of improper conduct in certain groups," he says. "For example, a disproportionate number of men are criminally prosecuted, but that doesn't necessarily mean there is an anti-male bias. It may be the case that men commit more crimes than women."

Although he admits that discrimi-

nation can occur, "Misbehavior is not evenly distributed among racial and ethnic groups," says Kent Scheidegger, legal director of the conservative Criminal Justice Legal Foundation in Sacramento, Calif. "It's possible they are being punished more because they are misbehaving more."

But researcher Skiba insists, "There's just no evidence of that whatsoever. There is pretty good evidence that this oversuspension is not the result of lower behavioral standards among black students," he says.

"There seems to be more going on than that."

In a recent study, Skiba found no difference between the punishments meted out to black and white students once the students are referred to the office. But black students were twice as likely to be referred to the office as white students were. "The real disparity was in classroom referrals," he says.

Black students were referred more often for minor, more subjective behaviors like loitering, disrespect, threats, excessive noise and a catchall category called "conduct interference," he found. Whites were referred for less-subjective behaviors, such as smoking, vandalism, obscene language or using drugs or alcohol. "These things could be culturally bound," Skiba says. "A white female teacher might not be culturally sensitive to the difference in styles of African-American male students."

A study by the Civil Rights Project at Harvard University corroborated Skiba's findings. "African-American and Latino children are constantly being suspended for the more discretionary offenses, such as 'defiance of authority' and 'disrespect of authority,'" it said. "These categories of conduct clearly provide more latitude for racial bias to play a part." [12]

The ACLU's Strossen argues that such "invidious discrimination" is probably occurring in the classroom, when the teacher decides who to refer to the office, just as it does when a policeman decides who to stop and frisk or a prosecutor decides who to prosecute. "Studies have demonstrably shown that with minimum-sentencing guidelines discrimination apparently occurs at the police and prosecutor levels," she says. "I assume the same thing happens in the schools."

Even if the punishment meted out is the same once an offender appears before a principal or a judge, she says, "We'll never know all of the infractions committed by white kids that teachers decide not to treat as an infraction, partly because they know the punishment is going to be so harsh."

"Schools are more willing to recognize mitigating circumstances if they perceive the student as having 'a real future' that would be destroyed by expulsion," said Terry Keleher, program director at the Applied Research Center, in Oakland, Calif., which studies race and social-change issues. [13]

Disparate treatment of disabled students under zero-tolerance policies is more confusing, but no less controversial. Some observers complain that federal law creates a dual system of punishment in which disabled children who bring guns to school are treated less harshly than non-disabled students caught with a weapon at school.

But parents and advocates for the disabled cite statistics showing that, in fact, disabled students are twice as likely as non-disabled students to be expelled or suspended. They say schools use zero tolerance to get rid of disabled students that are difficult to handle or are not performing as well as others. ∎

BACKGROUND

'We Need to Get Tough'

Presidential candidate Richard M. Nixon campaigned on "law and order" issues in the 1960s. Politicians in the '70s bragged of being "tough on crime." Then in the 1980s, as the government's "war on drugs" heated up, "zero tolerance" joined the lexicon.

The term probably first appeared in 1983, when the Navy cracked down on drug abusers. The Marines soon adopted a similar policy, and initiated random drug tests.

A year later, Congress passed the first mandatory-minimum sentencing law, specifying stiff, automatic penalties for drugs and firearms violations. Lawmakers also amended federal forfeiture laws, expanding the government's authority to seize private property suspected of being involved in commission of a crime.

By 1986, with the nation beset by crack cocaine and skyrocketing violence, President Ronald Reagan launched the "war on drugs," and Congress passed the Anti-Drug Abuse Act, which expanded the list of offenses covered by mandatory sentencing. [14]

The same year, Attorney General Edwin Meese III authorized Customs officials nationwide to seize the boats, automobiles, and passports of anyone crossing the border with even trace amounts of drugs.

Within months, angry citizens whose boats had been seized were testifying on Capitol Hill along with Customs and Coast Guard officials accused of trampling the rights and sometimes destroying the property of citizens, some later proved innocent.

But the administration continued on the attack. In May, Education Secretary William J. Bennett asked Congress to withhold federal education money from schools unless they adopted zero-tolerance expulsion policies for students using or dealing in drugs on school grounds.

"We need to get tough as hell and do it right now," Bennett told the House Select Committee on Narcotics Abuse and Control." [15]

Rep. E. Clay Shaw, R-Fla., supported Bennett's proposal, arguing, "We have to quit being bleeding hearts for every kid who's rotten to the core." [16]

But Bennett got little support from the rest of the Democratically controlled committee, which said it preferred drug-education programs to simple expulsion. "Are you suggesting that a junkie kicked out of school is no longer a junkie?" asked Chairman Charles B. Rangel, D-N.Y. [17]

Another section of the 1986 Anti-Drug Abuse Act contained the Drug-Free Schools and Communities Act, the precursor of today's Safe and Drug-Free Schools Act, the federal government's largest drug and violence-prevention activity. The act required schools to have policies prohibiting alcohol and drug use by youths.

"But it did not specify what was to happen once a kid was found possessing alcohol or drugs on school property," says the Education Department's Modzeleski, noting that the term "zero tolerance" does not appear in the act.

In 1990, the U.S. Customs Service discontinued its boat-impoundment program after a marijuana cigarette led to the seizure of a research vessel from the Woods Hole Oceanographic Institute.

Ironically, at about the same time that Customs was easing its policy, zero tolerance was catching on in the public schools. By late 1989, districts in California, New York and Kentucky had adopted zero-toler-

Chronology

1960s *Illegal drug trafficking skyrockets. Supreme Court recognizes free-speech rights for school students.*

1968
Mandatory drug testing begins for returning Vietnam War veterans.

1969
Supreme Court rules in *Tinker v. Des Moines Independent Community School District* that students' constitutional rights were violated when they were suspended for wearing black armbands to protest the Vietnam War.

———— • ————

1970s *Courts extend due-process protections to students and mandate equal education for the disabled.*

1971
President Richard M. Nixon declares the first "war on drugs."

1975
Supreme Court rules in *Goss v. Lopez* that students cannot be suspended without due process. Education for All Handicapped Children Act requires all children to be educated in the "least restrictive environment" possible.

———— • ————

1980s *Crack cocaine inundates inner cities, and homicide among juveniles, particularly young, black males, reaches epidemic proportions. First mass murders occur on school grounds.*

1982
An article in the *Atlantic* by researcher George Kelling espouses the "broken windows" theory of policing, providing the basis for later zero-tolerance tactics in cities and schools.

1983
Navy and Marines adopt zero-tolerance drug policy.

1984
Congress passes Comprehensive Crime Control Act, requiring a federal commission to develop mandatory-sentencing guidelines for federal judges. Congress mandates stiff penalties for drug and firearm offenses.

1986
President Ronald Reagan launches a second "war on drugs." Congress passes Anti-Drug Abuse Act, doubling the number of federal mandatory minimums in effect. Federal and state governments begin seizing boats, automobiles and homes of drug suspects.

Jan. 13, 1988
Supreme Court rules in *Hazelwood School District v. Kuhlmeier* that school officials can censor student expression for "legitimate pedagogical concerns."

Sept. 26, 1988
A 19-year-old gunman opens fire on a Greenwood, S.C., schoolyard, killing two and wounding nine.

1989
On Jan. 17, a man with an assault rifle kills six children and wounds 30 on a Stockton, Calif., playground.

1990s *Congress bans guns from school grounds; mass murders committed by students erupt at decade's end.*

1990
President George Bush signs Gun-Free School Zones Act.

1992-93
Fifty-five violent deaths occur at schools and school functions.

1993
Washington state mandates life imprisonment for repeat felons.

1994
California and 12 other states pass "three-strikes-and-you're-out" legislation. Congress passes Omnibus Crime Bill, which includes mandatory drug sentences, and the Gun-Free Schools Act.

1995
Supreme Court strikes down 1995 Gun-Free School Zones Act and upholds random drug testing of school athletes. Crime reverses its upward trend, except for homicides by teenage boys, which skyrockets.

1997-98
Students commit mass murder five times within eight months in rural schools; 13 students and faculty die and 47 are wounded.

April 20, 1999
Two teenage boys shoot and kill 13 people at Columbine High School in Littleton, Colo., and then commit suicide.

Feb. 29, 2000
Six-year-old Kayla Rolland is shot and killed by a classmate at an elementary school in Michigan.

Are Students Losing Legal Rights . . .

In Texas recently, a high school student was sent to juvenile jail for five days without a hearing after writing a Halloween horror story in which a teacher and some classmates were shot.

Constitutional scholar Jamin Raskin cites the "unbelievable and shocking" case as an example of due process being denied to a student because of a zero-tolerance policy.

In the 1970s and '80s, the war on drugs accustomed American students to such anti-drug tactics as warrantless drug testing, locker searches and drug-sniffing dogs nosing around their cars and bookbags.

But student rights eroded even faster in the '90s as schools embraced zero-tolerance discipline policies to address school violence, say legal scholars like Raskin, a professor at American University. Following a recent spate of mass murders at schools, lawmakers and school officials adopted zero tolerance for behavior that even implies violence. Now, students are being suspended for writing about death, suicide or murder or for drawing pictures of guns.

"Discipline codes should discourage some of the negative writing that goes on," says John Mitchell, deputy director of education issues for the American Federation of Teachers. "Schools shouldn't be compelled to display work that isn't uplifting."

Students have always had fewer First Amendment rights than other citizens, says Eugene Volokh, a law professor at the University of California at Los Angeles. "When you're talking about K-12 education, the government has much more authority than it does over private citizens," he says. But in the 1960s, the Supreme Court expanded those rights, a trend that some say has been dramatically reversed in the past two decades.

"From the Warren Court era to the Rehnquist Court era, there has been a progressive decline in constitutional protection for students' rights," says Raskin, author of *We the Students*, a new textbook on students' rights.

Others disagree. "I don't think students' rights have declined," says Edwin Darden, senior staff attorney for the National School Boards Association (NSBA). "There's been an evolution to try to balance the needs of school districts and the needs and rights of the students."

The courts have been "very thoughtful" about how to achieve that balance, Darden says. But constitutional rights don't exist in a vacuum, he says, and the courts have had to weigh schools' need to ensure the safety of all students against the rights of the individual. "The courts have often ruled in favor of the schools."

Raskin says the Supreme Court "aggressively defended" students' First Amendment rights its 1969 *Tinker v. Des Moines Independent Community School District* ruling. The court said students should not be prevented from wearing black armbands to protest the Vietnam War unless it would cause "material and substantial disruption of school activities or invasion of the rights of other students."

As Justice Abe Fortas wrote in the case: "Neither students nor teachers shed their constitutional rights to freedom of speech or expression at the schoolhouse gate."

But by the late 1980s, Raskin says, the reconstituted court's *Hazelwood School District v. Kuhlmeier* ruling upheld the authority of schools to censor student publications "for almost any reasonable purpose."

Raskin says another constitutional right being "violated all over the country by zero-tolerance policies" is the right to due process. In the years before zero tolerance, students had a right to hear and respond to the charges against them before being expelled or suspended. But now, Raskin says, "Students are automatically suspended without a hearing."

The tough, new policies reflect longstanding complaints by politicians that liberal court rulings allowed chaos to reign in classrooms because educators had to jump through procedural hoops to expel disruptive students. Many observers say the current crackdown is a backlash to those procedural excesses.

"The only due process right that the Supreme Court has given students is that they must be given some notice of the charge against them and some opportunity to respond," says Nadine Strossen, president of the American Civil Liberties Union (ACLU). "It can be completely informal, it can be verbal and it can be after the punishment has been meted out, and students have no right to a lawyer. To even call it 'due process' is an exaggeration.

"It's nothing compared with what you would get if you were accused of even a misdemeanor outside of the school," she says. "Yet the life-destroying consequences can be at least as great if you're talking about someone being thrown out of school."

However, students' rights have expanded in two areas, Raskin says. High school students may now sue their

ance expulsion policies for drugs or gang-related activity. By 1993, schools across the country had cracked down on tobacco, alcohol and disruptive activities, as well as drugs and weapons.

After an American Association of University Women survey showed that 81 percent of students in grades eight-11 said they had been sexually harassed at least once in school, many schools also instituted zero tolerance

for sexual harassment.

Zero tolerance was also becoming more popular with local lawmakers and soon was being applied to everything from pollution and trespassing to skateboarding, racial intoler-

... Or Getting More 'Care' From Schools?

school for student-on-student sexual harassment if the school knew about it and did nothing to stop it. And many state courts have ruled in recent years that corporal punishment is unlawful, he points out.

Legal experts predict that the next two frontiers for students'-rights litigation will involve what Raskin calls school "cyber-censors," and efforts by schools to extend their disciplinary authority to off-campus student behavior.

In the aftermath of the shootings at Columbine High School in Littleton, Colo., some schools are cracking down on students who put material on their home Web pages that criticizes or threatens school personnel.

Except for those posting bomb threats, students have generally won their court challenges to such policies, especially if it merely involved the right to criticize the school administration and caused no disruption in classes, Raskin says.

Darden says the courts will also be seeing more challenges of schools trying to discipline students for what they do during non-school hours. "It's the next big wave of school litigation over the next two years."

For instance the Texas legislature recently passed a law requiring the expulsion of any student who commits a felony or an assault, or distributes drugs or alcohol near school property. Many states are requiring that schools be notified when a student runs afoul of the law, even though it was not on school property or during school hours. Some of those students are summarily expelled or suspended.

Darden says these new laws are efforts by the school districts to tell students, "We care about the whole person. When you do things that are dangerous to yourself, like using drugs or alcohol, the school district cares about that and will not look the other way."

But others find them a disturbing trend. "It would be ridiculous for the school to get involved, unless perhaps the student was arrested for rape," says Kent Scheidegger, legal director of the conservative Criminal Justice Legal Foundation in Sacramento, Calif. "You wouldn't want a suspected rapist in the school. But arrested for marijuana possession? That doesn't make any sense. That should be a matter for parents and the juvenile courts. That's what they're there for."

Darden says it is often the parents who are "asking, begging and cajoling" the school districts to impose tough behavior standards off-campus. If the school is randomly testing kids for drugs, it's easier for a student to resist peer pressure, parents argue.

"Except for the most extreme circumstances, schools really have no rightful authority to discipline students for activity off-campus," says Peter Blauvelt, president of the National Alliance for Safe Schools (NASS). "I think you have to make a case that the child's presence in school causes an undue risk of violence to others at school if a student got caught smoking marijuana or drinking on Saturday night and the school wants to expel him, I think that's ridiculous," Blauvelt says.

"It's much easier for politicians to demand a crackdown on the most silly and imagined transgressions," Raskin says. "So we have some kid spending five days in juvenile detention for writing a ghost story."

John Whitehead, president of the Charlottesville, Va.-based Rutherford Institute, a conservative group dedicated to protecting civil liberties, worries about the long-term impact of zero-tolerance tactics. "You're teaching kids that they live in a totalitarian society," he says. "This generation has been raised being searched without a warrant, being strip-searched and having their urine tested without probable cause. You'll have a whole set of people who will be conditioned to promote order over rights.

"You also have a whole segment of society that is being repressed," Whitehead says. "They operate on a subterranean level, because they really don't have free speech. They have secret signals, eye movements and code words."

Further, he says, "Many kids are smoking as a way to rebel. And younger and younger kids are drinking. I think it's a way of shoving it into the faces of the adults."

He says much of the violence erupting among kids already is the result of repressed anger. "Sooner or later they will blow," he predicts.

Whitehead says adults are sending kids the wrong message with zero-tolerance policies. "The message kids are getting is that some crazy adult game is being played here, and that the rules are really stupid," he says. "The adults say they're teaching kids about 'justice' when they say they must treat every infraction the same. But how is it justice to treat someone with a pair of nail clippers the same as you treat someone with an Uzi?"

ance, homelessness and boom boxes.

'Broken-Windows' Approach

In 1990, President George Bush signed the Gun-Free School Zones Act into law, prohibiting the possession or discharge of a firearm near a public school. The act claimed Congress had the right to act under its power to regulate interstate commerce. But the Supreme Court disagreed, ruling in 1995 that Congress had exceeded its constitutional powers. By then, lawmakers had gone back to the drawing board and enacted the 1994 Gun-Free Schools Act, which tied enforcement to the federal government's spending power.

'Get Tough,' Younger Students Say

Middle-schoolers in Tustin, Calif., advocated tougher policies on alcohol and marijuana than local high school students.

1. When should students be suspended for marijuana or alcohol violations?

MS	HS	All	
72	41	55	A. Always.
24	50	38	B. In repeat or severe cases.
5	9	7	C. Never.

2. When should police be notified about marijuana or alcohol violations?

MS	HS	All	
63	34	49	A. Always.
32	53	42	B. In repeat or severe cases.
5	13	9	C. Never.

3. When should counseling be required for students with a marijuana or alcohol violation?

MS	HS	All	
57	38	47	A. Always.
36	48	42	B. In repeat or severe cases.
7	15	11	C. Never.

4. Should students be allowed to avoid transfer if they agree to random drug testing?

MS	HS	All	
33	44	39	A. Yes.
47	42	44	B. Sometimes, depending on the circumstances.
20	14	17	C. No.

Note: All totals do not add to 100 due to rounding.
Source: Tustin Unified School District, Orange County, Calif., February 2000

That prompted state legislatures to begin requiring local school districts to implement zero-tolerance policies for firearms and bombs. Many of the new laws also included anything that could be used as a weapon.

"There is no universal definition of a weapon," Modzeleski says. "A belt buckle is a weapon, a rat-tail comb is a weapon. So are box cutters and baseball bats."

Meanwhile, zero tolerance got a boost from *Fixing Broken Windows*, a 1996 book by George L. Kelling and Catherine M. Coles. They argue that ignoring minor problems in cit-ies, like broken windows or graffiti, eventually leads to an increase in serious crime.

Republican Mayor Rudolph W. Giuliani based his anti-crime program in New York City on the theory, adding panhandlers, graffiti and street peddlers to the proscribed list. His "broken-windows" policy was first outlined in a 1982 *Atlantic* article by Kelling.

After crime in New York declined dramatically, the policy was widely adopted. "Mayor after mayor has rediscovered that disorderly behavior creates fear and leads to serious crime," Kelling said. [18]

Is Violence Declining?

The string of recent school shootings has added to the perception that violence is increasing in schools. Nine mass homicides on school grounds in less than two years have left 29 dead. [19]

But education and juvenile-justice officials continue to insist that children are safer in schools than in their own homes. Except for the recent shootings, overall school violence has been fairly steady for the past 20 years. And according to the NCES survey, the behaviors that school principals list as "serious or moderate" discipline problems were not violent activities but tardiness (40 percent) and absenteeism (25 percent). Twenty-one percent of the principals listed fighting as a serious problem, but only 5 percent considered gangs serious, and 2 percent listed weapons possession or physical abuse of teachers. [20]

"Despite public perceptions to the contrary, the current data do not support the claim that there has been a dramatic, overall increase in school-based violence in recent years," said researcher Irwin Hyman. [21]

But Stephens of the school safety center says that just looking at official statistics on school violence is misleading. "We have redefined deviancy over the last couple of decades," he says. "In some schools, a fight is not reported unless there is blood on the floor.

"There is a disincentive for administrators to report crime in their schools," he says, because principals are afraid they will be blamed for doing an inappropriate job. To get a true picture of school violence, you must look at reported incidents, unreported incidents and underreported incidents."

"We've seen a tremendous growth in the number of alternative schools at the elementary level, because so many younger children are acting out violent behavior," Stephens says. "Some of the aggression that before was being experienced at the middle school and high school levels is being manifested in the elementary grades."

But Kathy Christie, a policy analyst at the Education Commission of the States, says she has not seen a huge jump in the number of alternative schools being built for elementary-grade students. ■

CURRENT SITUATION

Alternative Schools

The Clinton administration wants Congress to require all school districts to provide alternative education for any student expelled or suspended for disciplinary reasons. Under current federal law, that's required only if a child is disabled, and the Senate voted last May to rescind that requirement.

"It ought to be a basic American principle that no student should be punished by being denied an education," said Education Secretary Richard W. Riley after a Dec. 9 meeting with Jesse Jackson. Excluded students should receive "appropriate supervision, counseling and educational services so they can meet state [academic] standards."

But, according to the Education Commission of the States, only nine states require schools to provide alternative schooling, and it's optional in 25 states. In 14 states, no laws govern alternative services.

As a result, only 43 percent of the students expelled for carrying a fire-

arm to school in 1997 were sent to alternative schools. Law-enforcement groups complain that by not providing alternative services, schools are dumping their discipline problems onto the streets.

But even when suspended students get alternative education, the quality of the education they receive is sometimes questionable. "Usually they are warehouses — dumping grounds for the worst teachers, administrators and students," says George Washington University's Kingery. "There have been no evaluations of their quality."

An alternative school is defined as any school that addresses the needs of students that cannot be met in a traditional school. Other than that, there is no standard definition of what constitutes an alternative school. The Education Department is preparing a survey of the nation's more than 3,400 alternative schools — which serve 1 percent of the nation's youngsters — to determine their characteristics.

The quality of education in alternative schools "clearly is a civil rights issue if the kids who are there are disproportionately kids of color, and the schools are demonstrably of poor quality," says Mary Frances Berry, chairman of the Commission on Civil Rights.

Witnesses told the civil rights panel in February that some teachers and administrators — pressured by school boards to raise overall test scores or face pay cuts or dismissal — are using zero-tolerance policies to push out low achievers and learning-disabled students who perform poorly.

"The growing popularity of zero-tolerance school-discipline policies during a period of rapidly raised academic standards and high-stakes testing is not accidental," said Joan M. First, executive director of the National Coalition of Advocates for Students. "There are two ways to change standardized test scores. Ei-

ther children learn more, or the composition of the test pool changes. Zero tolerance effectively accomplishes the latter."

"With the new standardized tests, there's an awfully strong urge on the part of teachers and principals to get rid of students," agreed Cruz Reynoso, a law professor at the University of California at Los Angeles and vice chairman of the civil rights panel. "I've heard that from many sources in California."

NASSP General Counsel Steven Yurek admitted, "It is a very big issue for schools."

Others complained that by escalating the sheer number of minority students excluded from public education, zero-tolerance policies are reversing gains made since the Supreme Court's 1954 *Brown v. Board of Education* decision promised equal educational opportunities for all children.

"Zero-tolerance laws are challenging the whole concept of universal public education," says Ruth Zweifler, executive director of the Student Advocacy Center of Michigan. "Instead, we've moved to an, 'If they deserve it, then we'll give it to them' attitude."

Harsh zero-tolerance policies are "sweeping uncounted numbers of our most vulnerable and needy children into the streets," where they remain "uneducated, unserved and unsupervised," she said.

"If we find that what we have heard is verifiable across the board," Berry says, "the Education Department's Office of Civil Rights should investigate the situation in alternative schools. It ought to be taken up as a very serious issue."

The commission will discuss the issue further on April 14. "We don't want chaos and disorder to reign in the schools," Berry says, "but quite clearly there is something going on here regarding how kids of color and

Prohibited in Providence

Brass knuckles. Hand grenades. Mace. Toy guns. Students who bring those or other banned items to school face automatic expulsion in Providence, R.I., which passed a much more restrictive zero-tolerance policy than the federal Gun-Free Schools Act.

Federal law

- Guns
- Explosive devices
- Silencers and mufflers
- Bombs, grenades, rockets, missiles and mines

Providence policy

- Guns
- Explosive devices
- Silencers and mufflers
- Bombs, grenades, rockets, missiles and mines
- Realistic replicas of firearms
- Knives
- Razors
- Gas repellent, mace
- Martial-arts devices
- Objects that could inflict bodily harm: blackjacks, chains, clubs, brass knuckles, nightsticks, pipes, studded bracelets, etc.
- Any object that gives the appearance of any of the above.

Source: Applied Research Center, Feb. 18, 2000

---

disabled kids are dealt with under these discipline policies."

Amending IDEA

If Congress required all expelled or suspended students to be sent to alternative schools, it would resolve the controversy over the disparate treatment of disabled students under zero-tolerance policies.

Under the 1997 amendments to the Individuals with Disabilities Education Act (IDEA), special-education students — whose disabilities can range from stuttering to serious emotional disturbance — have extra protections from zero-tolerance policies. If a disabled child brings a weapon to school, he may be immediately removed from school and suspended for 10 days, during which time the school must determine whether the offense was a manifestation of his disability. If not, the student may be expelled for a year, the same as a non-disabled child. Unlike a non-disabled student, however, he must be given free alternative education.

The protections were designed to prevent schools from expelling disabled students just because they might be more difficult or expensive to educate.

If bringing the weapon to school was a manifestation of the child's disability, the school may let the child back into school after a 10-day suspension, or, if the school determines that the child is a danger to himself or the other students, the school may send him to an alternative school for 45 days. Then, the school can ask an independent hearing officer to determine whether the child is ready to return to school, a procedure that can be repeated indefinitely.

The 45-day reviews were put into the law so schools could not "just kick the student out and forget about him," says Lilliam Rangel-Diaz, a member of the National Council on Disabilities board. But the policy has generated a lot of resentment, especially among parents of regular-curriculum kids expelled without getting alternative education or review hearings every 45 days.

"IDEA overrides state and federal zero-tolerance-for-firearms laws," Lewis says. "They contradict one another. This policy ties the hands of school administrators, and it's creating a lot of problems."

School administrators complain that if a disabled student threatens a student or a teacher, they cannot expel him as they could a non-disabled student. And parents of general-education students are starting to realize that their kids have less protection than a disabled student does. "Now after a kid gets expelled, some parents are asking for retroactive coverage under IDEA," Lewis says.

Educators and parents are also upset about the cost of providing alternative services for expelled disabled students. "When you run alternative schools with an 8-to-1 student-to-teacher ratio, that comes at a cost to the other students who are sitting in bigger classes," said Edward Kelly, superintendent of schools in Prince William County, Virginia. "The good

At Issue:

Should disabled students be disciplined differently under zero-tolerance policies?

KEVIN P. DWYER
President, National Association of School Psychologists

WRITTEN FOR *THE CQ RESEARCHER*

*m*isguided efforts by some Congress members to amend the Individuals with Disabilities Education Act (IDEA) perpetuate the public's erroneous impression that the law creates a dual-discipline system that prevents schools from removing a child with a gun from school. Nothing could be further from the truth.

The law was amended in 1997 so that any gun-carrying child can be removed. Schools can expel a student with disabilities who brings a gun to school for one year — just as they do other students — if the behavior was not the result of the child's disability.

After removal, students also receive continued education in an alternative program. If it is determined that the behavior resulted from a student's disability, the law allows the child to be suspended for 10 days while determining if the student poses a danger. If so, the school can expel the student indefinitely, but the case must be reviewed every 45 days.

Congress included these rights to protect students with disabilities from discrimination. Students with disabilities often present challenges. Without due process, these students would be removed disproportionately by schools that decided providing services was too costly, time consuming or inconvenient. But Congress acknowledged that children with disabilities, like all children, have the right to a free, appropriate, public education.

Now some in Congress contend the alternative-education requirement should be dropped because other students don't receive such services. But withdrawing educational services from any student does not make our schools and streets safer.

Leaving any student free to roam the streets without supervision is a prescription for increasing crime. Research affirms that expelling troubled children without educational and mental-health services increases dropout rates, drug use and overall juvenile crime.

To get this message to Congress, we have developed a Safe Streets, Safe Schools effort — involving 50 education, mental-health, student-services and child-advocacy groups — to support providing alternative education and crisis-intervention for all students.

But that effort cannot fall upon the education community or the justice system alone. States and local jurisdictions must work together to fund and implement services for all students with challenging behavior.

To balance the movement toward zero tolerance for guns, drugs and violence in schools, we must also have zero tolerance for academic failure for all students.

SEN. JOHN ASHCROFT, R-MO.

WRITTEN FOR *THE CQ RESEARCHER*

*i*n light of the tragic school shootings, we must ask ourselves if federal education laws do all they can to promote school safety. America's classrooms must be safe and secure for students to get a world-class education.

Our general policy is commendable: Zero tolerance for weapons. Under the federal Gun-Free Schools Act, states receiving federal education funds were required to pass laws mandating an immediate, one-year expulsion for students who bring weapons to school.

Unfortunately, this policy does not apply to one out of every eight students subject to another federal law, the Individuals with Disabilities Education Act. Under IDEA, a student with a weapon typically is returned to the classroom in as few as 45 days. This category includes individuals who have serious emotional disturbances and behavior disorders. Schools have no power to expel these students if their disability caused them to bring a gun to school. If it didn't, schools can expel the student, but still must continue to provide full educational services.

Hence, schools are subject to a dangerous dual-discipline system that handcuffs them from removing violent students. It is deeply distressing that federal law requires that some who bring guns to schools be returned to a classroom filled with kids who want and deserve a safe and secure setting in which to learn.

Missouri teachers, parents, principals and superintendents have told me that we must do something in Washington to end this dual-discipline system that threatens the safety of children and invites a mass tragedy.

In response, I have authored the School Safety Act, which gives schools authority to remove any student who has a weapon at school. Congress voted overwhelmingly to include this provision in juvenile-justice legislation that now awaits conference committee action.

My legislation abolishes the dangerous double standard for weapons and returns control to where it belongs — local schools. Teachers, principals and superintendents care deeply about students with special needs. I trust these individuals to make the right decisions, including making special exceptions on a case-by-case basis. Dangerous and disruptive students are a small minority and pose a threat to all students.

A safe and orderly learning environment is critical to our children's success in school. Local schools must have the authority and flexibility to keep classrooms safe by being able to remove any student with a weapon from the classroom.

student is shortchanged." [22]

Administrators say their greater responsibility is to the 2,500 other students that attend a typical high school, rather than the one kid who is expelled.

Under the provision approved by the Senate last May, introduced by Sens. John Ashcroft, R-Mo., and Bill Frist, R-Tenn., disabled students who bring firearms to school would be treated the same as non-disabled students, regardless of whether or not the action resulted from their disability. Thus, if the state where the student lives is not required to provide educational services during the expulsion period, neither child would receive services.

"If you bring a gun or firearm to school, you should be treated the same, if you have a disability or no disability," Frist told fellow senators on May 20.

The amendment was attached to the juvenile-justice bill, which is not expected to go anywhere this year. However, Sens. Edward M. Kennedy, D-Mass., and Patrick J. Leahy, D-Vt., are expected to introduce an amendment to the education reauthorization bill this month requiring all expelled students to receive alternative education.

Dozens of advocacy groups support the amendment, including the two major teachers' unions and the National Parent-Teachers Association, as well as the Clinton administration. The bill would require the Education, Justice and Health and Human Services departments to share the cost of the alternative services.

The amendment is also supported by sheriffs, district attorneys and police and law enforcement groups like Fight Crime, Invest in Kids, which represents victims of violence.

"Giving a gun-toting kid an extended vacation from school and from all responsibility is soft on offenders and dangerous for everyone else," said the victims' group in opposing Ashcroft-Frist.

Supporters of mandatory alternative education often point to the tragic case of Kip Kinkel, the 14-year-old Oregon boy who was suspended for bringing a gun to school. He was not

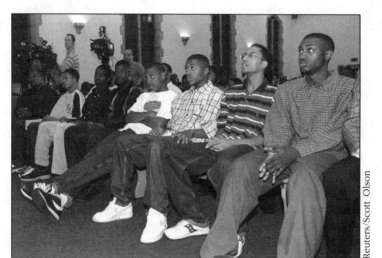

After several black high school students from Decatur, Ill., were suspended for two years for fighting at a football game, the Rev. Jesse Jackson and others said zero-tolerance policies unfairly target minorities.

Reuters/Scott Olson

required to attend alternative classes. He went home and killed his parents, then returned to school later to shoot and kill two students and wound 25.

Zero-Zero Tolerance

The administration also has proposed that Congress require any school receiving federal education funds to have "sound and equitable" discipline policies. Although neither the House nor the Senate has acted

on the proposal, school districts across the country are revisiting their zero-tolerance policies anyway, partly after pressure from parents.

"After all of the bad press, people are saying, 'Let's calm our jets a bit and think through this a little more,'" Newberry says.

But while some lawmakers are trying to make their laws less harsh, most are trying to broaden the definition of what is covered. "There has been a tremendous amount of activity in the state legislatures on this subject," says Christie of the Education Commission of the States.

Often legislators try to impose zero tolerance for drug and alcohol sales or consumption on school grounds. But the proposals usually don't make it through the legislature once lawmakers realize how damaging the consequences of long expulsions would be, she says.

"Zero-tolerance policies were initially put into place to ban lethal weapons from school grounds," she says. "Having a beer in your locker probably doesn't rate up there with carrying a weapon that could threaten the life of another student."

Some school districts are extending zero tolerance to cover off-campus behavior, punishing kids who get into trouble with the law on weekends, even for non-violent behavior like alcohol or marijuana use.

More and more schools are moving to ban images of guns on school grounds. Several school districts have taken rifles out of the hands of color guards, and one would not allow students re-enacting a Civil War battle to carry fake wooden muskets.

"Schools are reluctant to glorify

guns in any way right now," Tirozzi says. "You're seeing a knee-jerk Pavlovian response when people ban images of guns or weapons."

If a policy oversteps good sense, communities generally let their elected school board know about it, Resnick says. "Ninety-six percent of school board members in this country are elected. So there's a real opportunity for self-correction."

Tirozzi would like to see school boards limit their zero-tolerance policies to weapons, drugs and serious altercations, and return discretion to local superintendents. "Even the federal law mandates that for firearms superintendents should have discretion," he says.

The national associations representing elementary and secondary principals issued a joint statement in January asking school districts to consider three critical areas when reviewing zero-tolerance policies: the age of the child; fitting the punishment to the "crime" and ensuring that educational services are continued.

Blauvelt suggests that school boards should adopt the language in federal and state laws governing illegal drugs and weapons. "An aspirin is not a 'controlled and dangerous substance,'" he says. "Midol is not a 'controlled and dangerous substance.'"

Ferrandino of the elementary school principals association advises school boards to make sure policies are developed with community input and have reasonable penalties and allow for discretion. "There needs to be some sort of rationality and balance brought to the discussion," he says.

The National School Boards Association's Resnick agrees. "Hopefully, when you have a policy that can have as great an impact — positive and negative — on individual children as zero-tolerance policies can have, they are being developed with substantial community input," he says.

Mitchell of the AFT says school boards should be careful not to confuse zero-tolerance policies with discipline codes. Zero tolerance should be reserved for very serious offenses, he says. Less serious infractions should be covered under a discipline code, which allows for graduated consequences proportionate to the offense and punishes repeat offenses more severely than first-time offenses, he says. For instance, "A 'true weapon' should be covered by zero-tolerance policies," Mitchell says. "But a look-alike weapon should be covered by a school discipline policy."

The Rutherford Institute's Whitehead suggests that by relying on student courts for minor infractions, "You can get the decision out of the hands of one guy who's afraid of losing his job."

But most important, he says, zero-tolerance policies should only apply to "real offenses, like carrying real guns, real knives and real drugs — like cocaine — and not Alka-Seltzer."

Schools also should provide adequate due process and alternative educational services for expelled students, others say. "I don't know of any other situation in which an individual can be arrested, or put in jail or punished without some form of due process," Stephens, of the school safety center, says. "After all, we even have an appeal process for traffic tickets." ∎

OUTLOOK

Ebb and Flow

Educators predict that for the immediate future, the zero-tolerance pendulum will continue to swing back and forth. "It's cyclical," researcher Skiba says. "Every time there's another school shooting, you see a new round of ever-tougher zero-tolerance policies, followed in a few weeks by new community and parental outcries about violations of basic rights and common sense."

"Like any other reform issue, these things tend to ebb and flow," the Education Department's Modzeleski says. "Some places are already backing off from zero tolerance. We recommend that policies be reviewed on a regular basis."

George Washington's Kingery hopes that there will be "a little more reason" applied to zero-tolerance policies, and that the quality of alternative education will come under more scrutiny.

If zero tolerance is a backlash to judges and school administrators having broad discretion, says the University of California's Volokh. "Maybe there will be a backlash to the backlash. Maybe we will decide that we can't have a one-size-fits-all rule, and we should return discretion to the individual principals."

"Zero tolerance is now in the court of public opinion," Whitehead says. "All the major magazines have criticized it lately, and now even the teacher groups are saying, 'Let's have some reason.'"

But most agree that schools will not entirely abandon strict discipline, and that the public will continue to support zero tolerance for extreme acts involving guns, violence and drugs.

The NEA has launched a public-education campaign to get school districts to think in terms of a comprehensive, community-generated school-safety program that addresses the entire education system, including physical plant, teacher training, early elementary intervention, effective mental-health programs, crisis intervention and conflict resolution.

"We must move from a knee-jerk reaction to one in which we are willing to invest a lot of dollars over the long term," the NEA's Newberry says. "Until school boards come up with money and creative plans to address these larger issues in a comprehensive way, we're not really going to solve the problem."

Ferrandino of the elementary school principals' group says many school districts are trying to make schools smaller and gentler places. "Since these school shootings began, we have learned that there's much that both the schools and communities can do to create an environment where students can feel they belong and are valued as individuals," he says. Among other things, principals are trying to reduce class size and student anonymity. Other schools have developed community relationships with social-service agencies and are getting parents more involved in the schools.

"I think it is quickly being recognized that smaller might be better," Ferrandino says.

Others advocate more after-school and youth-development programs, both of which are more expensive and require long-term commitments — and time — from adults.

Sadly, two weeks before Kayla Rolland was shot in Michigan, several experts tied the future of zero tolerance to what the nation decides to do about guns. "Handgun availability is part of what is driving this ridiculous response on the part of the schools," Newberry says.

"I would love to say that within 10 years we won't need policies like zero tolerance," Tirozzi says. "By then, I would hope we will have gotten weapons out of the hands of youngsters, parents will be doing a better job in the household and we will have changed the kind of things that are projected onto movie screens. But unless and until this society comes to grips with its love affair with violence, and as long as children can easily obtain weapons, these problems will continue to come into the schoolhouse.

"When society zeroes out violence,

FOR MORE INFORMATION

National Association of Elementary School Principals, 1615 Duke St., Alexandria, Va. 22314-3483; (703) 684-3345; www.naesp.org. This association of elementary and middle school principals conducts workshops for members on federal and state policies and programs.

National Association of Secondary School Principals, 1904 Association Dr., Reston, Va. 20191-1537; (703) 860-0200; www.nassp.org. This group, which includes college-level teachers of secondary education, conducts training for members and serves as an information clearinghouse.

National School Boards Association, 1680 Duke St., Alexandria, Va. 22314; (703)683-7590; www.nsba.org. This federation of school board associations monitors legislation and regulations affecting public-education funding, local governance and education quality.

National School Safety Center, 141 Duesenberg Dr., Suite 11, Westlake Village, Calif. 91362; (805) 373-9977; www.nssc1.org. The center was created by presidential directive in 1984 to meet the growing need for additional training and preparation in the area of school crime and violence prevention.

we'll be happy to zero out zero tolerance," he says. ■

Notes

[1] Of the 100,000 students expelled nationwide during the 1997-98 school year, 3,930 were expelled for bringing a firearm to school under the Gun-Free Schools Act. That was a 31 percent drop from the previous year's total, according to Department of Education statistics.

[2] The statistics are from an unpublished study by Kingery, "Suspension and Expulsion: New Directions."

[3] See *Dothan City Board of Education v. V.M.H.*

[4] Quoted in "The Intolerance of Zero Tolerance," Intellectual Capital.com, Aug. 19, 1999.

[5] Robert C. Johnson, "Decatur Furor Sparks Wider Policy Debate," *Education Week,* Nov. 24, 1999.

[6] "The Fight's Not Over, *The New Republic,* Dec. 6, 1999.

[7] "National Survey of Teens, Teachers and Principals," National Center on Addiction and Substance Abuse, Columbia University, 1998.

[8] "Violence and Discipline Problems in U.S. Public Schools: 1996-1997," National Center for Education Statistics, 1998.

[9] Russ Skiba and Reece Peterson, "The Dark Side of Zero Tolerance: Can Punishment

Lead to Safe Schools?" *The Kappan,* January 1999.

[10] For details, see Kathy Koch, "Drug Testing, *The CQ Researcher,* Nov. 20, 1998, p. 1014.

[11] The unpublished study was conducted by the Applied Research Center, in Oakland, Calif.

[12] "Education Denied: The Negative Impact of Zero Tolerance Policies," The Civil Rights Project at Harvard, February 2000.

[13] Keleher testified before the U.S. Civil Rights Commission on Feb. 18, 1999.

[14] For background, see Margaret Edwards, "Mandatory Sentencing," *The CQ Researcher,* May 26, 1995, pp. 465-488.

[15] "Zero tolerance on drugs urged," *Houston Chronicle,* May 21, 1986.

[16] James J. Kilpatrick, "Get tough with kids who use, sell drugs," *Houston Chronicle,* June 17, 1986.

[17] *Houston Chronicle, op. cit.,* May 21.

[18] Harry Bruinius, "In Giulianiville, it's a case of law vs. order," *The Christian Science Monitor,* Nov. 9, 1999.

[19] For background, see Kathy Koch, "School Violence," *The CQ Researcher,* Oct. 9, 1998, pp. 881-904.

[20] Violence and Discipline Problems in U.S. Public Schools, 1996-1997, The National Center for Education Statistics, February, 1998.

[21] Quoted in Skiba and Peterson, *op. cit.*

[22] Dennis Cauchon, "Zero-tolerance policies lack flexibility," *USA Today,* April 13, 1999.

Bibliography

Selected Sources Used

Books

Kelling, George L., and Catherine Coles, *Fixing Broken Windows: Restoring Order and Reducing Crime in Our Communities*, Martin Kessler Books, 1996.

The Rutgers University professor and his co-author argue that ignoring minor problems in cities, like broken windows or graffiti, eventually leads to an increase in serious crime. Kelling first outlined the approach in a 1982 *Atlantic* magazine article.

Raskin, Jamin B., *We the Students: The High School in the High Court*, Congressional Quarterly, 2000.

An American University constitutional law professor outlines precedent-setting Supreme Court cases involving drug testing, locker searches, school newspaper censorship, sexual harassment and free speech.

Articles

"Zero tolerance on drugs urged," *Houston Chronicle*, May 21, 1986.

Education Secretary William Bennett becomes the first official to ask Congress to withhold federal education funds unless schools adopt "zero-tolerance" expulsion policies for drug dealing on school grounds.

Baxter, Bethany, "The Intolerance of Zero Tolerance," Intellectual Capital.com, Aug. 19, 1999.

A consultant to colleges argues that school officials do not model good judgment by setting up zero-tolerance policies that treat all offenses equally harshly.

Cloud, John, "The Columbine Effect," *Time*, Dec. 6, 1999.

Zero tolerance sounds like a good way to treat violence in schools, but experts say it may have gone too far.

Grier, Peter, and Gail Russell Chaddock, "Schools get tough as threats continue," *The Christian Science Monitor*, Nov. 5, 1999.

Educators are struggling with how to implement get-tough safety rules meant to stop student shootings.

Johnson, Dirk, "Schools' New Watchword: Zero Tolerance," *The New York Times*, Dec. 1, 1999.

This overview looks at how zero-tolerance school discipline has replaced more traditional punishment.

Skiba, Russ, and Reece Peterson, "The Dark Side of Zero Tolerance: Can Punishment Lead to Safe Schools?" *The Kappan*, January 1999.

The authors argue that increasingly broad interpretations of zero tolerance have resulted in a near epidemic of suspensions for seemingly trivial events, increasing the likelihood that excluded students will get involved in drugs and gangs.

Wing, Bob, and Terry Keleher, "Zero Tolerance: An Interview with Jesse Jackson on Race and School Discipline," *Colorlines*, spring 2000.

Jackson contends that zero-tolerance polices disproportionately target minority students.

Reports and Studies

Keleher, Terry, Applied Research Center, March 1999.

In a survey of 12 large school districts across the country, the public-policy institute found that black students are three to five times more likely to be expelled than white students in some districts.

Kingery, Paul, "Suspension and Expulsion: New Directions," Hamilton Fish Institute, unpublished 1999 study.

Kingery found that expulsions and suspensions are rising nationwide and that longer and permanent expulsions are at an all-time high.

National Center on Addiction and Substance Abuse, "National Survey of Teens, Teachers and Principals," 1998.

The Columbia University research center found that 85 percent of principals believe zero-tolerance policies keep drugs out of schools.

National Center for Education Statistics, "Violence and Discipline Problems in U.S. Public Schools: 1996-1997," 1998.

This survey of more than 1,000 school principals found mixed and minor improvements in school discipline and drug problems.

The Civil Rights Project at Harvard, "Education Denied: The Negative Impact of Zero Tolerance Policies," February 2000.

A briefing paper prepared for the U.S. Civil Rights Commission argues that zero-tolerance policies are having a disproportionate impact on African-American and Latino children.

U.S. Department of Education, "Report on State Implementation of the Gun-Free Schools Act," August 1999.

This annual report shows that in the 1997-98 school year, 3,930 students were expelled for bringing a firearm to school, a 31 percent drop from the previous year.

How to Write a Research Paper

This guide to writing a research paper is arranged in five parts: the first section outlines six steps that will help you write a paper—from getting ready to choose a topic to writing and revising. The second part discusses library research, and the third and fourth give tips on using the Web to conduct research. Finally, you will find a list of links to useful online resources. The Internet is constantly changing. Be aware that some of the resources noted here may no longer be available; however, you should be able to find most of them and what is included here will give you a good idea of the information that is available.

Six Steps to Writing a Research Paper

Step 1 Getting Started

Goal: Preparing for the assignment and getting ready to choose a topic

UNDERSTAND THE ASSIGNMENT. Read over the instructions for the assignment to make sure you fully understand what the instructor has in mind and on what basis you will be graded.

CONSIDER THE PROCESS YOU'LL USE. The paper is your final *product,* but a research paper involves an extensive *process* before you can generate the product. If you focus too quickly on the end product, you may miss some of the important research steps and find yourself writing a paper

Adapted, with permission, from *A+ Research and Writing for High School and College Students,* copyright 1997 by Kathryn L. Schwartz. Published by the Internet Public Library: http://www.ipl.org.

without enough understanding of the topic. Browse over the rest of the steps suggested here to get an idea of the process and think about how you'll approach each step. Start a journal or notebook and begin jotting notes about not only "what" you plan to do but also "how" you plan to do it.

SET YOUR DEADLINES FOR EACH STEP OF THE ASSIGNMENT. Ideally, you will have at least four weeks from the date it's assigned to complete a research paper of seven or eight pages (2,000 to 2,500 words). Shorter papers requiring fairly simple research (four or five pages—1,500 words) may not require four weeks' "lead time," while a fifteen-page or longer paper might be a semester-long project.

THINK ABOUT POSSIBLE TOPICS: The word "topic" is used variably by many teachers of writing and research to mean anything from the very general "subject matter" to the very specific "thesis statement." Here, the term *topic* is broadly defined, while *focus* means a narrower perspective on the topic, and *thesis* statement is the main point of your paper, which cannot be determined until after research and analysis is complete.

INFO SEARCH—BROWSE, READ, RELAX. Start by thumbing through the textbooks or course pack for the class in which your paper was assigned. Browse the table of contents, chapter headings and subheadings to get an overview of the subject matter. Visit your library and browse in the catalog and reference room to find out what sources are held by the library that may relate to your class. Browse some of the subject-indexed sources on the Internet with the same purpose.

RELATE YOUR PRIOR EXPERIENCE AND LEARNING. The process of successful research and writing involves build-

ing on what you know. You don't need to know a *lot* about a subject to use it as your topic, but choosing one you're totally unfamiliar with could be a mistake. It may take so much time and effort to become informed about the subject that you don't really have time to get into the depth required by your assignment.

JOT DOWN YOUR QUESTIONS AND IDEAS ABOUT POSSIBLE TOPICS. Use your notebook to starting recording questions that interest you or ideas for possible topics.

You'll end up with a list of ideas and musings, some of which are obviously ridiculous and not reasonable topics for your paper, but don't worry about that at this point. Think about things that interest you and that build upon some experience or knowledge you have or build upon things you're presently learning in class.

BRAINSTORM, ALONE AND WITH OTHERS. Toss ideas around in your mind. Bounce ideas off of your classmates, your teacher or your siblings and parents to get their reactions and ideas. Many times another person will have a fresh perspective you might not have thought of, or something they say will trigger an idea for you.

Step 2 Discovering and Choosing a Topic

Goal: Discovering and choosing a topic for your research

INFO SEARCH—READ FOR OVERVIEW OF VARIOUS TOPICS. Use the notes you've made and the thinking you've done so far to select some areas for general reading. Use the library's reference room—encyclopedias, dictionaries, almanacs—to get an overview of possible topics (even if your instructor has told you that you can't use an encyclopedia as a reference—that's not important at this stage).

Explore CD-ROM tools in your library, like newspaper and magazine indexes, searching with key words representing your topic ideas. Explore the Internet by using several of the resources organized by subject.

Remember to keep your concept of topic rather broad at this stage—you can look for a focus later, after you know something about the topic.

CONTINUE THINKING AND JOTTING DOWN QUESTIONS AND IDEAS IN YOUR NOTEBOOK. As you read, ideas and questions may strike you—write them down, or you'll lose track of them. Look for issues that interest you, that arouse your curiosity or your passion. Consider the audience for your research paper: what kinds of things have been discussed in class that seemed to interest the class and the instructor? What kinds of issues were touched upon but could use further study and elaboration?

INFO SURVEY—WHAT PRINT AND ELECTRONIC RESOURCES ARE AVAILABLE? When you've narrowed your choices down, make a quick survey of the research resources that will be available to you on each potential topic. How much information seems to be available in your library's catalog? If it's a current topic, is there information in newspaper and magazine indexes and are those newspapers and magazines held by your library? Is there much authoritative information on your topic on the Internet? Is the available information slanted to one side of an issue versus another? How much work will it take to get the information you need if you choose a particular topic?

TRY DIFFERENT TOPICS ON FOR "SIZE." The topic you choose should "fit" in several important respects: your interests and knowledge, the purpose of the assignment, the type of paper

(report, issue, argument), the length of the paper. Don't worry too much about having a broad topic at this point. Look for topic ideas at Researchpaper.com (http://www.researchpaper.com/) or in your library. Ask the reference librarian if the library has books of suggested topics like Kathryn Lamm's *10,000 Ideas for Term Papers, Projects, Reports & Speeches* (New York: Macmillan, 1995).

Step 3   Looking for and Forming a Focus

Goal: Exploring your topic; finding and forming a focus for your research

INFO SEARCH—EXPLORING YOUR TOPIC. Before you can decide on a focus, you need to explore your topic, to become informed about the topic, to build on your knowledge and experience. You'll be locating books, articles, videos, Internet and other resources about your topic and reading to learn! You're looking for an issue, an aspect, a perspective on which to focus your research paper.

This is the first step in which you'll probably be checking books out of the library. Encyclopedias won't be much help here. You're looking for treatments of your topic that are either more comprehensive or more specific than an encyclopedic treatment, with various authors' summaries, analyses and opinions. But, until you've chosen a focus, you're not really on a mission of gathering information. If you gather information on the topic as a whole, you'll waste a lot of time doing it and have way too much to sort through when you are ready to write your paper. Resist the temptation to "gather" until you've chosen a focus. Now you'll be using the library's online catalog, online indexes and the Web search engines along with the reference room and

the subject-based Web directories.

INFO SEARCH—PRELIMINARY NOTE TAKING. As you read, start taking notes of what you're learning about your topic—concepts, issues, problems, areas where experts agree or disagree. Keep track of the bibliographic references for the information you're using, and write down a note or two of what's contained in the book, article, Website, etc. There's nothing more frustrating than knowing you read something earlier about a particular point and not being able to locate it again when you decide it's something you need.

Find out what kind of citations are required by your instructor and make sure you're recording what you'll need to do your bibliography.

PURPOSEFUL THINKING ABOUT POSSIBLE FOCUSES. While you're learning about your topic, intentionally look for possible focuses in the material. You could spend enormous amounts of time reading, especially about an interesting topic, without being any closer to a focus unless you purposefully keep that goal in your mind while you read.

CHOOSING A FOCUS OR COMBINING THEMES TO FORM A FOCUS. Try your choices of focus on for "size" as you did your topic. Which ones fit the assignment, the size, scope and type of the paper? Think about which of your possible focuses has the best chance for making a successful paper. If you find several themes within your topic that separately are too small to support the entire paper, can they be combined to form a focus?

Step 4   Gathering Information

Goal: Gathering information that clarifies and supports your focus

INFO SEARCH—FINDING, COLLECTING AND RECORDING. This is the step most people think of when they think of "library research." It's a hunt for information in any available form (book, periodical, CD, video, Internet) which is pertinent to your chosen focus. Once you know the focus of your research, there are lots of tools and strategies to help you find and collect the information you need.

Your information search should be focused and specific, but pay careful attention to serendipity (finding, by chance, valuable things you weren't even looking for). Keep your mind open to continue learning about your focused topic.

Now is the time to carefully record your sources in the bibliographic format required by your instructor. Every piece of information you collect should have bibliographic information written down before you leave the library. You should also pay attention to the quality of the information you find, especially if you're using information you find on the Internet. Now is also the time to learn the details of using search engines. Many of the sources you will want to use are online, whether in the library or on the Internet.

THINK ABOUT CLARIFYING OR REFINING YOUR FOCUS. As you gather information about your focused topic, you may find new information that prompts you to refine, clarify, extend or narrow your focus. Stay flexible and adjust your information search to account for the changes, widening or narrowing your search, or heading down a slightly different path to follow a new lead.

START ORGANIZING YOUR NOTES. Start organizing your notes into logical groups. You may notice a gap in your research, or a more heavy weighting to one aspect of the subject than what you had intended. Starting to organize as you gather information can save an extra trip to the library. It's better to find the gap

now instead of the night before your paper is due.

THINK ABOUT WHAT YOUR THESIS STATEMENT WILL BE. The thesis statement is the main point of your paper. The type of thesis statement you'll be making depends a lot on what type of paper you're writing—a report, an issue analysis, an advocacy paper or another type. As you gather specific information and refine your focus, intentionally look for a main point to your findings. Sometimes, a thesis emerges very obviously from the material, and other times you may struggle to bring together the parts into a sensible whole. The tricky part is knowing when to stop gathering information—when do you have enough, and of the right kind? Seeking a main point as you research will help you know when you're done.

Step 5   Preparing to Write

Goal: Analyzing and organizing your information and forming a thesis statement

ANALYZE AND ORGANIZE YOUR INFORMATION. The word "analyze" means to break something down into its parts. A meaningful analysis identifies the parts and demonstrates how they relate to each other. You may have information from different sources that examines different aspects of your topic. By breaking down the information, you may be able to see relationships between the different sources and form them into a whole concept. When you're trying to make sense of the information coming out of your research process, you often have to look at it from different perspectives and sometimes have to step back and try to get a "big picture" view. Some ways to do this are to try out different organization patterns: compare and contrast, advantages and disadvantages, starting from a narrow premise and building on it,

cause and effect, logical sequence.

CONSTRUCT A THESIS STATEMENT AND TRY IT ON FOR "SIZE." Before beginning to write the paper, write the thesis statement. Boil down the main point of your paper to a single statement. Sharon Williams and Laura Reidy at the Hamilton College site (http://www.hamilton.edu/academic/Resource/WC/Intro_Thesis.html) give this explanation of the thesis statement:

A well-written thesis statement, usually expressed in one sentence, is the most important sentence in your entire paper. It should both summarize for your reader the position you will be arguing and set up the pattern of organization you will use in your discussion. A thesis sentence is not a statement of accepted fact; it is the position that needs the proof you will provide in your argument. Your thesis should reflect the full scope of your argument—no more and no less; beware of writing a thesis statement that is too broad to be defended within the scope of your paper.

Another way to summarize the nature and function of the thesis statement is that it is a single sentence, usually in the first paragraph of the paper, which:

- declares the position you are taking in your paper,
- sets up the way you will organize your discussion, and
- points to the conclusion you will draw.

WEED OUT IRRELEVANT INFORMATION. Now that you have all those wonderful notes and citations from your research, you're going to have to get rid of some of them! No matter how profound and interesting the information is, if it doesn't relate to and support the thesis you've chosen, don't try to cram it into the paper—just set it aside. You'll have an easier time writing if you do this weeding before you start.

Appendix

INFO SEARCH—FILL IN THE GAPS. Once you've identified which of your research notes you'll use, you may see some gaps where you need an additional support for a point you want to make. Leave enough time in your writing plan for an extra trip to the library, just in case.

Step 6   Writing the Paper

Goal: Writing, revising and finalizing the paper

THINK ABOUT THE ASSIGNMENT, THE AUDIENCE AND THE PURPOSE. To prepare for writing, go over once more the requirements of the assignment to make sure you focus your writing efforts on what's expected by your instructor. Consider the purpose of the paper, either as set forth in the assignment, or as stated in your thesis statement—are you trying to persuade, to inform, to evaluate, to summarize?

- Who is your audience and how will that affect your paper?
- What prior knowledge can you assume the audience has about the topic?
- What style and tone of writing are required by the audience and the assignment—informal, scholarly, first-person reporting, dramatized?

PREPARE AN OUTLINE. Try to get a "model" outline for the type of paper you're writing, or look at examples of good papers to see how they were organized. The Roane State Community College Online Writing Lab (Jennifer Jordan-Henley) gives an example of an outline for a paper written to describe a problem. See http://www2.rscc.cc.tn.us/~jordan_jj/OWL/Research.html:

- Introduction
  Statement of the Problem
  Thesis Sentence
- Body: Paragraphs 1 and 2
  History of the Problem (Include,

perhaps, past attempts at solutions. Work in sources.)
- Body: Paragraphs 3 and 4
  Extent of the Problem (Who is affected? How bad is it? Work in sources.)
- Body: Paragraphs 5 and 6
  Repercussions of the Problem (Work in sources.)
- Body: Paragraphs 7 and 8
  Future solutions (not necessarily your own. More sources.)
- Conclusion
  Summarize your findings

WRITE THE ROUGH DRAFT—VISIT THE OWLS. Here's where the Online Writing Labs, or OWLs, excel—there are many dozens of great articles on every aspect of writing your paper. The *Links to Online Resources* pages (p. 163) have classified these by topic so that you can browse easily and pick out articles you want to read. The entire *Links for Writing* section will be helpful, and specifically the sections on:

- Title, introduction and conclusion
- Writing style and technique
- Grammar and punctuation

KNOW HOW TO USE YOUR SOURCE MATERIALS AND CITE THEM. See the section *Citing Sources* on the Links page (p. 163). There's also a nice section on using sources in the middle of the article entitled "Writing a General Research Paper" (http://www2.rscc.cc.tn.us/~jordan_jj/OWL/Research.html) from the Roane State Community College Online Writing Lab (Henley, 1996). The section, "What Happens When the Sources Seem to be Writing My Paper For Me?" describes how to break up long quotations and how to cite an author multiple times without letting the author take over your paper, and it links to both the MLA and the APA style requirements for partial quotations, full quotations, indented quotations, in-text quotations, and paraphrasing.

HAVE OTHERS READ AND CRITIQUE THE PAPER. Read your paper out loud, to yourself. See if the arguments are coherent, logical and conclusive when read aloud. Have several experienced people read and critique your paper. If your school has a writing lab, use the tutors or helpers there as critics.

REVISE AND PROOFREAD. See the "Revision Checklist" section of the article *The Research Paper* (http://www.chesapeake.edu/Writingcenter/respaper.html) from Chesapeake College. The checklist asks some general questions to help you step back and take a look at the overall content and structure of the paper, then drills down to paragraphs, sentences and words for a closer examination of the writing style. Almost all the OWLs have very large sections on grammar, sentence and paragraph structure, writing style, proofreading, revising and common errors.

Browse some of the larger OWLs like Purdue University and University of Victoria and see the linked articles on *Revising and rewriting* (p. 163).

Learning to Research in the Library

Get to know your library

Libraries build their collections based on what they think their patrons will need, so the collections of reference materials, fiction and non-fiction will differ between a public and an academic library. Be aware of what kind of collection you're working with, and make arrangements to visit a different library if necessary.

Learn to browse—understand the classification scheme in your library

A library's classification scheme is a system by which books are organized to be placed on the shelves.

Browsing the shelves is an important step when you're trying to get ideas for your research project, so it's worth the effort to become familiar with your library's system.

Most libraries in the U.S. use either the Dewey Decimal system or Library of Congress system, while Britain uses the UDC and other countries use various systems. All of the systems attempt to "co-locate" books with similar subject matter. In a smaller library, many times you can bypass the catalog as a starting point and go directly to the shelves for a first look at your topic, so long as you have a chart of the classification scheme as a guide.

Remember, though, that a book can have only one location in a library. Some books cover more than one subject and the cataloguer has to choose one place to locate the book. Also, non-book materials such as videos and films, will be located in a different section of the building and could be missed by simply shelf-browsing the book collection.

Learn how online library catalogs work

A library catalog is a listing of all the items held by a particular library. A cataloguer examines the item (book, video, map, audio tape, CD, etc.) and decides how it will be described in the library's catalog and under what subject it will be classified. When the item is entered into the library's online catalog database, information is entered into different fields, which are then searchable by users.

Library catalogs usually treat a book as a single "item" and catalog it that way, even if it might be a book of poetry or a book of essays by different authors. You can't find a reference to a particular poem in the library catalog, nor to a particular essay within a book of essays. The same is true of magazines, journals and newspapers. The library catalog will tell you if the library keeps a particular periodical in its collection, but will not list all the articles within the periodical, nor will it necessarily even list all the issues of the periodical which are kept. There are other publications in the reference room which will help you retrieve these individual items, but usually not the library catalog.

Most catalogs are searchable by author, title, subject and keyword. Some of the important things you need to know about the information in those fields are discussed below.

SEARCHING THE CATALOG BY SUBJECT AND KEYWORD. The subject field of a catalog record contains only the words or phrases used by the cataloguer when assigning a subject heading. If the library is using Library of Congress Subject Headings (LCSH), for example, the subject heading for a book about how playing football affects the players' bodies would probably be assigned the subject heading "Football—physiological aspects." Unless you type in that entire phrase as your search term, you won't find the book by searching the subject field.

Subject field searching can be very helpful, but you must find out how the subject you're looking for is worded by using the subject manuals or getting help from the reference librarian. Once you zero in on an appropriate subject heading, a search in the catalog will give you a list of all the items in the library's collection categorized under that heading, so you can browse the collection online. Note also that most items are classified under one or two *very specific* subject headings, rather than under many subjects. The keyword field of a library catalog generally searches several fields in the database record—the author, title and description fields. The description is any information about the catalogued item which may have been entered by the cataloguer. *This is not the full text of the book, nor is it an abstract (summary) of the book but rather a short paragraph containing information the cataloguer thought would be helpful to a user.* This is *not* like searching for keywords in an indexed database like Alta Vista on the Internet, where every word in a document has been recorded.

For this reason, keyword searching alone could miss an item pertinent to your research project if the keyword you use was not included in the short paragraph written by the cataloguer. It's best to use a combination of keyword searching and subject-field searching to make a comprehensive search of the library catalog.

SEARCHING OTHER LIBRARIES' CATALOGS. There are lots of library catalogs on the Internet—but so what? You can search the catalog of a library in Timbuktu, but that doesn't get you the book. Remember that library catalogs do not have full text of books and documents but are just a database with descriptions of the library's holdings. There are a few, and will be more, actual online libraries where you can go to read or search full text documents. Just don't confuse these special resources with a library catalog, which is very different.

Find out how to search for journals and newspapers at your library

Most libraries have either print, CD-ROM or online (either in the library or sometimes on the Web) indexes of magazine, journal and newspaper articles (referred to as periodicals) available for users. Some of these are abstracts of the articles, which are short summaries written to describe the article's contents in enough detail so that a reader can decide whether or not to seek out the full text. Some of these sources may be in the form of full text, where the entire articles have been entered into the database.

The databases will include particular periodicals published within a span of time (for example, a popular newspaper index goes back 36 months for certain major newspapers). Know what the database you're searching contains and whether it's represented as abstract or full text.

Note that these resources, whether print or digital, contain information about periodicals which may not be held by your library. If the database does not have full text articles, you may find an article right on point to your topic, but that particular newspaper or journal may not be in your library's collection. Check out your options with the reference desk if you need an article that's not in your library's collection.

Bibliography surfing

Web surfing is finding an interesting Web page and then using the hyperlinks on that page to jump to other pages. If you find the first page interesting, chances are you'll also be interested in the pages the author has chosen to link to. Librarians and researchers have been doing this for a long time, in the print medium. It's a valuable tool for identifying sources on your chosen topic.

What you do is use the bibliography provided at the end of an encyclopedia article, journal article or book that you've found particularly pertinent to your topic and follow the bibliographic references much as you would hyperlinks on the Web. Since you're locating items that influenced the author of the original article and to which he or she referred, they're likely to be "on point" to your topic. Then use the bibliography at the end of *those* cited articles to find even *more* items, and so on.

Consult the reference librarian for advice

Several times above, you've been advised to consult the reference librarian. Reference librarians can help save you a lot of time because they know their library's collection very well—both the reference collection and the nonfiction collection—and can often tell you "off the top of their heads" whether or not the library has a particular item you're looking for. They are also skilled searchers, both of the library's catalog and of online resources such as CD-ROM, online databases and the Internet. In addition, they're trained in teaching others to use these resources and are glad to do so.

Learn about search syntax and professional search techniques

To be successful at any kind of online searching, you need to know something about how computer searching works. At this time, much of the burden is on the user to intelligently construct a search strategy, taking into account the peculiarities of the particular database and search software.

Learning to Research on the Web

Cyberspace is not like your library

When your search term in one of the popular search engines brings back 130,000 hits, you still wonder if the *one* thing you're looking for will be among them. This can be an enormous problem when you're trying to do serious research on the Internet. Too much information is almost worse than too little, because it takes so much time to sort through

it to see if there's anything useful. The rest of this section will give you some pointers to help you become an effective Internet researcher.

Get to know the reference sources on the Internet

Finding reference material on the Web can be a lot more difficult than walking into the Reference Room in your local library.

The subject-classified Web directories described below will provide you with your main source of links to reference materials on the Web. In addition, many public and academic libraries, like the Internet Public Library (http://www.ipl.org), have put together lists of links to Web sites, categorized by subject. The difficulty is finding Web sites that contain the same kind of substantive content you'd find in a library. See the links to *Reference sources on the Web* (p. 163) for a list of some Web-based reference materials.

Understand how search engines work

Search engines are software tools that allow a user to ask for a list of Web pages containing certain words or phrases from an automated search index. The automated search index is a database containing some or all of the words appearing on the Web pages that have been indexed. The search engines send out a software program known as a spider, crawler or robot. The spider follows hyperlinks from page to page around the Web, gathering and bringing information back to the search engine to be indexed.

Most search engines index all the text found on a Web page, except for words too common to index, such as *a, and, in, to, the* and so on. When a user submits a query, the search engine looks for Web pages containing the words, combinations, or phrases asked for by the user. Engines may be programmed to look for an exact match or a close match (for example, the plural of the word submitted by the user). They may rank the hits as to how close the match is to the words submitted by the user.

One important thing to remember about search engines is this: once the engine and the spider have been programmed, the process is totally automated. No human being examines the information returned by the spider to see what subject it might be about or whether the words on the Web page adequately reflect the actual main point of the page.

Another important fact is that all the search engines are different. They each index differently and treat users' queries differently. The burden is on the searcher to learn how to use the features of each search engine.

Know the difference between a search engine and a directory

A search engine lets you seek out specific words and phrases in Web pages. A directory is more like a subject catalog in the library—a human being has determined the main point of a Web page and has categorized it based on a classification scheme of topics and subtopics used by that directory. Many of the search engines have also developed browsable subject catalogues, and most of the directories also have a search engine, so the distinction between them is blurring.

Jack Solock, special librarian at InterNIC Net Scout, classifies Web directories into categories based on the amount of human intervention (see "Searching the Internet Part II: Subject Catalogs, Annotated Directories, and Subject Guides" at http://rs.internic.net/nic-support/nicnews/

oct96/enduser.html). The categories he uses are subject catalogs, annotated directories and subject guides.

A subject catalog classifies Web pages into subject categories and uses excerpts from the Web page as a short description. An annotated directory divides sites by subject but also contains analysis of the site by an editor, librarian or subject specialist, who writes a description to assist the user. A subject guide attempts to provide a selection of sites relating to a particular subject that represent high quality resources, thus representing the highest level of human intervention of the three types because it involves building a collection of sites to represent a subject area.

Mr. Solock categorizes the following resources:

- Yahoo, BUBL and Galaxy as *subject catalogs,*
- Magellan, Lycos Top 5% and InterNIC Directory of Directories as *annotated directories* and
- Argus Clearinghouse and the WWW Virtual Library as *subject guides.*

Learn about search syntax and professional search techniques

To be successful at any kind of online searching, you need to know something about how computer searching works. At this time, much of the burden is on the user to intelligently construct a search strategy, taking into account the peculiarities of the particular database and search software.

Learn some essential browser skills

Know how to use your browser for finding your way around, finding your way back to places you've been before and for "note-taking" as you

gather information for your paper. A large part of effective research on the Web is figuring out how to stay on track and not waste time—the "browsing" and "surfing" metaphors are fine for leisure time spent on the Web, but not when you're under time pressure to finish your research paper.

URLs. UNDERSTAND THE CONSTRUCTION OF A URL. Sometimes a hyperlink will take you to a URL such as http://www.sampleurl.com/files/howto.html. You should know that the page "howto.html" is part of a site called "www.sampleurl.com." If this page turns out to be a "not found" error, or doesn't have a link to the site's home page, you can try typing in the location box "http://www.sampleurl.com/" or "http://www.sampleurl.com/files/" to see if you can find a menu or table of contents. Sometimes a file has been moved or its name has changed, but the site itself still has content useful to you—this is a way to find out.

If there's a tilde (~) in the URL, you're probably looking at someone's personal page on a larger site. For example "http://www.bigsite.com/~jonesj/home.html" refers to a page at www.bigsite.com where J. Jones has some server space in which to post Web pages.

NAVIGATION. Be sure you can use your browser's "Go" list, "History" list, "Back" button and "Location" box where the URL can be typed in. In Web research, you're constantly following links through to other pages then wanting to jump back a few steps to start off in a different direction. If you're using a computer at home rather than sharing one at school, check the settings in your "Cache" or "History list" to see how long the places you've visited will be retained in history. This will determine how long the links will show as having been visited before. Usually, you want to set this period of time to cover the full time frame of your research project so you'll be able to tell which Web sites you've been to before.

BOOKMARKS OR FAVORITES. Before you start a research session, make a new folder in your bookmarks or favorites area and set that folder as the one to receive new bookmark additions. You might name it with the current date, so you later can identify in which research session the bookmarks were made. Remember you can make a bookmark for a page you haven't yet visited by holding the mouse over the link and getting the popup menu (by either pressing the mouse button or right clicking, depending on what flavor computer you have) to "Add bookmark" or "Add to favorites." Before you sign off your research session, go back and weed out any bookmarks that turned out to be uninteresting so you don't have a bunch of irrelevant material to deal with later. Later you can move these bookmarks around into different folders as you organize information for writing your paper—find out how to do that in your browser.

PRINTING FROM THE BROWSER. Sometimes you'll want to print information from a Web site. The main thing to remember is to make sure the Page Setup is set to print out the page title, URL, and the date. You'll be unable to use the material if you can't remember later where it came from.

"SAVING AS" A FILE. Know how to temporarily save the contents of a Web page as a file on your hard drive or a floppy disk and later open it in your browser by using the "file open" feature. You can save the page you're currently viewing or one which is hyperlinked from that page, from the "File" menu or the popup menu accessed by the mouse held over the hyperlink.

COPYING AND PASTING TO A WORD PROCESSOR. You can take quotes from Web pages by opening up a word

processing document and keeping it open while you use your browser. When you find text you want to save, drag the mouse over it and "copy" it, then open up your word processing document and "paste" it. Be sure to also copy and paste the URL and page title, and to record the date, so you know where the information came from.

BE PREPARED TO CITE YOUR WEB REFERENCES. Find out what form of bibliographic references your instructor requires. Both the MLA and APA bibliographic formats have developed rules for citing sources on CD-ROM and the Internet. Instructions for citing electronic sources are available at many libraries, including the Purdue University Online Writing Lab (http://owl.english.purdue.edu/Files/110.html).

Skills for Online Searching

There are many sources on the Web to help you learn search skills. Many of the concepts for using Web search engines also apply to searching online library catalogs and CD-ROMs. This section of the manual will get you started and point you to other online sources where you can learn more.

Learn how search syntax works

Search syntax is a set of rules describing how users can query the database being searched. Sophisticated syntax makes for a better search, one where the items retrieved are mostly relevant to the searcher's need and important items are not missed. It allows a user to look for combinations of terms, exclude other terms, look for various forms of a word, include synonyms, search for phrases rather than single words. The

main tools of search syntax are these:

BOOLEAN LOGIC. Boolean logic allows the use of AND, OR and NOT to search for items containing both terms, either term, or a term only if not accompanied by another term. The links below and all the Web search engines "search help" have a lot of good examples of Boolean logic. Tip: NOT can be dangerous. Let's say you want to search for items about Mexico, but not New Mexico, so you use NOT to exclude the word *New* from your retrieved set. This would prevent you from retrieving an article about *New regulations in Mexico* because it contained the word *New,* though that wasn't what you intended.

WILDCARDS AND TRUNCATION. This involves substituting symbols for certain letters of a word so that the search engine will retrieve items with any letter in that spot in the word. The syntax may allow a symbol in the middle of a word (wildcard) or only at the end of the word (truncation). This feature makes it easier to search for related word groups, like *woman* and *women* by using a wildcard such as *wom*n*. Truncation can be useful to search for a group of words like *invest, investor, investors, investing, investment, investments* by submitting *invest* rather than typing in all those terms separated by OR's. The only problem is that *invest** will also retrieve *investigate, investigated, investigator, investigation, investigating.* The trick, then is to combine terms with an AND such as *invest** AND *stock* or bond* or financ* or money* to try and narrow your retrieved set to the kind of documents you're looking for.

PHRASE SEARCHING. Many concepts are represented by a phrase rather than a single word. In order to successfully search for a term like *library school* it's important that the search engine allow syntax for phrase searching. Otherwise, instead of get-

LINKS TO ONLINE RESOURCES

http://www.ipl.org/teen/aplus/links.htm
Go online to link to over a hundred Web pages that will help you with your research and writing project.

Links for Research

Reference sources on the Web
http://www.ipl.org/teen/aplus/referenceweb.htm
A chart of some of the online reference books available free on the Web

Web directories and subject-classified resources
http://www.ipl.org/teen/aplus/linksdirect.htm
Yahoo, Argus, IPL et al.

Search engines and their "search help" pages
http://www.ipl.org/teen/aplus/linksengines.htm
Alta Vista, Excite, Lycos et al.

Other links for learning to research
http://www.ipl.org/teen/aplus/linksother.htm
Online articles, online library and research instruction

Links for Writing

OWLs on the Web
http://www.ipl.org/teen/aplus/linksowls.htm
Links to Online Writing Labs (OWLs) "handouts"

OWL Handouts by Topic:

Common types of papers
http://www.ipl.org/teen/aplus/linkscommon.htm
Research papers; persuasive essays; narrative essays; cause/effect essays; how to write summaries and more

Papers on special subjects
http://www.ipl.org/teen/aplus/linksspecial.htm
Film, drama and book reviews; writing about poetry; scientific and lab reports; abstracts and others

Planning and starting the writing assignment
http://www.ipl.org/teen/aplus/linksplanning.htm
The writing process; ideas; journal writing; overcoming obstacles

The topic
http://www.ipl.org/teen/aplus/linkstopic.htm
Several articles from the OWLs

Title, introduction and conclusion
http://www.ipl.org/teen/aplus/linkstitle.htm
Several articles from the OWLs

Thesis statement
http://www.ipl.org/teen/aplus/linksthesis.htm
Articles from many points of view

Organizing information
http:///www.ipl.org/teen/aplus/linksorganizing.htm
Taking notes; outlining; organizing by cubing, mapping and more

Writing style and technique
http://www.ipl.org/teen/aplus/linkswritingstyle.htm
Audience and tone; logic and developing arguments; sentences, words and phrases; paragraphs; coherence, clarity, conciseness; transitions; gender-fair writing; writing on the computer other style and technique issues

Citing sources
http://www.ipl.org/teen/aplus/linkciting.htm
Paraphrasing, summarizing and plagiarism; using quotations; styles of citation

Grammar and punctuation
http://www.ipl.org/teen/aplus/linksgrammar.htm
Links to grammar handbooks

Revising and rewriting
http://www.ipl.org/teen/aplus/linksrevising.htm
How to proofread, edit and revise; short proofreading and editing checklists; critiques and peer review

ting documents about library schools you could be getting documents about school libraries or documents where the word *library* and *school* both appear but have nothing to do with a library school.

PROXIMITY. This allows the user to find documents only if the search terms appear near each other, within so many words or paragraphs, or adjacent to each other. It's a pretty sophisticated tool and can be tricky to use skillfully. Many times you can accomplish about the same result using phrase searching.

CAPITALIZATION. When searching for proper names, search syntax that will distinguish capital from lower case letters will help narrow the search. In other cases, you would want to make sure the search engine isn't looking for a particular pattern of capitalization, and many search engines let you choose which of these options to use.

FIELD SEARCHING. All database records are divided up into fields. Almost all search engines in CD-ROM or online library products and the more sophisticated Web search engines allow users to search for terms appearing in a particular field. This can help immensely when you're looking for a very specific item. Say that you're looking for a psychology paper by a professor from the University of Michigan and all you remember about the paper is that it had something about Freud and Jung in its title. If you think it may be on the Web, you can do a search in Alta Vista, searching for *Freud* AND *Jung* and limit your search to the *umich.edu* domain, which gives you a pretty good chance of finding it, if it's there.

Make sure you know what content you're searching

The content of the database will affect your search strategy and the search syntax you use to retrieve documents. Some of the different databases you'll encounter in your library and online research are:

REPRESENTATION OR SUMMARY OF A DOCUMENT. If a document has been summarized, like a library catalog entry where certain features like title and author have been recorded along with a sentence or two of description, don't expect to retrieve the document by looking for keywords in the text. A search is only searching what's in the database—the representation, not the document itself.

INDEX AND ABSTRACT OF A DOCUMENT. When a document like a journal article has been indexed and an abstract written, a human indexer has helped organize the document for easy retrieval. He or she has chosen some words, phrases and concepts that represent the subject matter of the document and has attached those to the database record as "descriptors." The specific terms usually come from a book of terms used by that database producer, to promote consistency between indexers.

The indexer, or possibly the author of the article, has written an abstract or summary of the article's content that is included in the database. Again, it's important to realize that you're not searching the entire text of the document but someone's representation of the document. If you can zero in on some of the database's descriptors that accurately describe the topic you're looking for, you can easily retrieve all the articles with the same descriptors. If you do a keyword search in this type of database without checking the permissible descriptors, you're hoping that the indexer will have used your keyword in the summary or that the author will have used it in the title of the article.

FULL TEXT OF A DOCUMENT. Searching full text documents gives you a good chance of retrieving the document you want, provided you can think of some key words and phrases that would have been included in the text. The problem is retrieving too many documents when you're looking for something particular, because common words and concepts can appear in documents irrelevant to your topic. This is one of the problems with Internet search engines that index the full text of Web pages. The more skilled you can become in your use of search syntax, the greater will be your success in finding relevant information in a full text database.

Index

Index

Index